The Injury Fact Book

The Injury
Fact Book Second Edition

SUSAN P. BAKER
BRIAN O'NEILL
MARVIN J. GINSBURG
GUOHUA LI

New York   Oxford
OXFORD UNIVERSITY PRESS
1992

Oxford University Press

Oxford   New York   Toronto
Delhi   Bombay   Calcutta   Madras   Karachi
Petaling Jaya   Singapore   Hong Kong   Tokyo
Nairobi   Dar es Salaam   Cape Town
Melbourne   Auckland

and associated companies in
Berlin   Ibadan

Library of Congress Cataloging-in-Publication Data
The Injury fact book / Susan P. Baker . . . [et. al.].—2nd ed.
Rev. ed. of: The injury fact book / Susan P. Baker, Brian O'Neill, Ronald S. Karpf.
p.   cm. Includes bibliographical references and index.
ISBN 0-19-506194-2
1. Wounds and injuries—United States—Statistics.
2. Accidents—United States—Statistics.
3. Mortality—United States—Statistics.
I. Baker, Susan P.   II. Baker, Susan P.   Injury fact book.
RD93.8.I54   1992
362.1′971′00973021—dc20
91-7727

Printing 9 8 7 6 5 4 3 2

Printed in the United States of America
on acid-free paper

Foreword

The United States has an injury problem. Each year, one in four Americans sustains an injury serious enough to warrant medical treatment or to restrict activity for at least a day. A conservative estimate of the lifetime cost of injuries sustained in a single year (1985) in the United States is $158 billion dollars. Since publication of the first edition of *The Injury Fact Book* in 1984, those costs have exceeded one trillion dollars.

The first step in developing effective solutions to the injury problem is to provide an accurate description of what that problem is. We need clarity in the definition of terms, access to current and historical data, research findings with citations of sources, sufficient detail about risk factors and at-risk populations, and a simple, graphic presentation of facts. The "we" in this context are all of us who need injury facts and figures as the raw material of our daily work.

The injury problem presents a challenge to the organizer of its facts. Injuries have traditionally been categorized by intent (unintentional, homicidal, suicidal). Alternative categories are type of injury (e.g., spinal cord, brain, fracture) or cause (e.g., firearm, motor vehicle). Some researchers favor categories by population at risk (children, adolescents, the elderly, minorities). Because sources of data are different, descriptions sometimes are confined to a single level of severity, such as fatal injuries or injuries requiring hospitalization. Other descriptions focus on the setting of the injury event (e.g., work, recreation). The requirements of simplicity and clarity demand hard choices from those who describe the injury problem.

Professor Susan Baker makes these hard choices. She is the consummate describer of the fatal injury problem, dating back to the late 1960s and to her desk at the medical examiner's office in Baltimore. Attracted by the wealth of information available in medical examiner reports, she was able to describe patterns in the causes of fatal injuries and make suggestions for preventive action, primarily focusing upon specific environmental changes.

During the 1970s and 1980s, Professor Baker and colleagues at The John Hopkins School of Public Health refined research in the injury field and enlarged the "pool" of injury researchers through the education of graduate students. At the same time, Dr. William Haddon, Jr., Brian O'Neill, and other colleagues at the Insurance Institute for Highway Safety worked to identify, evaluate, and develop ways to reduce human and economic damage associated with the use of motor vehicles.

Drawing on this combined experience, Susan Baker, Brian O'Neill, and Ronald Karpf compiled the first edition of *The Injury Fact Book*. Its graphs and tables, organized by cause of injury and based on mortality statistics, were supplemented with findings from research on both fatal and nonfatal injuries. Implications for prevention strategies were embedded in every chapter.

The Injury Fact Book became our "almanac," one of those dog-eared volumes kept in a sheltered place on the reference shelf, lest it disappear permanently in the arms of someone borrowing it "just for a second." It works for us. It provides material for media briefings, testimony before legislative committees, class lectures, and grant proposals. It is what it says it is—a compendium of injury facts, an invaluable asset to those who are asked constantly by mail or telephone about details of specific injury problems. It is a time-saver for those providing this extremely time-consuming service.

The second edition of *The Injury Fact Book* again teams Susan Baker with Brian O'Neill and adds two new authors, Marvin Ginsburg and Guohua Li. Maintaining the structure of the original, this edition presents mortality data for the years 1980–1986. The aggregation of seven years of data allows computation of rates for important subgroups, such as age-specific rates for Asians and Native Americans. When combined, the data in the two editions span a full decade. Time trends are analyzed and reported. In fact, for most categories of injury, the rates for 1984–1986, when compared to rates for 1977–1979, are lower. There are exceptions, however, such as a dramatic increase in the death rates for bicyclists over the age of twenty.

Chapters on sports and recreation, aviation, and large trucks have been added, and the chapter on machinery has been expanded to include all occupational injuries. Through its extensive references—double those of the previous edition—the second edition of *The Injury Fact Book* continues to be a treasure trove of references for investigators who wish to pursue questions addressed in published studies and reviews.

One measure of influence of a publication is the number of times a work is cited by other authors. This frequency of citation is documented in the *Science Citation Index* and the *Social Science Citation Index*. The titles of the fifty-two citations in the most recent annual indexes (1989) were reviewed, to get a measure of the relevance of *The Injury Fact Book* to the broad range of issues addressed by injury researchers.

The list of authors citing the book reads like a "who's who" in the injury field. The titles of the articles cover the full range of the injury problem. Some articles focus on high-risk populations (e.g., "Predicting traffic injuries in childhood: A cohort analysis," "Motor trauma in geriatric patients," "Injury mortality in New Mexico's American Indians, Hispanics, and non-Hispanic whites, 1968–1982"). Others focus on a type of injury (e.g., "Unusually low mortality of penetrating wounds of the chest—12 years' experience," "Time trends in the incidence of hospitalized ocular trauma," "Epidemiology of chest trauma").

Many articles focus on a cause of injury in a specified state or region (e.g., "Unintentional firearm death in California," "Effects of the 65-MPH speed limit on rural interstate fatalities in New Mexico," "Employment status and the frequency and causes of burn injuries in New England"). The specificity of these articles is in line with the book's emphasis on state and regional differences. These are presented by means of U.S. maps with states shaded according to cause-specific injury rates. Evidence of the book's relevance to the international community of injury researchers is found in citations from abroad (e.g., "Injury mortality and morbidity in New Zealand," "Unintentional injuries among elderly people—incidence, causes, severity, costs" [Sweden]).

The variety of articles citing *The Injury Fact Book* bears testimony not only to the usefulness of the book but also to the way the injury research field itself has matured. Our research questions in the latter half of the 1980s have become more tightly framed, our research methods more sophisticated, our interventions more informed by data and previous experience, our evaluations less pro forma. The findings of many of the studies that cite the first edition of *The Injury Fact Book* are themselves discussed and referenced in its second edition. Thus, *The Injury Fact Book* has played a vital facilitating role in the evolution of injury research over the past six years. The cycle is sure to be repeated.

Director   Elizabeth McLoughlin, Sc.D.
San Francisco Injury Prevention
Research Center

Foreword to the First Edition

Injuries are the leading cause of death in the United States from the first year of life to age 44. An incalculable cause of human suffering, injuries are also a major source of medical costs and losses to the economy. Yet the subject is largely unknown territory, even to professionals concerned with impairments to the health of the American people and ways in which the quality of life in the United States can be improved. Only rarely do colleges or universities teach the scientific aspects of injuries—except with respect to the treatment of the injured.

This is not because of lack of knowledge. Since about 1940, what is now termed "injury control" has evolved rapidly from the prescientific folklore that still dominates much popular thinking about the causes, prevention, and amelioration of injuries to a mature scientific field with sophisticated research methods, a practical theoretical base, an extensive body of empirical knowledge, and increasing examples of the successful control of the human damage.

In these respects, injuries and their prevention are the last of the great human plagues to be the subject of scientific inquiry and understanding. But, unlike the situation in the case of infectious, cardiovascular, and neoplastic diseases, until the preparation of this book there has been no body of truly competent, comprehensive information giving, so to speak, the statistical lay of the land in the case of the many kinds of injuries.

Most of the basic analyses had never even been done before the authors meticulously performed them using a variety of governmental and other sources. Analyzed by cause, age, sex, race, socioeconomic status, urbanization, geography, time, and other variables, the results of this book, together with those the authors have drawn from other works, will constitute the indispensable statistical reference on injuries for years to come. The book will also undoubtedly be the source to which graduate students and others turn for injury research information, since the reasons for many of the trauma distributions it documents are, as yet, only poorly understood.

Since in many respects the authors have broken entirely new ground, many of the results they report will surprise, and in some cases shock, even specialists in the field. For example:

Death rates from drowning are higher at ages one and two than at any other age, and remain high throughout the preschool period.

State death rates from motor vehicle crashes correlate closely with death rates in the same states from other unintentional injuries.

The death rate per freight ton-mile varies a thousandfold, depending on the transportation mode employed. The lowest death rates are for freight moved by pipeline and marine transport, the highest for freight moved by highway.

Firearm suicide rates decrease and non-firearm suicide rates increase with increased socioeconomic status.

Per capita, Asians have by far the lowest motor vehicle death rates. Native Americans have by far the highest.

During World War II, more than 20,000 U.S. military personnel died in plane crashes in the continental United States.

With only four known exceptions, all male injury death rates greatly exceed those of females. The exceptions are deaths from falls on the same level (the rates for which are about equal), deaths from barbiturates and psychotherapeutic drugs, and deaths from strangulation, which show marked female excesses compared to males.

Although it was not the authors' intent to discuss injury theory, research, or prevention, their statistics are laced with incisive comments about the wide variations in incidence, explanations of many of the findings, and references to relevant work. In the process, they have also documented the substantial success of several injury control efforts.

An example is provided by childhood poisonings: "Since 1960, poisoning deaths among children younger than 5 years have decreased dramatically. The rate for poisoning by solids and liquids was 2.2 per 100,000 in 1960 and 0.5 in 1980 .... Between 1960 and 1980, the number of deaths from lead poisoning dropped from 78 to 2. Deaths from kerosene and other petroleum products dropped from 48 to 9, while those from aspirin dropped from 144 to 12 .... An especially steep decline in childhood poisoning death rates occurred after childproof packaging was required on all drugs and medications beginning in 1973. The 50 percent decrease in poisoning by all drugs and medications in the first three years (1973–1976) was substantially greater than the decrease in poisonings by other solids and liquids, most of which were not required to be packaged in childproof containers .... During 1968–1979, the period analyzed for most causes of death in this book, the 80 percent decline in poisoning death rates for children ages 1–4 exceeded that for any other major cause of childhood injury death."

In 1930, 348 people died in elevator failures. With improved elevator designs and government regulations and inspections, such deaths, despite huge increases in elevator use, have become so rare that they are no longer recorded separately in the nation's vital statistics.

The dramatic change in injury deaths, whether inadvertent or deliberate, that can result from correcting an environmental hazard is also illustrated by what happened when coal gas (which had a higher carbon monoxide content) was replaced by natural gas. In 1947, domestic piped gas caused about 1,000 unintentional deaths and was the agent in some 1,200 suicides. In 1980, after the change to natural gas, the corresponding totals were only 61 and 23 deaths, a decrease of more than 90 percent.

Despite such examples, the injury picture presented in this book is generally grim. It resembles the situation in the history of infectious diseases before the sanitary revolution and subsequent preventive and therapeutic measures. In contrast, the magnitude and characteristics of the injury problem documented in this book make it clear that the country and the relevant professions have a huge amount of catching up to do to bring injury control to the level of success already achieved with the infectious diseases and the level being approached with respect to malignancies and afflictions of the cardiovascular system. The data in the book are a baseline against which that objective will long be measured. Thorough familiarity with this book will long be necessary for professional literacy in the fields with which it deals and in those to which it relates. In addition, the data and commentary this book provides will long be invaluable resources for insurers, public health workers, and, in fact, for everyone concerned with the occurrence, reduction, and cost of injuries of all kinds.

William Haddon, Jr., M.D.

Dr. Haddon was the first head of the National Highway Traffic Safety Administration and was President of the Insurance Institute for Highway Safety from 1969 until his death in 1985.

Preface

Great changes have characterized the field of injury prevention since the first edition of *The Injury Fact Book* was published in 1984.

First is the sheer number of health professionals now actively engaged in the battle against injury. More than 800 came to the 1991 National Injury Control Conference, and attendance is standing-room-only at our scientific sessions of the American Public Health Association.

Second is our ability to attract doctoral students committed to specializing in injury prevention. People grounded in epidemiology, public health practice, education, nursing, medicine, law, engineering, psychology, and other disciplines are essential to our growth and advancement—but those with added training in injury prevention will have the greatest ability to effectively reduce injuries.

Third is the burgeoning literature. Dr. McLoughlin, in her foreword to this edition, describes the explosion of journal articles. Equally impressive is the number of relevant new books. Teaching is now far easier as a result of the textbooks, and more exciting with each landmark research paper.

Last, but hardly least, is the increased public demand for action. Fewer people tolerate bad designs and manmade environments that invite injury, and many understand that blaming the victim leads only to more victims. A good example of this new awareness is that in the past most automakers held the view that "safety doesn't sell," but virtually all automakers now promote the advantages of their cars' safety features, such as air bags and antilock brakes. Perhaps most important, interest in injury prevention now motivates increasing numbers of legislators, members of the media, professional organizations, and others who shape the decisions that determine the public's risk of injury.

Unchanged is our great debt to the pioneers who placed the study and control of injuries on a solid, scientific basis. In particular, William Haddon, Jr., emphasized the role of various forms of energy as the etiologic agents of injury and developed useful frameworks for conceptualizing strategies to prevent injuries. He was a passionate advocate for changes in the policies and environments that determine the burden of injury on mankind.

The Injury Fact Book has been written in the hope that it will be an instrument of those still-needed changes. The Insurance Institute for Highway Safety provided essential resources, both human and financial. The

National Center for Health Statistics and the National Highway Traffic Safety Administration collected and made available data for most of the analyses.

With my co-authors, Brian O'Neill, Marvin Ginsburg, and Guohua Li, I wish to thank all those whose hard work has enabled us to complete our task. In particular, Sharon Rasmussen at the Insurance Institute for Highway Safety and Diane Reintzell, my secretary, have given high priority to ensuring the excellence of our product.

Susan P. Baker, M.P.H.

Abbreviations

AMA	American Medical Association
ATV	All-terrain vehicle
BAC	Blood Alcohol Concentration
BLS	Bureau of Labor Statistics
CDC	Centers for Disease Control
CPR	Cardiopulmonary resuscitation
CPSC	Consumer Product Safety Commission
DSR	Division of Safety Research
FARS	Fatal Accident Reporting System
FBI	Federal Bureau of Investigation
FDA	Food and Drug Administration
FHWA	Federal Highway Administration
GAO	General Accounting Office
ICD	International Classification of Diseases
IIHS	Insurance Institute for Highway Safety
IIP	Industrial Index of Production
MSA	Metropolitan Statistical Area
NASS	National Accident Sampling System
NCHS	National Center for Health Statistics
NEISS	National Electronic Injury Surveillance System
NHIS	National Health Interview Survey
NHTSA	National Highway Traffic Safety Administration
NIOSH	National Institute of Occupational Safety and Health
NRC	National Research Council
NSC	National Safety Council
NTOF	National Traumatic Occupational Fatality
NTSB	National Transportation Safety Board
OSHA	Occupational Safety and Health Administration
SIDS	Sudden Infant Death Syndrome
USCG	United States Coast Guard
USMC	United States Marine Corps
WHO	World Health Organization

Contents

The Injury Fact Book

1

Introduction

Injuries are the most serious public health problem facing developed societies. They take a heavy toll among people of all ages and cause the majority of deaths among children and young adults in the United States. Once overshadowed by more common causes of death and illness, injuries have grown in relative importance as many diseases have been controlled. Throughout the world, they are now the leading cause of death during half of the human lifespan (Barss et al. 1991).

Injury is important not only in relation to other health conditions but also in the absolute magnitude of the problem. More than six million people alive today in the United States can be expected to die from injuries (Whitfield et al. 1983). The risk of injury while traveling, working, playing, or even sleeping is so great that most people sustain a significant injury at some time during their lives. Few escape the tragedy of a fatal or permanently disabling injury to a relative or friend. Nevertheless, this widespread human damage too often is taken for granted, in the erroneous belief that injuries occur by chance and are the result of unpreventable "accidents."

Comparatively little public attention is given to injuries and their prevention except during the aftermath of a disaster, even though on an average day the number of injury deaths in the United States is several times the toll of a major airliner crash. The amount of scientific attention directed to the injury problem is small in relation to the attention and resources accorded many other health problems (National Academy of Sciences 1985).

EPIDEMIOLOGY AND PREVENTION

The occurrence of injuries is largely determined by characteristics of the environment and the many products we use in work, recreation, and travel. Modifying man-made systems and products is often more feasible than altering the behavior of each individual. Failure to recognize the difficulty of "improving" behavior has often led to failure to apply more effective alternative countermeasures to the injury problem.

Specific injuries differ greatly in their distribution in space, time, and populations. The incidence and severity of injury are influenced by demographic factors such as age, sex, race, and occupation as well as by economic, temporal, and geographic effects (Figure 1-1). The influence of these

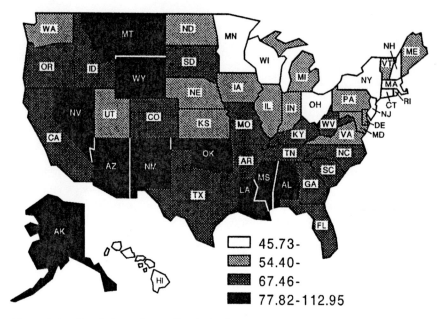

45.73-
54.40-
67.46-
77.82-112.95

Figure 1-1.   Death Rates from All Injuries by State, per 100,000 Population, 1980–
1986

factors is so great that death rates from many injuries differ enormously
among various groups of people. For example, the homicide rate in the
United States is 24 times as high for black men aged 25–29 as for Asian
women of the same age; the risk of dying in an airplane crash is 45 times as
great for residents of Alaska as for residents of Massachusetts; and the
death rate from occupational injury among truck drivers is 48 times the rate
for laundry operators (Leigh 1987).

     Injuries are caused by acute exposure to physical agents such as mechan-
ical energy, heat, electricity, chemicals, and ionizing radiation interacting
with the body in amounts or at rates that exceed the threshold of human
tolerance (Gibson 1961; Haddon 1963). In some cases (for example, drowning and frostbite), injuries result from the sudden lack of essential agents
such as oxygen or heat. About three-fourths of all injuries, including most
from vehicle crashes, falls, sports, and shootings, are caused by mechanical
energy (Figure 1-2).

     Although there are no sharp scientific distinctions between injury and
disease, injuries usually are perceived almost immediately after contact with
the causal agent (Haddon 1980). Because injuries and the events leading to
them are generally more obvious and closer together in time than are
diseases and the events that precede them, the role of human behavior is
often erroneously assumed to be more important to injury causation than to
disease causation. In fact, human behavior is important to both. For example, wearing shoes and cooking food are behaviors that can influence
susceptibility to disease—but the behavioral element often goes unnoticed

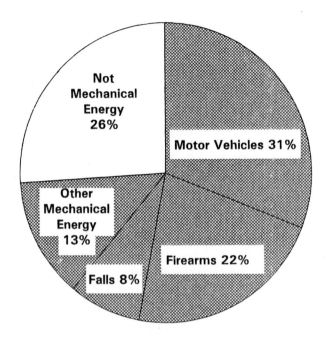

Figure 1-2. Percentage of All Injury Deaths Caused by Mechanical Energy, 1986

because symptoms of hookworm or amebic dysentery may not be apparent until months after a person walked barefoot in dirt infested with hookworm larvae or ate uncooked vegetables containing amebic cysts. There is no basis for the widespread assumption that modifying human behavior is any more important in preventing injuries than diseases (Haddon and Baker 1981).

ORGANIZATION OF THE BOOK

This book includes detailed information on many of the factors surrounding injuries—the man-made systems and products involved, the groups of people at greatest risk, and effective ways to protect people from injuries. The circumstances under which injuries occur, the etiologic agents, and the characteristics of the people involved are examined. Chapter 2 summarizes the importance of injuries in relation to other prominent health problems. Subsequent chapters describe injury mortality and, in cases where good population-based studies are available, nonfatal injuries.

The organization of the book is influenced by the International Classification of Diseases (ICD) codes, which determine the availability of most national mortality data on injuries. Since these codes are subdivided according to apparent "intent" of injury (i.e., unintentional, suicidal, or homicidal), Chapters 3-6 are organized on the basis of intent. Chapters 7-21 are organized on the basis of injury etiology; the chapter on poisoning, for example, includes details on suicidal as well as unintentional poisonings. To minimize repetition, the reader is sometimes referred to other chapters.

The analyses in Chapters 3–15 are primarily of injury deaths during 1980–1986, the most recent years for which detailed mortality data were available in mid-1989 for deaths other than those related to motor vehicles. In many instances the text and tables have been further updated with 1988 mortality data. Most of these data were collected by the U.S. Department of Health and Human Services, National Center for Health Statistics (NCHS).

Chapters 16–21 present data on deaths from motor vehicle-related injuries, based primarily on the Fatal Accident Reporting System (FARS) of the U.S. Department of Transportation, National Highway Traffic Safety Administration (NHTSA). The U.S. Bureau of the Census population estimates for 1980–1986 provided denominators for rates throughout the book. Further details on data sources may be found in the Appendix, which also provides a wealth of statistics on 69 categories of injury.

The scientific foundation for injury research was laid almost three decades ago by William Haddon and his colleagues in their comprehensive review and analysis of the injury studies available at that time (Haddon et al. 1964). The literature on injury research and prevention has grown rapidly in recent years and is comprehensively described elsewhere (Baker 1989; Barss et al. 1991; Haddon 1980; Haddon and Baker 1981; National Academy of Sciences 1985; National Committee for Injury Prevention and Control 1989; Rice et al. 1989; Robertson 1983, in press; Waller 1985; Wilson et al. 1991).

The purpose of this second edition of *The Injury Fact Book* is not only to present more recent data but also to further improve understanding of the nature and magnitude of the injury problem in the United States. Most of the analyses presented here were conducted for this book and are not presented elsewhere. To highlight changes since the first edition was published, where appropriate, comparisons are drawn for the periods 1977–1979 and 1984–1986.

This book provides a detailed documentation of the injury problem in the United States. The facts are presented to improve understanding of which groups of people are likely to be injured and how, and to encourage work on solutions to the injury problem.

REFERENCES

Baker, S.P. (1989). Injury science comes of age. *Journal of the American Medical Association* 262:2284–2285.

Barss, P., G.S. Smith, D. Mohan, and S.P. Baker (1991). *Injuries to adults in developing countries: Epidemiology and policy*. Washington, DC: The World Bank, pp. 1–132.

Gibson, J.J. (1961). The contribution of experimental psychology to the formulation of the problem of safety—A brief for basic research. In *Behavioral approaches to accident research.* New York: Association for the Aid of Crippled Children, pp. 77–89.

Haddon, W., Jr. (1963). A note concerning accident theory and research with special reference to motor vehicle accidents. *Annals of the New York Academy of Science* 107:635–646.

Haddon, W., Jr. (1980). Advances in the epidemiology of injuries as a basis for public policy. *Public Health Reports* 95:411–421.

Haddon, W., Jr., and S.P. Baker (1981). Injury control. In D. Clark and B. MacMahon (eds.), *Preventive and community medicine.* Boston: Little, Brown, pp. 109–140.

Haddon, W., Jr., E.A. Suchman, and D. Klein (1964). *Accident research: Methods and approaches.* New York: Harper & Row.

Leigh, J.P. (1987). Estimates of the probability of job-related death in 347 occupations. *Journal of Occupational Medicine* 29:510–519.

National Academy of Sciences (1985). *Injury in America.* Washington, DC: National Academy Press.

National Committee for Injury Prevention and Control (1989). *Injury prevention: Meeting the challenge.* New York: Oxford University Press. (Published as a supplement to the *American Journal of Preventive Medicine*, Vol. 5, No. 3.)

Rice, D.P., E.J. MacKenzie, and associates (1989). *Cost of injury in the United States: A report to Congress.* San Francisco: Institute for Health and Aging, University of California and Injury Prevention Center, The Johns Hopkins University.

Robertson, L.S. (1983). *Injuries: Causes, control strategies, and public policy.* Lexington, MA: Lexington Books.

Robertson, L.S. (in press). *Injury epidemiology.* New York: Oxford University Press.

Waller, J.A. (1985). *Injury control: A guide to the causes and prevention of trauma.* Lexington, MA: Lexington Books.

Whitfield, R., P. Zador, and D. Fife (1983). *The accident deaths to be expected among the cohort alive in 1979.* Washington, DC: Insurance Institute for Highway Safety.

Wilson, M.H., S.P. Baker, S.P. Teret, S. Shock, and J. Garbarino (1991). *Saving children: A guide to injury prevention.* New York: Oxford University Press.

2

Injuries in Relation to
Other Health Problems

This chapter documents the importance of injuries in relation to other health problems. Health expenditures in the United States in recent years have been rising much faster than the gross national product. Increasingly, policymakers and health professionals recognize that the resources needed for health care are limited and that available resources must be used more efficiently. Allocations of resources for research and for prevention and treatment of disease and injury should be made on the basis of the relative importance of various causes of morbidity and mortality in the population and the potential for effective intervention.

INJURIES AS A CAUSE OF DEATH

Mortality data are commonly used to describe and compare public health problems, in part because deaths are well defined and detailed data are available. Most of the analyses presented in this book focus on mortality. In keeping with standard public health practice, results are generally summarized by death rates, defined as the number of deaths per 100,000 population each year.

One death out of every 14 in the United States results from injury. Injuries are the third leading cause of death, claiming 150,000 lives each year. In 1988, the death rate for injuries (62 per 100,000 people) was surpassed only by the rates for heart disease and cancer (NCHS 1990a).

For more than four decades of life—specifically, ages 1–44—injuries are the leading cause of death (Figure 2-1; NCHS 1990a). As is true of cancer and other disease groups, injuries include a number of subgroups. One subgroup of injuries, those related to motor vehicles, is the most common cause of death for ages 1–34. Fatal motor vehicle injuries outnumber by 125 to 1 deaths from cystic fibrosis, a disease that is the object of considerable public concern.

The age-specific death rates for injuries far surpass those for cancer and heart disease for ages 1–44 (Figure 2-2; NCHS 1990). From age 1 through 4, injuries cause almost half of all deaths and result in more than three times

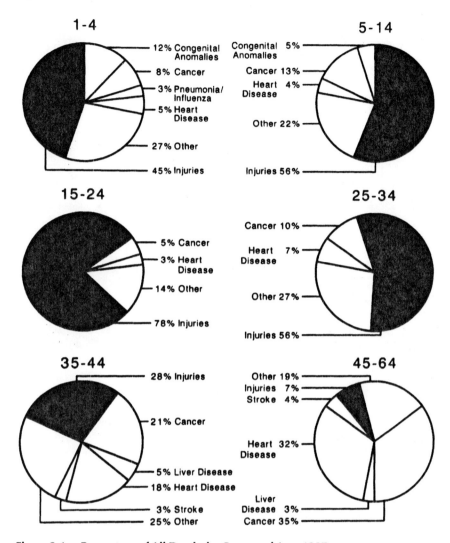

Figure 2-1. Percentage of All Deaths by Cause and Age, 1987

the number of deaths from congenital anomalies, the second leading cause. Injury deaths exceed deaths from all other causes combined from age 5 through 34 and are most prominent at ages 15–24, when they cause 78 percent of all deaths. From age 35 through 44, they continue to outnumber deaths from any other single cause (NCHS 1990a).

After age 45, injuries account for fewer deaths than several other health problems, such as heart disease, cancer, and stroke. Despite the decrease in the proportion of deaths due to injury, the death rate from injuries is actually higher among the elderly than among younger people. In absolute numbers, injuries remain important throughout life. For example, each year some 30,000 people aged 65 or older die from injuries (NCHS 1990a).

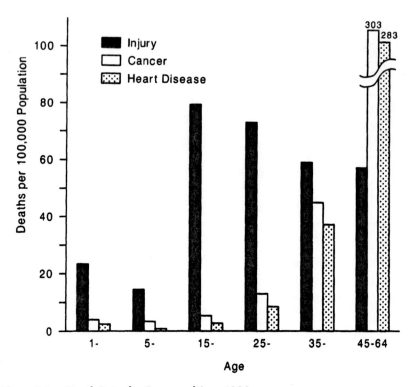

Figure 2-2.   Death Rates by Cause and Age, 1986

Children less than 1 year old are often omitted from published injury statistics, even though injury deaths during the first year of life now are twice the number of deaths from pneumonia and are outranked only by congenital anomalies and perinatal conditions.

TRENDS IN MORTALITY FROM INJURIES AND OTHER CAUSES

Injuries have always been a serious problem, but until the 1940s their importance was overshadowed by the prominence of many infectious diseases. In 1910, the death rates from three major disease groups—tuberculosis, influenza/pneumonia, and gastroenteritis—were higher than the death rate from injuries (Figure 2-3). By 1980, however, death rates from tuberculosis and gastrointestinal disorders had declined by 99 percent and deaths from influenza/pneumonia by 85 percent, whereas the injury death rate had declined by only about 30 percent during these seven decades. Injuries presently are responsible for more than twice as many deaths as are influenza and pneumonia.

Trends in childhood deaths during this century vividly illustrate the success of disease prevention and amelioration, which have long been based on scientific approaches, in contrast with injury prevention, which only

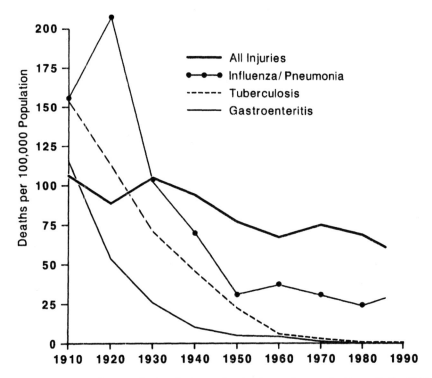

Figure 2-3. Death Rates from Injuries and Infectious Diseases by Year, 1910–1986

recently has been treated scientifically. In 1930, deaths from diseases among children aged 1–4 were eight times as common as injury deaths, but by 1980 the death rate from diseases had decreased almost to the level of the injury rate, which had declined by less than half (Figure 2-4). For ages 15–24, the injury death rate by 1986 was three and a half times the death rate from diseases, whereas the opposite was true in 1930.

SOCIETAL COSTS

Mortality comparisons, useful as they are for policymakers, illustrate only one part of the nation's health burden. Nonfatal health problems are also significant because of the large number of people involved and the demands they place on the health care system. In addition, as in the case of deaths, nonfatal injuries cause suffering and inconvenience to involved individuals and their families and associates. Comparing the relative impact of health problems is a complex matter because of the difficulty of assessing the seriousness of quite different health problems, for example, a serious brain injury versus breast cancer, as well as the substantially different outcomes that can result. One comparative approach involves computing the societal costs associated with health problems and thus using dollars as a basis for

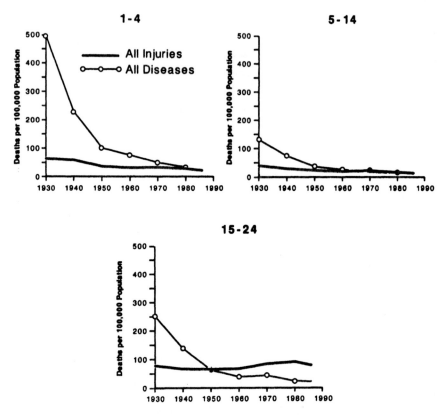

Figure 2-4. Death Rates from All Diseases and Injuries by Year and Age Group, 1930–1986

comparison. Comparisons of the impact of health problems in economic terms must always be treated with caution because effects such as pain, grief, and family or social disruption cannot be measured in these terms. However, key effects such as loss of productivity (indirect costs to society) and the use of medical and other resources (direct costs) can be measured and compared in dollars for various health problems.

A study of motor vehicle crash injuries occurring in 1975 found their total societal cost to be second only to the cost of cancer (Figure 2-5; Hartunian et al. 1980, 1981). The direct costs (expenditures for goods and services) resulting from motor vehicle crash injuries were approximately twice the direct costs of coronary heart disease. Indirect costs (loss of potential earnings) are especially high for injuries because the average age at which fatal or disabling injury occurs is much lower than the corresponding ages for most major diseases.

A major component of indirect costs is the loss of productivity associated with premature death. For convenience, deaths prior to age 70 are sometimes called premature, and the number of years of life that would

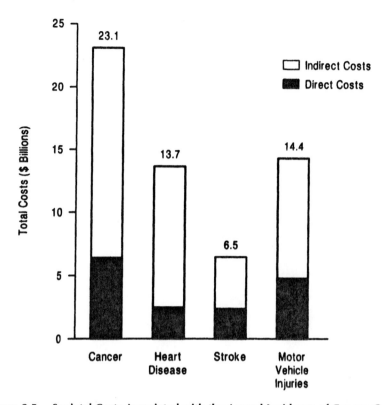

Figure 2-5.   Societal Costs Associated with the Annual Incidence of Cancer, Coronary Heart Disease, Stroke, and Motor Vehicle Injuries, 1975 (*Source:* N.S. Hartunian, C.N. Smart, and M.S. Thompson, The incidence and economic costs of cancer, motor vehicle injuries, coronary heart disease and stroke: A Comparative analysis. *American Journal of Public Health* 70 (1980): 1258. Reprinted with the permission of the publisher.)

have remained are considered years of life lost prematurely. For each cause, the difference between age 70 and the age at death can be used to calculate the total number of years of life lost because of death prior to age 70. There are 4.3 million potential years of life lost prematurely each year because of injuries, compared with less than 3 million each for cancer and heart disease and about 0.4 million each for AIDS and cerebrovascular disease (stroke) (Figure 2-6). Even when injury deaths from homicide and suicide are not included, the remaining unintentional injury deaths result in a greater loss than for any single disease.

A recent report to Congress carefully documented the cost to society of injury (Rice, MacKenzie, and associates 1989). In this analysis, years of life lost per death were based on average life expectancy at the time of death. Discounting lifetime earnings at 6 percent, the total lifetime costs of all injuries that occurred during 1985 were estimated at $158 billion. Lifetime costs per death were almost four times the losses for cancer and more than

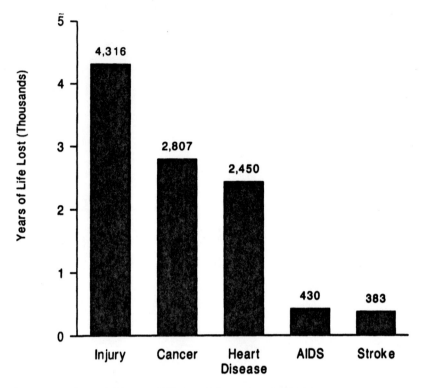

Figure 2-6.   Potential Years of Life Lost Prior to Age 70, 1987

six times the losses for cardiovascular disease (heart disease and stroke) (Figure 2-7). The rationale for government research and programs to reduce injuries is further strengthened by the fact that more than one-fourth (28 percent) of the direct cost of injuries is borne by federal, state, and local governments. In marked contrast to societal burdens, total federal research expenditures for injury were estimated at $160 million, compared with National Cancer Institute obligations of $1,400 million and National Heart, Lung, and Blood Institute obligations of $930 million.

PHYSICIAN CONTACTS

Another measure of the burden that nonfatal injuries place on society is the utilization of physicians for treatment. Injuries result in 114 million physician contacts annually, almost as many as for respiratory conditions (118 million), the leading cause of such visits (NCHS 1987).

Hospital emergency department visits are an important component of medical care. More than 25 percent of *all* emergency room or hospital clinic visits are for the treatment of injuries (NCHS 1983). The annual cost of emergency room care of the injured is $2.6 billion (Rice, MacKenzie, and

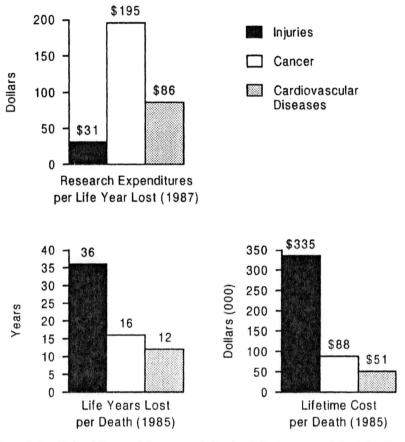

Figure 2-7. Federal Research Investment, Productivity Losses, and Costs by Cause of Death, 1985 (*Source:* D.P. Rice, E.J. MacKenzie, and associates, *Cost of injury in the United States: A report to Congress.* San Francisco: Institute for Health and Aging, University of California and Injury Prevention Center, The Johns Hopkins University, 1989, p. 69.)

associates 1989). The cost of care in nursing homes is an additional $2.5 billion, primarily for injury from falls.

HOSPITAL ADMISSIONS

The number of people who are admitted to hospitals for treatment provides another basis for comparing health problems in terms of the resources utilized. Injuries result in 2.8 million hospital admissions each year, almost one of every 10 admissions at short-stay hospitals. For all ages combined, injury admissions are outranked only by diseases of the circulatory, digestive, and respiratory systems (Table 2-1). In 1988, there were 1.6 million

Table 2-1.   Number of Discharges from Short-Stay Hospitals
for Eight Leading Causes, 1988[a]

Condition	Number	Percentage
Diseases of circulatory system	5,296	17
Diseases of digestive system	3,268	11
Diseases of respiratory system	2,937	9
Injuries	2,817	9
Diseases of genitourinary system	2,204	7
Neoplasms	2,098	7
Diseases of musculoskeletal system and connective tissues	1,647	5
Mental disorders	1,559	5
Other	9,320	30
Total	31,146	100

Source: National Center for Health Statistics, 1988 Summary: National Hospital Discharge Survey. *Advance Data* 185(1990):4–8.

[a]Discharges from nonfederal hospitals where the average stay is less than 30 days. Excludes newborn infants.

injury admissions for people younger than 45 years, making injuries the leading cause of hospital admissions for this age group (NCHS 1990b).

REFERENCES

Hartunian, N.S., C.N. Smart, and M.S. Thompson (1980). The incidence and economic costs of cancer, motor vehicle injuries, coronary heart disease, and stroke: A comparative analysis. *American Journal of Public Health* 70:1249–1260.

Hartunian, N.S., C.N. Smart, and M.S. Thompson (1981). *The incidence and economic costs of major health impairments: A comparative analysis of cancer, motor vehicle injuries, coronary heart disease and stroke*. Lexington, MA: Lexington Books.

National Center for Health Statistics (1983). Physician visits: Volume and interval since last visit, United States 1980. *Vital and Health Statistics* 10:27, 58–59.

National Center for Health Statistics (1987). Physician contacts by sociodemographic and health characteristics. United States, 1982–1983. *Vital and Health Statistics* 10(161):31.

National Center for Health Statistics (1990a). Advance report of final mortality statistics, 1988. *Monthly Vital Statistics Report* 39(7):22–25.

National Center for Health Statistics (1990b). 1988 summary: National Hospital Discharge Survey. *Advance Data* 185:4–8.

Rice, D.P., E.J. MacKenzie, and associates (1989). *Cost of injury in the United States: A report to Congress*. San Francisco: Institute for Health and Aging, University of California and Injury Prevention Center, The Johns Hopkins University.

3

Overview of Injury Mortality

Unlike diseases, injuries are often classified on the basis of the behaviors and events that preceded them and the imputed intent of the people involved. The commonly used major subdivisions of injury deaths are homicide, suicide, and unintentional (accidental).[1] Although the events leading to intentional and unintentional injuries may differ widely, the mechanisms of injury and the injuries themselves are typically similar. For example, ingesting a toxic substance produces the same outcome even though the spectrum of behavior can range from completely unintentional, as when a person is not aware of the presence or nature of a drug or its potential effect, to overtly suicidal self-poisoning. In addition, many of the basic preventive strategies are the same. Reductions in the carbon monoxide content of cooking and heating gas in England reduced both unintentional and suicidal deaths without corresponding increases in suicide by other means (Alphey and Leach 1974; Hassall and Trethowan 1972). Similarly, the crashworthy fuel systems that have virtually eliminated postcrash fire deaths in Army helicopters are equally effective regardless of whether a crash occurs on training maneuvers or as a result of combat (Springate et al. 1989).

Almost 153,000 Americans died of injuries in 1988. Of these deaths, 64 percent were classed as unintentional and 34 percent as intentional; for the remaining 2 percent the intent was unknown (Figure 3-1). Unintentional injury deaths included approximately 49,000 resulting from motor vehicle crashes and 48,000 from other events. Of approximately 52,000 intentional injury deaths, 30,000 were classified as suicide and 22,000 as homicide or legal intervention (people killed by law-enforcement agents in the line of duty). An additional 3,000 deaths (predominantly by poisoning, shooting, or drowning) were of undetermined intent (NCHS 1990).

AGE AND SEX

The death rate from injuries varies greatly with age (Figure 3-2). It is highest for ages 75 and older; for ages 75–84 it is twice the overall rate for all ages combined. For ages 85 and older the death rate is almost 300 per 100,000 population. The lowest injury death rate is for ages 5–14. The next age group, 15–24, has a particularly high death rate. The shape of the curve for

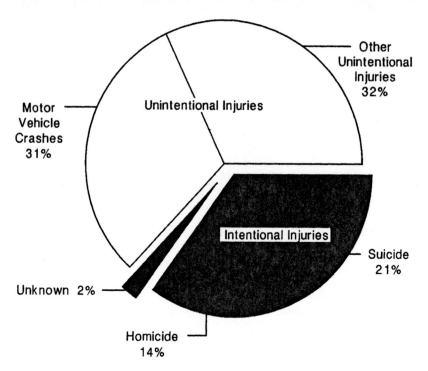

Figure 3-1. Percentage of Injury Deaths by Manner of Death, 1986

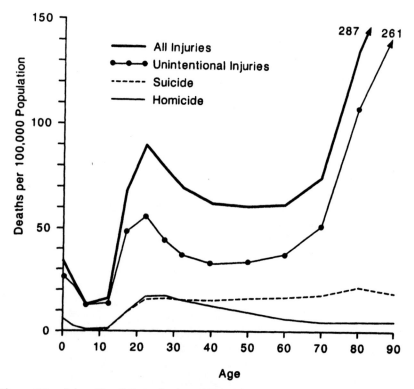

Figure 3-2. Injury Death Rates by Age, 1980–1986

all fatal injuries combined is largely determined by the high death rates from unintentional injuries among young children, young adults, and the elderly.

The homicide rate is highest for ages 20–29, but among adults the suicide rate for both sexes combined shows little variation with age.

In addition to differences by age, injury death rates also vary by sex (Figure 3-3; note that to facilitate comparisons, the vertical scales for the three parts of this figure differ). Males have much higher rates in each category of injury death. For unintentional injury, male death rates have one peak in the 20–24 age group and another among the elderly. For suicide, there are also two peaks, one at ages 20–29 and a higher peak in the 75 and older age group. For homicide, the single peak occurs at ages 20–29.

Among women, the highest suicide rates occur at about age 50. (That many women experience menopause at this age suggests a potential avenue of research.) For unintentional injury and homicide, peaks occur among women at ages 15–19 and 20–24, respectively. These peaks are at slightly younger ages than the corresponding peaks for men, possibly because in

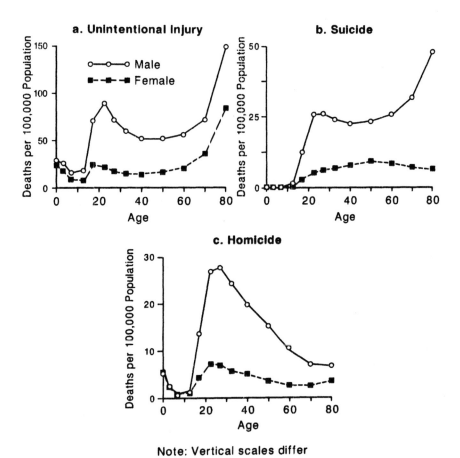

Note: Vertical scales differ

Figure 3-3.   Death Rates from Unintentional Injury, Suicide, and Homicide by Age and Sex, 1980–1986

many social relationships women are generally somewhat younger than men.

The overall death rate for unintentional injuries for males is more than twice as high as for females (59 versus 25 per 100,000 population). In the case of intentional injuries, male rates are more than three times as high as female rates (19 versus 5 per 100,000 population for suicides and 14 versus 4 for homicides). The higher rates for males in large part reflect differences in the likelihood of risk-taking activities. These differences may be partly innate and partly a result of societal expectations; for example, hazardous jobs are typically performed by men, and in many groups men are expected to drink more alcohol than women.

Within each of the three major categories of injury, the ratios of male to female death rates vary widely depending on the specific cause of injury (Figure 3-4). For example, the male to female ratio ranges from about 1 to 2 for homicide by strangling to 29 to 1 for falls from ladders and scaffolds. In the case of firearm deaths classified as legal intervention, no females were killed during 1980–1986.

For some types of fatal injury, the sex ratios are similar regardless of intent. For example, the male to female ratios for deaths from firearms are 6.5 to 1, 5.7 to 1, and 4.8 to 1 for unintentional injury, suicide, and homicide, respectively; and the ratios for cutting are 4.5 to 1 and 3.5 to 1 for unintentional injury and suicide, respectively.

Unlike death rates, the nonfatal injury rates for males are only slightly higher than for females. Based on estimates from the National Health Interview Survey (NHIS), injuries that are medically treated or result in at least one day of restricted activity occur annually at a rate of about 370 per 1,000 males and 259 per 1,000 females, a ratio of 1.4 to 1 (NCHS 1985). Since male injury death rates are more than twice the female rates, the smaller differences in the nonfatal injury rates indicate that injuries to males on average are more severe than those to females.

The best estimates of the per capita incidence of injuries that are serious enough to result in emergency room visits come from the Northeastern Ohio Trauma Study (Barancik et al. 1983). These injuries are somewhat more serious than injuries reported in surveys, and the male to female ratio (1.6 to 1) is slightly higher, with incidence rates of 244 per 1,000 males and 148 per 1,000 females. Male rates exceed female rates until about age 60 (Figure 3-5). Among older people, the rate is slightly higher among females than males, largely because of falls (Iskrant and Joliet 1968). For both sexes, injury rates are highest at ages 15–24. In contrast to the age-related pattern for fatal injuries and hospital admissions, for which the rates are highest among the elderly, the rates for injuries treated in hospital emergency rooms are lowest after age 65.

The number of deaths occurring for every 1,000 injuries treated in hospital emergency rooms shows a very different pattern with age from the population-based injury and death rates (Figure 3-5). The ratios of deaths per 1,000 injuries are higher among young adults than children, indicating

Ratio	Unintentional Injury	Suicide	Homicide
29:1	Fall, ladder/scaffold		
23:1	Machinery		
19:1	Electric current		
16:1	Struck by falling object		
14:1	Drowning, boat-related		
11:1	Motorcyclist		
9:1	Caught/crushed		
7:1	Explosion Lightning Collision, object/person Pedestrian, train Firearm		
6:1	Fall, building/structure Poisoning, opiates	Firearm	
5:1	Aircraft Bicyclist Drowning, non-boat Cutting/piercing	Hanging	Firearm
4:1	Motor vehicle exhaust Poisoning, alcohol	Cutting/piercing	Cutting/stabbing
3:1	Suffocation Excessive cold Pedestrian, traffic Motor vehicle occupant	Motor vehicle exhaust	
2:1	Fall, different level Pedestrian, non-traffic Poisoning, tranquilizers Natural disaster Housefire	Jumping	Other
1.5:1	Exposure/neglect Aspiration, food Excessive heat Fall, stairs Poisoning, barbiturates Aspiration, non-food	Drowning	
1:1	Clothing, ignition Fall, same level Poisoning, antidepressants	Poisoning, solid/liquid	
1:2			Strangulation

Figure 3-4.   Male to Female Ratios of Death Rates by Cause, 1980–1986

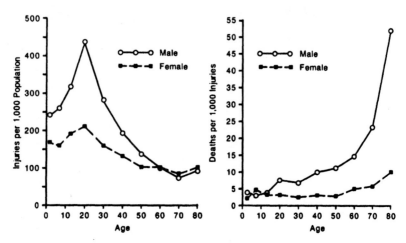

Figure 3-5. Rates of Injuries Requiring Emergency Room Visits by Age and Sex, and Ratios of Deaths to Injuries, Northeastern Ohio, 1977 (*Source:* D. Fife, J. I. Barancik, and B.F. Chatterjee, Northeastern Ohio Trauma Study: II. Injury rates by age, sex, and cause. *American Journal of Public Health* 74 (1984): 475, 476. Reprinted with the permission of the publisher.)

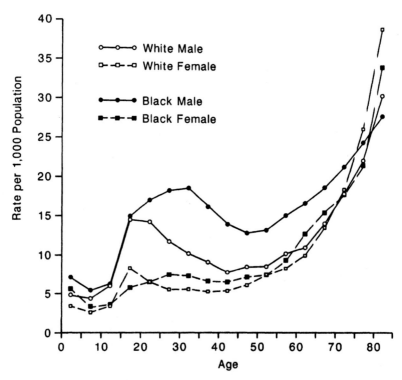

Figure 3-6. Short-Stay Hospital Discharge Rates for Injuries by Age, Race, and Sex, Maryland 1988

that the injuries sustained are, on average, more severe after age 15. The increase in deaths at ages 16 and older in large part reflects increasing involvement in serious motor vehicle crashes. Large increases in the number of deaths per 1,000 injuries among the elderly reflect their greater likelihood of serious complications and poorer prognosis after injury.

As with fatalities, the elderly also have the highest rates of hospitalization for injuries at acute-care (short-stay) hospitals (Figure 3-6). These rates are due to higher rates of admissions for fractures of the limbs—especially hip fractures, which are primarily fractures of the neck of the femur and intertrochanteral fractures (Figure 3-7; see also Chapter 10). Hospitalization rates for intracranial and other internal injuries, lacerations, and dislocations are highest at ages 15-24, and sprains of the back and neck are most prominent at ages 35-44. Fractures of the arm resulting in hospital admission have high rates at ages 5-14 as well as among the elderly. These rates are determined not only by the incidence of the respective injuries but also by factors (such as age and injury severity) that influence the likelihood of admission after injury. Nevertheless, the shapes of the curves shown in Figure 3-7 for various fracture groups are roughly similar to the curves for

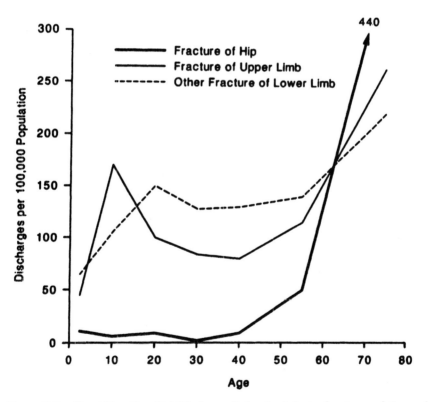

Figure 3-7.   Short-Stay Hospital Discharge Rates for Injuries by Age and Type of Injury, NCHS Hospital Discharge Survey, 1981

incidence rates based on x-rays rather than hospitalization (Buhr and Cooke 1959).

RACE AND PER CAPITA INCOME

Injury death rates vary substantially among racial and economic groups. Native Americans (Indians, Eskimos, and Aleuts) have the highest death rates from unintentional injury; blacks have the highest homicide rates; and whites and Native Americans have the highest suicide rates (Figure 3-8). Asian Americans (Chinese, Japanese, Koreans, Hawaiians, Filipinos, and Guamanians) have the lowest rates of death from unintentional injury and homicide. Blacks have the lowest suicide rate, which is slightly lower than the rate for Asians. As a proportion of all deaths, injuries are most important among Native Americans, among whom they account for 63 percent of all deaths at ages 1–44 (Indian Health Service 1990).

The relative importance of the leading causes of injury death differs among the racial groups (Table 3-1). For each race, motor vehicles, suicide,

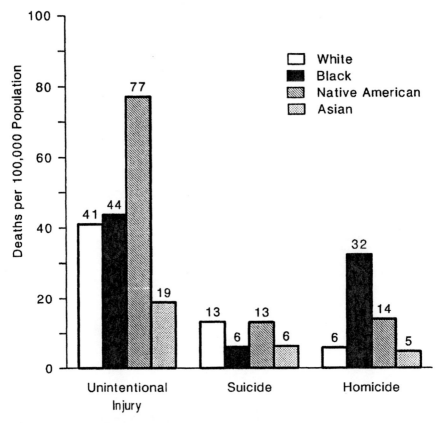

Figure 3-8. Death Rates from Unintentional Injury, Suicide, and Homicide by Race, 1980–1986

Table 3-1. Leading Causes of Injury Death by Race, 1980–1986

Rank	Race	Rate	Race	Rate
	White		*Black*	
1	Motor vehicle	20.42	Homicide	32.36
2	Suicide	13.23	Motor vehicle	16.88
3	Homicide	5.91	Suicide	6.09
4	Falls	5.52	Fires/burns	5.52
5	Drowning	2.34	Drowning	4.22
6	Fires/burns	1.87	Falls	3.66
7	Poisoning—solids/liquids	1.49	Poisoning—solids/liquids	2.34
8	Aspiration—food	0.77	Aspiration—nonfood	0.99
9	Firearm (unintentional)	0.71	Excessive cold	0.95
10	Aircraft	0.68	Firearm (unintentional)	0.93
	Native American		*Asian*	
1	Motor vehicle	41.97	Motor vehicle	10.82
2	Homicide	14.01	Suicide	6.31
3	Suicide	13.11	Homicide	4.83
4	Drowning	6.92	Drowning	2.09
5	Fires/burns	3.82	Falls	1.72
6	Falls	3.70	Fires/burns	0.65
7	Excessive cold	2.61	Poisoning—solids/liquids	0.37
8	Firearm (unintentional)	2.33	Aspiration—food	0.34
9	Poisoning—solids/liquids	2.28	Aspiration—nonfood	0.25
10	Exposure, neglect	1.41	Aircraft	0.19

and homicide lead the list, but in varying order; the next three causes are falls, drowning, and fires in varying order. Excessive cold, however, is an important problem for Native Americans, with a death rate that is 10 times that for whites. The importance of cold as a cause of death for Native Americans is not limited to the northern states and Alaska. It is an important cause in mountain states, for example, New Mexico, where excessive cold is the fourth leading cause of injury death in Native American males but does not rank among the 10 leading causes for white males (Sewell et al. 1989).

Rates of hospital admission for injuries were calculated for whites and blacks in Maryland (Figure 3-6). The peaks seen among whites of both sexes at ages 15–24 are not as pronounced for black males and are. absent for black females. For all ages less than 80, admission rates are highest for black males.

National mortality data do not include information on individual economic status, but considerable evidence indicates that injury rates vary substantially among different economic groups (Barancik and Shapiro 1976; Mierley and Baker 1983; Wise 1983). For example, injury death rates in Maine are exceptionally high for children in low-income families; compared with other children, death rates from fire are five times as high, and drowning rates are four times as high (Nersesian et al. 1985).

In this book, analyses of injury rates by economic group have been made on the basis of the per capita income of the area of residence of each fatally injured individual. For unintentional injuries, the death rate varies inversely with per capita income, decreasing from 61 per 100,000 in the lowest-income areas to 27 in the highest-income areas (Figure 3-9). This relationship holds for both motor vehicle and non-motor-vehicle unintentional injuries. For suicide, there is little relationship between death rate and per capita income; for homicide, residents of the wealthiest areas have much lower rates than those in other areas.

Some of the differences among races in injury rates may be related to economic status. Both blacks and whites have an inverse relationship between income levels and death rates: The higher the income level, the lower the death rate (Baker et al. 1984). Asians have the lowest death rates in all income groups and, as with other races, show an inverse relationship between death rate and per capita income.

Native Americans, with the highest death rates overall, have especially high rates in low-income areas. Unlike the other racial groups, the trend of lower death rates in high-income areas is reversed for Native Americans, in part because many Native Americans live in Alaska, where both per capita income and injury death rates are extremely high (Baker et al. 1984).

URBAN/RURAL AND GEOGRAPHIC DIFFERENCES

The U.S. population was subdivided into five groups for the purpose of comparisons on the basis of place of residence (Table 3-2). Counties that are

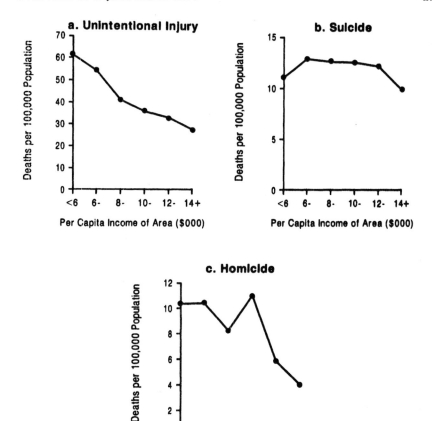

Note: Vertical scales differ

Figure 3-9. Death Rates from Unintentional Injury, Suicide, and Homicide by Per Capita Income of Area of Residence, 1980–1986

part of the U.S. Census Bureau's Metropolitan Statistical Areas (MSAs)[2] were divided into three groups, and counties not part of MSAs were divided into two groups. This categorization permitted the calculation of death rates for the most rural and the most urban areas, as well as for three intermediate areas. As with rates calculated by per capita income, death rates calculated by place of residence are based on the residence of the decedent, not the place of injury.

Unintentional injury death rates are highest in rural areas (Figure 3-10). This is true for both motor vehicle and non-motor-vehicle injury. For these categories combined, the rate for the most rural areas is more than 50 percent greater than that for the central cities (60 versus 39 per 100,000 population). Homicide rates, however, are several times as high in central cities as in other areas. Suicide shows the least variation by place of residence.

Table 3-2. Population Subdivisions Used for Analyses by Place of Residence

Designation	Description	Number of Counties	Average Population 1980–1986
Central cities	Central counties of metropolitan areas of 1 million population or more	54	58,423,000
Metropolitan > 1 million	Fringe counties of metropolitan areas of 1 million population or more	173	38,792,000
Metropolitan < 1 million	Other counties in metropolitan areas	487	72,053,000
Nonmetropolitan	Nonmetropolitan counties either adjacent to a metropolitan area or having a settlement with at least 2,500 persons	1,826	51,615,000
Rural remote	Not adjacent to a metropolitan area and having no settlement as large as 2,500 persons	557	3,974,000

Source: Based on codes prepared by the Economic Development Division, Economic Research Service, U.S. Department of Agriculture.

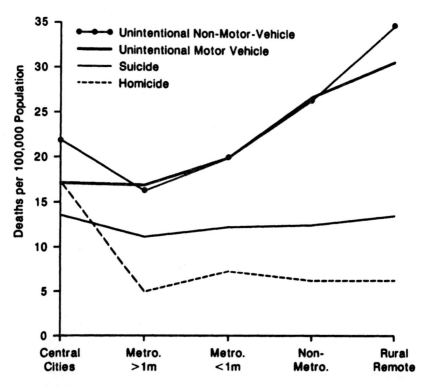

Figure 3-10. Death Rates from Unintentional Injury, Suicide, and Homicide by Place of Residence, 1980–1986

In general, income is lowest in rural areas; for 1980–1986, 85 percent of all residents of counties with a per capita income below $6,000 lived in rural counties that were not part of an MSA. When income and place of residence are considered jointly, however, it has been shown that economic differences do not account for the higher death rates for unintentional injuries in rural counties. The most rural areas have high death rates regardless of income category (Figure 3-11).

Ratios of death rates in remote rural areas to those in central cities range from 1 to 83 for suicide by jumping to 23 to 1 for natural disasters (Figure 3-12). The differences shown in Figure 3-12 underscore the importance of the physical environment in determining injury death rates. High buildings and illicit drugs, for example, are especially present in large cities, whereas farm machinery and firearms are especially prevalent in rural areas.

In addition to urban/rural variations, pronounced geographic patterns characterize injury death rates (Figure 3-13). Rates from unintentional injuries and suicides tend to be high in the West and South, while suicide rates are highest in the West and homicide rates are highest in the South. The death rates for unintentional injury range from a low of 30 in Rhode Island and Hawaii to a high of 84 in Alaska; for suicide, from a low of 8 in New

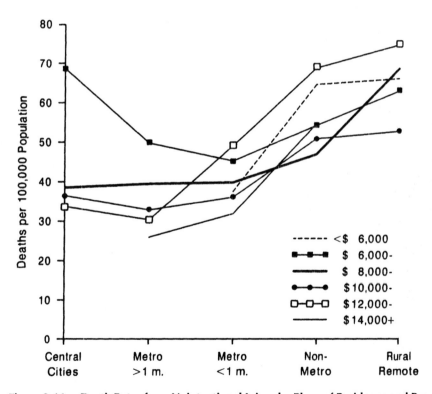

Figure 3-11.   Death Rates from Unintentional Injury by Place of Residence and Per Capita Income of Area of Residence, 1980–1986

Ratio	Unintentional Injury	Suicide	Homicide
23:1	Natural disaster		
15:1	Drowning, boat-related		
8:1	Machinery		
6:1	Aircraft		
	Lightning		
5:1	Exposure, neglect		
4:1	Firearm		
	Struck by falling object		
	Excessive cold		
3:1	Electric current		
	Motor vehicle occupant		
	Drowning, non-boat		
2:1	Caught/crushed		
	Pedestrian, non-traffic		
	Collision, object/person		
	Housefire		
	Explosion		
1.5:1	Cutting/piercing		
	Motor vehicle exhaust	Firearm	
	Poisoning, alcohol		
	Fall, same level		
	Suffocation		
	Excessive heat		
1:1------	----------------	------------	------------
	Aspiration, food		
	Aspiration, non-food	Motor vehicle exhaust	
	Fall, different level	Drowning	
	Pedestrian, train	Hanging	
1:2	Motorcyclist	Cutting/piercing	
	Poisoning, tranquilizers		
	Pedestrian, traffic		
	Clothing, ignition		
	Fall, building/structure		
	Bicyclist		
	Fall, stairs		
	Fall, ladder/scaffold		
1:3	Poisoning, antidepressants		Firearm
1:4	Poisoning, barbiturates	Poisoning, solids/liquids	Other
1:5			Strangulation
			Cutting/stabbing
1:20	Poisoning, opiates		
1:83		Jumping	

Figure 3-12.   Rural to Urban Ratios of Injury Death Rates by Cause, 1980–1986

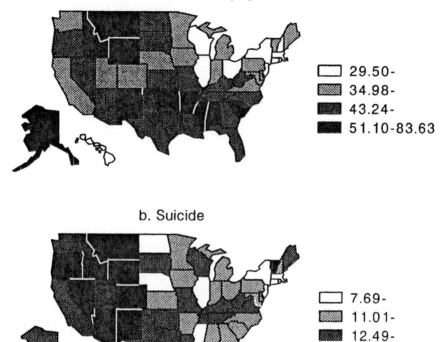

a. Unintentional Injury

☐	29.50-
▨	34.98-
▓	43.24-
■	51.10-83.63

b. Suicide

☐	7.69-
▨	11.01-
▓	12.49-
■	14.98-24.79

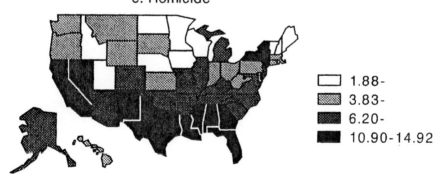

c. Homicide

☐	1.88-
▨	3.83-
▓	6.20-
■	10.90-14.92

Figure 3-13. Death Rates from Unintentional Injury, Suicide, and Homicide by State, per 100,000 Population, 1980–1986

Jersey and New York to 25 in Nevada; and for homicide, from less than 2 in North Dakota and New Hampshire to 15 in Louisiana and Texas (Washington, D.C., has an even higher rate, 28 per 100,000, but is not included in the comparisons among states). The magnitude of these differences reflects the great diversity among the states in population characteristics and exposure to hazards. Many of these relationships will be discussed in later chapters in connection with specific causes of death. Detailed state-specific data for childhood injury have been published elsewhere (Baker and Waller 1989).

State-specific death rates, like other death rates presented in this book, have not been adjusted for age or other population characteristics that may differ from state to state, as is often done with health statistics. Except for falls, the age-adjusted death rates for most injuries differ very little from the actual (unadjusted) death rates (Iskrant and Joliet 1968). In contrast, for most causes of injury there are fourfold to twentyfold differences in death rates among the various states. Age adjustment would not change the patterns illustrated and would only slightly increase or reduce the differences in the actual rates. The use of unadjusted rates permits others to replicate the analyses in this book and portrays the actual rates of death in various population subgroups. Age-adjusted rates for major categories of injury deaths have also been calculated and mapped by county (Devine et al. 1991).

TEMPORAL VARIATION

With the exception of suicides, injury deaths occur most frequently on weekends, peaking on Saturdays (Figure 3-14). Suicides show less variation

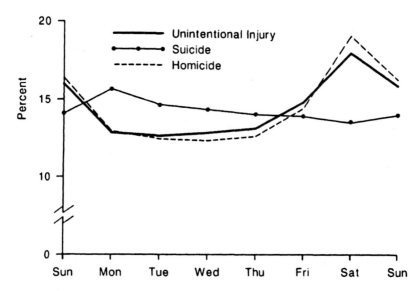

Figure 3-14.   Percentage of Deaths from Unintentional Injury, Suicide, and Homicide by Day of Week, 1980–1986

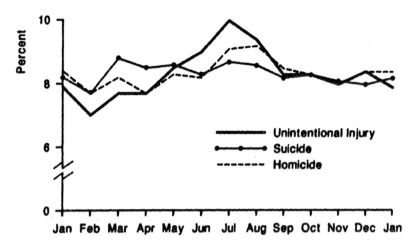

Figure 3-15.   Percentage of Deaths from Unintentional Injury, Suicide, and Homicide by Month, 1980–1986

by day of week than the other major injury groups. The greatest numbers occur on Mondays, the fewest on Thursdays through Sundays.

Seasonal variation is most pronounced for unintentional injuries, with July the peak month (Figure 3-15). Several major causes of death contribute to this summer peak, including drowning and motorcycle crashes. (As with later figures showing month of death, Figure 3-15 does not adjust for the number of days in each month during the years studied. Such adjustment would tend to reduce slightly some of the monthly variation shown in this graph.)

HISTORICAL TRENDS

Throughout most of this century, the death rate from injuries has declined. Most of this decline has occurred in the general category of unintentional injury deaths not related to motor vehicle crashes (Figure 3-16). Although the non-motor-vehicle injury per capita death rate declined by 76 percent between 1910 and 1986, the death rate from motor vehicle crashes increased approximately tenfold between 1910 and 1930 and has decreased by about 25 percent since that time. The homicide rate varied from a low of about 6 in 1910 to a high of more than 11 in 1980, with an earlier peak during the 1930s. In contrast, the suicide rate has shown less fluctuation.

Comparison of injury death rates during 1984–1986 with rates during 1977–1979 reveals that the rate for unintentional injury declined by 15 percent, the rate for homicide declined by 7 percent, and the rate for suicide increased by 2 percent (Table 3-3). Much larger differences in the percentage change were seen among the subcategories of injury causes.

When the economy is depressed, suicides and homicides reportedly increase and motor vehicle deaths decrease (Brenner 1976). The national

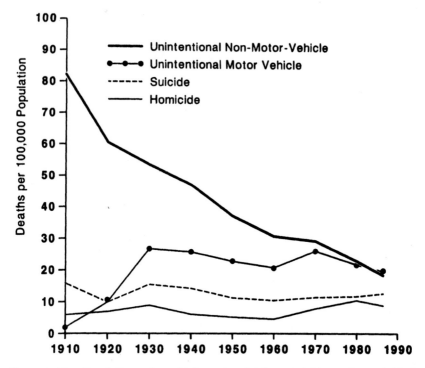

Figure 3-16. Death Rates from Unintentional Injury, Suicide, and Homicide by Year, 1910–1986

economic indicator most commonly used to quantify these associations has been the Federal Reserve Board Industrial Index of Production (IIP), which since 1950 has been strongly correlated with the annual number of motor vehicle deaths. Virtually every drop in the index during this period has been accompanied by a reduction in motor vehicle deaths (Figure 3-17). It is important to note that this correlation is not due to increases or decreases in vehicle mileage. During the 1981–1982 economic slowdown, vehicle mileage increased while motor vehicle deaths declined in parallel with the economy. A correlation is also seen between the IIP and homicide but not as consistently as with motor vehicle deaths. To date, no empirical research has adequately explained the causal mechanisms producing the correlations between injury death rates and economic indicators. Partyka (1984) reported that fatality trends from 1960 through 1982 appear consistent with changes in the numbers of unemployed workers, employed workers, and people not available for the labor force.

Trends in nonfatal injury rates are harder to identify than mortality trends because of the relative lack of detailed, consistently recorded data. For hospitalized injuries in Maryland, discharge rates decreased between 1981 and 1988, with the most notable changes seen for white males aged 15–

Table 3-3. Percentage Change in Injury Death Rates by Cause, 1984–1986 Compared with 1977–1979

Percentage Change	Unintentional	Percentage Change	Intentional
− 15	All unintentional injuries	2	Suicide
278	Cocaine poisoning	15	Hanging
143	Opiate poisoning	9	Motor vehicle exhaust
68	Aspiration—nonfood	6	Firearm
14	Excessive cold	0	Cutting/piercing
12	Solids/liquids excluding opiates	− 3	Nonfirearm, total
		− 20	Drowning
2	Motorcyclist	− 21	Poisoning by solids/liquids
0	Pedestrian—train	− 23	Jumping
0	Excessive heat		
0	Bicyclist	− 7	Homicide
− 5	Suffocation	8	Strangulation
− 13	Natural disaster	7	Other (beating, etc.)
− 16	Motor vehicle occupant	7	Nonfirearm, total
− 16	Pedestrian	5	Cutting/stabbing
− 17	Cutting/piercing	− 15	Firearm
− 18	Falls		
− 19	Housefires	− 11	Legal intervention
− 20	Aspiration—food		
− 21	Firearm		
− 22	Pedestrian—nontraffic		
− 23	Electric current		
− 24	Struck by falling object		
− 26	Drowning		
− 28	Farm machinery		
− 29	Collision with object or person		
− 29	Caught/crushed		
− 31	Other machinery		
− 32	Aircraft		
− 35	Explosion		
− 38	Motor vehicle exhaust		
− 40	Clothing ignition		
− 40	Motor vehicle—train		
− 43	Exposure, neglect		

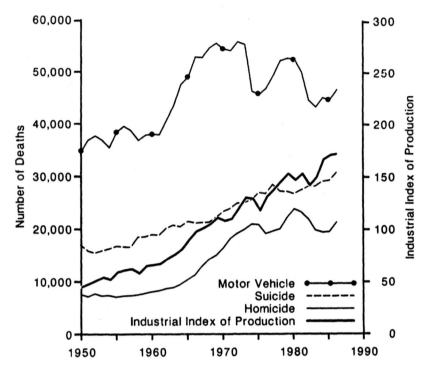

Figure 3-17. Federal Reserve Board Industrial Index of Production and Deaths from Motor Vehicle Crashes, Suicide, and Homicide by Year, 1950–1986

29, whose rates decreased by about 20 percent. Comparison of Figure 3-6 with the corresponding data in Baker et al. (1984) reveals that rates for black males did not show a similar decrease; rather, their hospitalization rates surpassed those for white males, which previously had been higher for ages 15–24.

NOTES

1. The word "accident" erroneously implies that injuries occur by chance and cannot be foreseen or prevented. In much scientific work the descriptor "accident" is gradually being replaced by more appropriate terms, such as "unintentional injury," descriptions of the injuries (e.g., "fractured tibia"), or specification of the injury-producing event, such as a motor vehicle crash.

2. A MSA is a large population nucleus together with adjacent communities that have a high degree of economic and social integration. Areas qualify for establishment as a new MSA by containing either a central city of 50,000 population or a Census Bureau-defined urban area of 50,000 with a total metropolitan population of at least 100,000 (75,000 in New England).

REFERENCES

Alphey, R.S., and S.J. Leach (1974). Accidental death in the home. *Royal Society of Health Journal* 3:97–102, 144.

Baker, S.P., and A.E. Waller (1989). *Childhood injury state-by state mortality facts.* Baltimore, MD: Johns Hopkins Injury Prevention Center.

Baker, S.P., B. O'Neill, and R. Karpf (1984). *The injury fact book.* Lexington, MA: Lexington Books.

Barancik, J.I., and M.A. Shapiro (1976). *Pittsburgh Burn Study. Pittsburgh and Allegheny County, Pennsylvania, 1 June 1970–15 April 1971.* Washington, DC: U.S. Consumer Product Safety Commission.

Barancik, J.I., B.F. Chatterjee, Y.C. Greene, E.M. Michenzi, and D. Fife (1983). Northeastern Ohio Trauma Study: I. Magnitude of the problem. *American Journal of Public Health* 73:746–751.

Brenner, M.H. (1976). Estimating the social costs of national economic policy: Implications for mental and physical health, and criminal aggression. In *Achieving the goals of the Employment Act of 1946 thirtieth anniversary review. Volume 1: Employment. A study prepared for the Joint Economic Committee, Congress of the United States.* Washington, DC: U.S. Government Printing Office.

Buhr, A.J., and A.M. Cooke (1959). Fracture patterns. *Lancet* 1:531–536.

Devine, O.J., J.L. Annest, M.L. Kirk, P. Holmgreen, and S.S. Emrich (1991). *Injury mortality atlas of the United States 1979–1987.* Atlanta, GA: Centers for Disease Control.

Fife, D., J.I. Barancik, and B.F. Chatterjee (1984). Northeastern Ohio Trauma Study: II. Injury rates by age, sex, and cause. *American Journal of Public Health* 74:473–478.

Hassall, C., and W.H. Trethowan (1972). Suicide in Birmingham. *British Medical Journal* 1:717–718.

Indian Health Service (1990). Injuries among Native American Indians and Alaska natives 1990. Rockville, MD: U.S. Department of Health and Human Services.

Iskrant, A.P., and P.V. Joliet (1968). *Accidents and homicide.* Cambridge, MA: Harvard University Press.

Mierley, M.C., and S.P. Baker (1983). Fatal house fires in an urban population. *Journal of the American Medical Association* 249:1466–1468.

National Center for Health Statistics (1985). Persons injured and disability days due to injuries. United States 1980–1981. *Vital and Health Statistics* 10(149).

National Center for Health Statistics (1990). Advance report of final mortality statistics, 1988. *Monthly Vital Statistics Report* 39(7):23.

Nersesian, W.S., M.R. Petit, R. Shaper, D. Lemieux, and E. Naor (1985). Childhood death and poverty. A study of all childhood deaths in Maine, 1976 to 1980. *Pediatrics* 75:41–50.

Partyka, S.C. (1984). Simple models of fatality trends using employment and population data. *Accident Analysis and Prevention* 16:211–222.

Sewell, C.M., T.M. Becker, C.L. Wiggins, C.R. Key, H.F. Hull, and J.M. Samet (1989). Injury mortality in New Mexico's American Indians, Hispanics, and non-Hispanic whites, 1958 to 1982. *Western Journal of Medicine* 150:708–713.

Springate, C.S., R.R. McMeekin, and C.J. Ruehle (1989). Fire deaths in aircraft
without the crashworthy fuel system. *Aviation Space & Environmental Medicine* 60(10):B35–38.

Wise, P.H. (1983). Differential childhood mortality in Boston (abstract). *American Journal of Diseases of Children* 137:538.

4

Unintentional Injury

Unintentional injuries cause about 100,000 deaths annually and are the fourth leading cause of death in the United States. Table 4-1 shows the numbers of deaths from the 20 leading causes of unintentional injury death. Motor vehicle crashes, falls, poisoning, fires, and drowning cause more than three-fourths of all deaths from unintentional injuries.

Table 4-1.   Twenty Leading Causes of Unintentional Injury Death, 1988

Rank	Cause	Number of Deaths
1	Motor vehicle crashes—traffic	48,024
2	Falls	12,096
3	Poisoning by solids/liquids	5,353
4	Fires and burns	5,087
5	Drowning	4,966
6	Aspiration—nonfood	2,230
7	Aspiration—food	1,575
8	Firearm	1,501
9	Machinery	1,176
10	Aircraft	1,012
11	Suffocation	956
12	Poisoning by gas/vapor	873
13	Excessive cold	846
14	Struck by falling object	835
15	Electric current	714
16	Pedestrian—train	470
17	Excessive heat	454
18	Pedestrian—nontraffic	380
19	Collision with object/person	239
20	Exposure, neglect	199

AGE AND SEX

The relative importance of various causes of fatal injury varies substantially with age (Table 4-2). Motor vehicle crashes are the most frequent cause of fatal injury for ages 1–74, and falls are the most frequent cause for ages 75 and older. Drowning is the second leading cause of unintentional injury death for ages 1–44 and the third leading cause for all ages combined. Falls account for almost one-fifth of all unintentional injury deaths among females, compared with one-tenth among males (Figure 4-1).

The proportions of injury deaths show the most important causes among specific groups of people but do not tell which groups have the highest mortality *rates* per 100,000 population. For example, firearms cause 6.4 percent of all unintentional injury deaths at ages 10–14 compared with 2.6 percent at ages 15–19, but the death *rate* from this cause is highest among 15–19-year-olds. Analysis of the various causes of death for ages 15–19 shows that the high injury death rates from many other causes eclipse unintentional deaths from firearms, despite the high death rate from this cause relative to other ages.

The death rates by age for all unintentional injuries combined form a J-shaped curve with an intermediate peak at ages 20–24 (Figure 3-2). The shape of this curve, however, does not hold for individual causes of fatal injury. Mortality patterns for 12 categories of unintentional injury by age and sex exhibit widely differing patterns (Figure 4-2).

Some causes of death (e.g., deaths from firearms) have one especially high-risk age group (Figure 4-2e). The more complex patterns (e.g., deaths from poisoning by solids and liquids) usually reflect the composite nature of a group of injury deaths (Figure 4-2i). In this case, poisoning deaths from

Table 4-2.   Percentage of Unintentional Injury Deaths by Age and Cause, 1980–1986

Cause	Age						
	0–	5–	15–	25–	35–	55–	75+
Motor vehicle crashes	26.9	52.1	75.3	60.4	50.7	30.8	19.5
Aircraft	0.3	0.6	0.6	1.8	2.8	0.2	0.0
Poisoning	2.4	1.3	3.4	11.6	10.2	3.5	2.6
Falls	3.0	1.3	2.0	3.1	6.4	25.4	40.5
Housefires	19.2	9.6	1.7	2.8	3.6	4.5	3.6
Drowning	19.6	15.4	6.7	6.3	5.7	2.6	1.6
Aspiration	7.3	1.2	0.4	0.9	2.2	8.4	10.4
Suffocation	6.5	2.3	0.7	1.0	0.8	0.4	0.4
Other and unspecified	14.8	16.2	9.2	12.1	17.6	24.2	21.4
Total	100.0	100.0	100.0	100.0	100.0	100.0	100.0

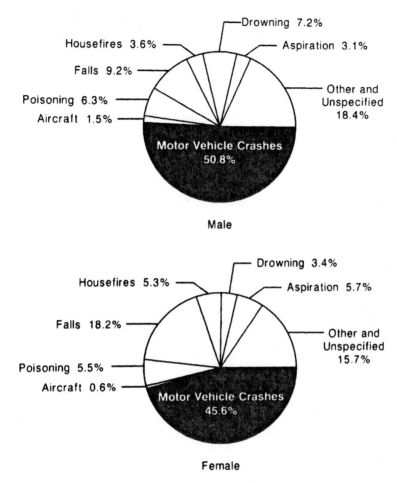

Figure 4-1. Percentage of Unintentional Injury Deaths by Sex and Cause, 1980–1986

several groups of toxic substances with distinctive age and sex patterns are included. (Chapter 15 presents more detailed information on poisoning.)

Compared with other types of unintentional injury, deaths from natural disasters (e.g., floods, earthquakes, and tornados) have less dramatic age- and sex-related patterns (Figure 4-2l), presumably because people of both sexes and all ages are more similar in exposure than is the case with other injury causes. The somewhat higher death rate among the elderly from disasters probably reflects their reduced ability to escape such situations, greater susceptibility to injury (i.e., lower injury threshold), and higher case fatality rates when they are injured. Elderly people have the highest death rates from many causes, including pedestrian injuries, excessive cold, falls, fires and burns, and farm machinery (Figure 4-2). Among people aged 70 or

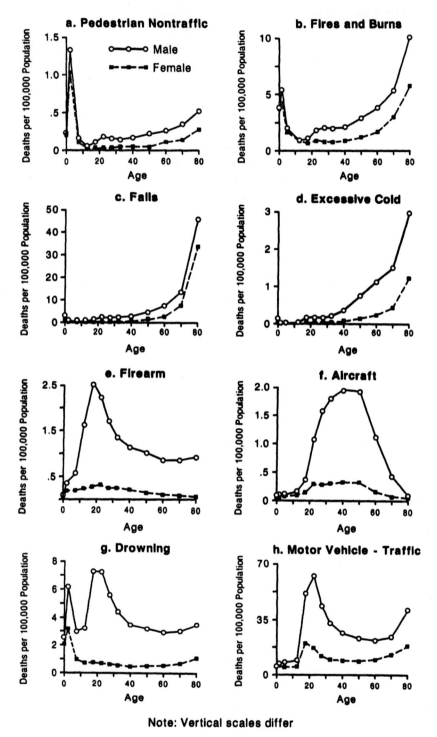

Note: Vertical scales differ

Figure 4-2.   Death Rates from Unintentional Injury by Age, Sex, and Cause, 1980–1986

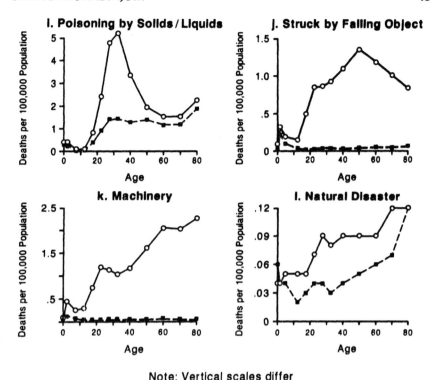

I. Poisoning by Solids/Liquids

J. Struck by Falling Object

k. Machinery

l. Natural Disaster

Note: Vertical scales differ

Figure 4.2.   *Continued*

older, the extremely steep rise in fatal falls is substantially greater than the increase in deaths from any other cause (Figure 4-3).

The higher injury death rates among the elderly result from a combination of factors, including decreasing ability to perceive and avoid hazards such as moving automobiles; musculoskeletal, proprioceptive, and other changes that increase their likelihood of falling; greater likelihood of injury when subjected to a given force; and poorer outcome following injury (Baker 1975; Haddon et al. 1961; Hogue 1982).

The importance of exposure (the opportunity of being injured) as a factor in death rates is suggested by the decline after age 70 or 80 in death rates from some causes. Machinery-related deaths in men decline sharply after age 75; about one-half involve tractors. For most causes of death that are typically work-related, such as deaths from falling objects, the death rate is relatively high throughout the working ages (Figure 4-2j; see also Chapter 9).

High death rates in the 15–24 age group (e.g., from firearms, drownings, and motor vehicles) are partly due to increasing use by males, beginning in their early teens, of alcohol and potentially lethal products such as guns and motorcycles. The role of cultural patterns of expected behavior (e.g., what is

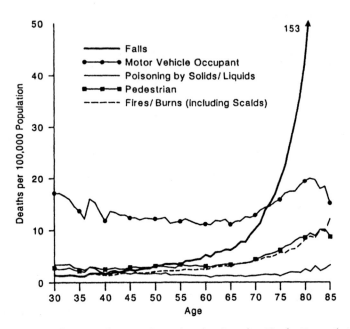

Figure 4-3. Death Rates from Unintentional Injury by Single Year of Age and Cause for Ages 30–85, 1980–1986

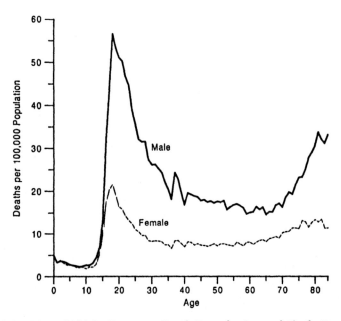

Figure 4-4. Motor Vehicle Occupant Death Rates by Sex and Single Year of Age, 1980–1986

regarded as appropriate behavior by young men compared with that for young women) has not been adequately explored.

An increase in death rates from many causes begins at about age 10. Motor vehicle occupant death rates begin increasing very steeply at age 13, peaking at 18 and then declining until the late sixties (Figure 4-4). No other causes of unintentional injury death exhibit such pronounced age effects. Among males, drownings peak at age 18 and motorcyclist and pedestrian deaths at age 21, but these peaks are less pronounced (Figure 4-5). Death

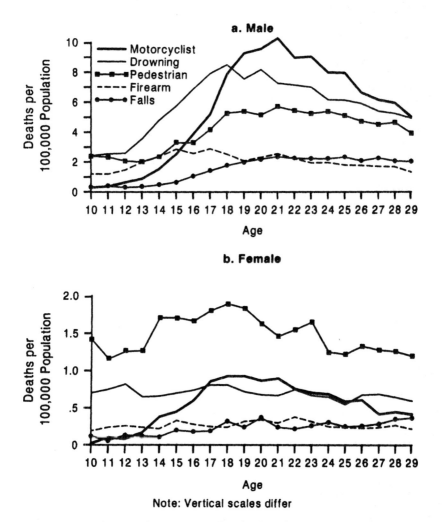

Figure 4-5.   Death Rates from Unintentional Injury by Age, Sex, and Cause, for Ages 10–29, 1980–1986; Excludes Motor Vehicle Occupants

rates from falls are high at ages 19–25 but, unlike many injuries, do not change markedly thereafter until about age 65, when they begin to increase dramatically. Firearm deaths are unusual in having the highest death rate at about age 15.

Rates for females are much lower and show less dramatic peaks at slightly younger ages than is the case for males (Figure 4-5). As shown in Figure 4-4, the motor vehicle occupant death rate, which is highest at age 18 for females, is an exception to this pattern.

The patterns of death rates during early childhood reflect various aspects of physical and mental development that influence susceptibility to injury: recognition of hazards, curiosity, ability to perform certain tasks (for example, opening a gate or riding a bicycle), and need for supervision. High death rates among very young children are partly due to their inability to recognize hazards and protect themselves. An example is a child who is struck by a vehicle in a driveway or other off-road place. Such deaths occur predominantly in the first year or two of life, and they are the only major type of injury death for which the rate is highest among young children (Figure 4-2a).

Figure 4-6 shows specific age patterns for 10 causes of unintentional injury deaths during the preteen years. Aspiration, suffocation, falls, and motor vehicle occupant deaths decrease after the first year of life, as do nontraffic pedestrian deaths (see Chapter 19). Pedestrian deaths in traffic peak at age 6 and then decline. Deaths from some of these causes increase again during the teenage years.

During childhood, there is little difference between the sexes in motor vehicle occupant deaths, probably reflecting the fact that in this case, unlike many other causes of injury, children have little influence over their exposure to risk. The ratio of male to female deaths is especially high for

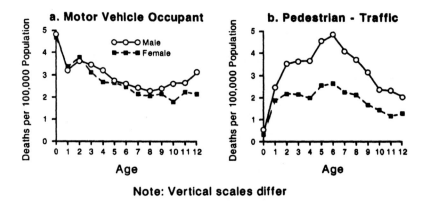

Note: Vertical scales differ

Figure 4-6. Death Rates from Unintentional Injury by Age, Sex, and Cause, for Ages 0–12, 1980–1986

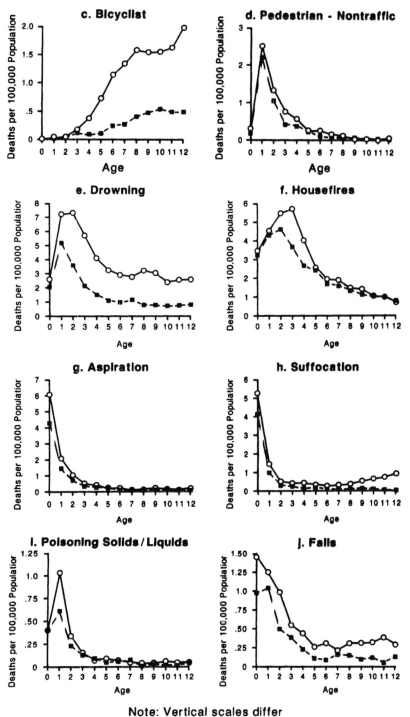

Note: Vertical scales differ

Figure 4.6. *Continued*

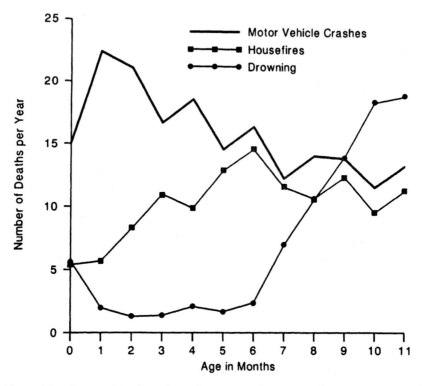

Figure 4-7. Average Number of Deaths per Year from Housefires, Drowning, and Motor Vehicle Crashes by Month of Age, for Ages 0–11 Months, 1980–1986

drowning, bicycling, and pedestrian deaths in traffic; these deaths result from activities the child is more likely to have initiated. For nonfatal injuries treated in emergency departments, higher rates among male children are evident beginning in the first year of life (Rivara 1982). As in the case of teenagers and young adults, sex differences in injury rates among young children raise questions regarding societal norms and parental expectations in influencing their activities and behaviors, as well as the role of innate biological differences.

During the first year of life, the major causes of injury death differ in their distribution by month of age (Figure 4-7). Motor vehicle occupant deaths are most common at age 1–2 months. Drowning rates are high in the first month of life, possibly reflecting the inclusion of some unidentified homicides,[1] and then increase markedly beginning at age 7 months, when many infants start to crawl. Housefire death rates are lowest for the young-est babies, perhaps because families with infants are less likely to be sound asleep during the early morning hours when most housefires occur (see Chapter 12). Deaths coded as aspiration and suffocation, the other major categories of fatal unintentional injury during infancy, occur primarily during the first 5 months (see Chapter 14).

RACE AND PER CAPITA INCOME

There are differences by race not only in overall death rates from unintentional injuries (Figure 3-8) but also in age-specific patterns (Figure 4-8). Native Americans have the highest rates at all ages. Whites have the second highest rates at ages 15–24, and blacks have the second highest rates at other ages. Unlike rates for other races, those for blacks do not peak between ages 15 and 24, and they increase after age 25.

Motor vehicles are the major cause of fatal unintentional injury for each racial group, but the relative importance of other causes differs (Figure 4-9). Falls are the second leading cause of unintentional death among whites. Drownings are second or third among each racial group. Among blacks, the death rate from housefires is even higher than the drowning rate. (See Table 3-1 for details on other major causes of death for each racial group.)

Death rates are high in low-income areas for most categories of unintentional injury (Figure 4-10). Causes of death with this pattern include exces-

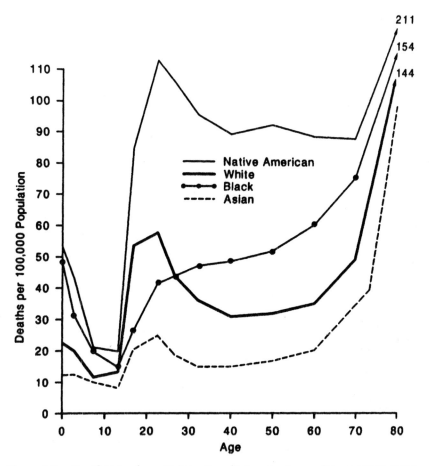

Figure 4-8. Death Rates from Unintentional Injury by Age and Race, 1980–1986

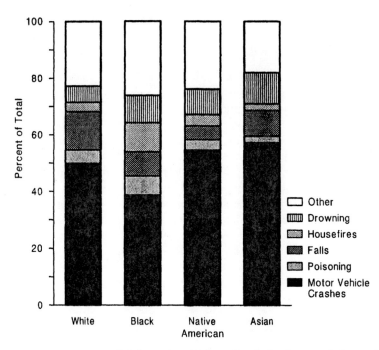

Figure 4-9. Percentage of Unintentional Injury Deaths by Race and Cause, 1980–1986

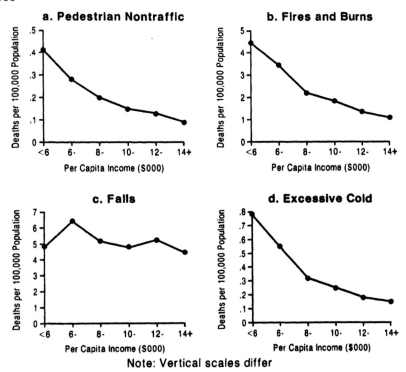

Note: Vertical scales differ

Figure 4-10. Death Rates from Unintentional Injury by Per Capita Income of Area of Residence and Cause, 1980–1986

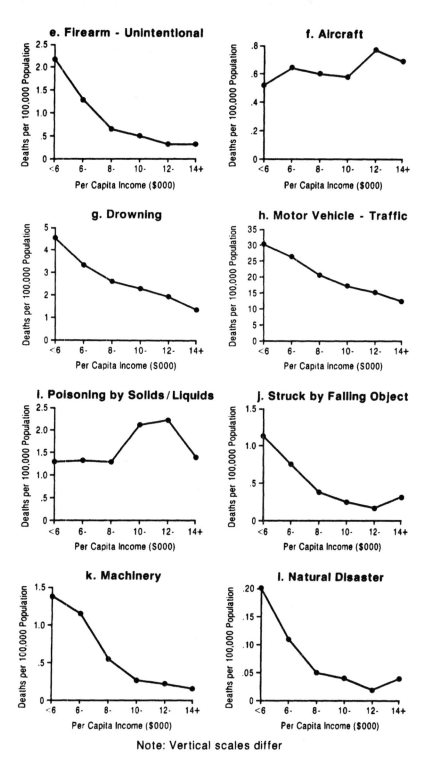

Note: Vertical scales differ

Figure 4.10.   *Continued*

sive cold, fires, firearms, machinery, falling objects, and aspiration of nonfood objects (not shown). The pattern of high death rates in low-income areas from natural disasters may reflect housing that provides less protection against tornados and is more likely to be located in floodplains. Death rates from falls decline only slightly with income.

URBAN/RURAL AND GEOGRAPHIC DIFFERENCES

For most unintentional injuries, death rates are highest in the more rural areas (Figure 4-11). These high rates are in part related to exposure to certain causes of injury among people living or working on farms. Although farm workers constitute only 4 percent of U.S. workers (Bureau of the Census 1988), 35 percent of all deaths identified as machinery-related occur on farms, as do 5 percent of deaths from electricity and 9 percent from falling objects (Table 4-3). The most common sources of fatal injury on farms, other than machinery and road vehicles, are drowning, falling objects, and firearms.

Injury deaths on farms are not limited to adult workers. Farm machinery death rates are also high among young children; for ages 4–5 years, the

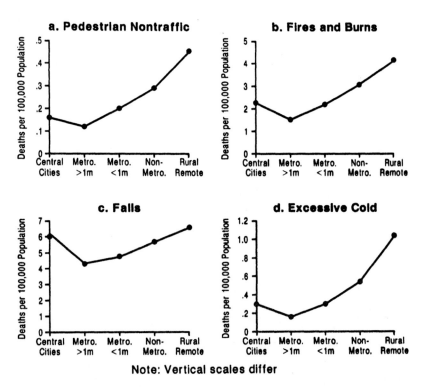

Note: Vertical scales differ

Figure 4-11. Death Rates from Unintentional Injury by Place of Residence and Cause, 1980–1986

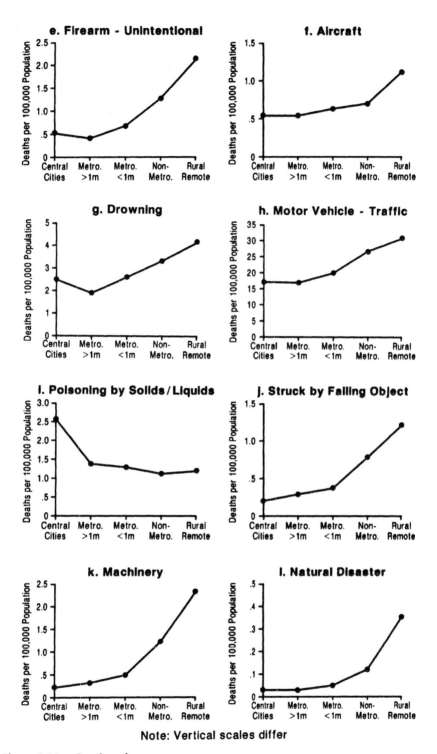

Note: Vertical scales differ

Figure 4.11.   *Continued*

53

Table 4-3. Percentage of Unintentional Injury Deaths by Place of Injury and Cause, 1980–1986

Cause	Home	Resident Institution	Public Building	Recreation/ Sport	Farm	Industrial/ Mine	Other	Unspecified	Total
Drowning	12.4	0.4	1.0	14.6	1.9	1.3	53.8	14.6	100.0
Motor vehicle exhaust	45.4	0.0	3.2	0.8	1.4	12.8	22.9	13.5	100.0
Other gas/vapor	45.8	0.2	2.0	1.5	1.6	5.4	10.0	33.5	100.0
Falls	39.6	11.9	3.1	0.8	0.4	2.4	9.1	32.7	100.0
Fires and burns	87.9	1.0	1.7	0.1	0.4	1.5	2.6	4.8	100.0
Firearm	42.9	0.1	2.3	0.8	4.1	0.4	17.8	31.6	100.0
Lightning	11.6	0.8	3.0	14.3	8.6	2.4	29.5	29.8	100.0
Suffocation	48.3	5.1	1.7	0.5	3.1	6.9	10.6	23.8	100.0
Falling object	25.5	0.3	4.4	1.1	8.9	20.1	26.2	13.5	100.0
Collision with object or person	20.9	3.0	6.6	11.2	3.1	17.9	21.1	16.2	100.0
Caught/crushed	20.8	3.0	6.2	0.9	5.3	29.0	23.8	11.0	100.0
Machinery	8.6	0.2	1.4	0.8	35.4	24.4	14.5	14.7	100.0
Explosion	30.2	0.2	5.8	1.1	1.9	32.6	14.1	14.1	100.0
Electric current	25.5	0.3	3.9	1.1	4.7	24.3	12.7	27.5	100.0

number of these deaths is similar to the number from falls. This is remarkable, because virtually all young children are exposed at some time to the possibility of falls whereas only 2 percent live on farms (Bureau of the Census 1988). Major causes of farm machinery deaths among young children are being run over by tractors and falling from tractors, on which they are often carried as passengers (McKnight 1984). In addition to tractors, encounters with farm wagons, combines, and forklifts are involved in many deaths and severe injuries in the under-20 age group (Rivara 1985). Entanglement in augers and power take-off shafts also causes serious injuries to young children.

Pronounced geographic variation characterizes unintentional injury deaths (Figure 4-12). The high death rates from many causes in southern and mountain states reflect the fact that much of their population lives in rural areas, where injury death rates tend to be high. For falls, the death rates are highest in the northern half of the country, an unexplained pattern that persists when death rates are age adjusted. As in the case of urban/rural differences, these dramatic regional variations illustrate the importance of the environment as a determinant of injury death rates.

There is a generally unrecognized correlation between state death rates from motor vehicle injuries and those from other unintentional injuries (Figure 4-13). This close correlation suggests common factors in the initiating circumstances (for example, high alcoholism rates would influence the incidence of most categories of injuries) and in access to emergency care. In many of the states with high death rates from motor vehicle and other unintentional injuries, much of the population lives far from major medical centers; this is especially true in Alaska, which has the highest death rate from unintentional injuries. If the rates plotted in Figure 4-13 were for travel and nontravel injury deaths, Alaska would fall much closer to the line for other states, since a substantial portion of the injury deaths in that state result from airplane crashes and water transport.

The high rates of injury death in Alaska cannot be explained by the age distribution of its residents. Age-adjusted death rates for all United States counties or groups of counties place Alaska in the upper 25th percentile for seven of the eight major categories of injury, including homicide and suicide (Devine et al. 1991). Motor vehicle-related injuries are the single exception to this pattern.

TEMPORAL VARIATION

Most causes of death from unintentional injury have weekend peaks, generally coinciding with increased social and recreational activity and greater alcohol use (Figure 4-14). The data analyzed are based on date of death rather than date of injury; consequently, they may obscure temporal differences in the occurrence of injuries that usually are not rapidly fatal, which is especially true in the case of falls.

a. Motor Vehicle - Traffic

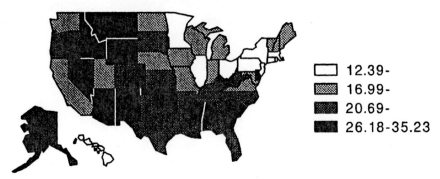

☐ 12.39-
▨ 16.99-
▦ 20.69-
■ 26.18-35.23

b. Non-Motor-Vehicle - Unintentional

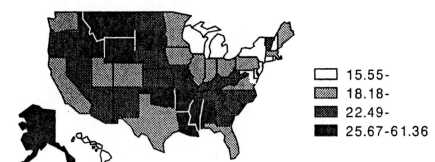

☐ 15.55-
▨ 18.18-
▦ 22.49-
■ 25.67-61.36

c. Falls

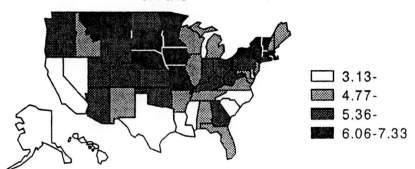

☐ 3.13-
▨ 4.77-
▦ 5.36-
■ 6.06-7.33

Figure 4-12. Death Rates from Unintentional Injury by State and Cause, per 100,000 Population, 1980–1986

d. Drowning

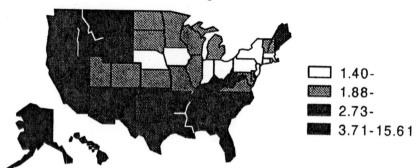

☐	1.40-
▨	1.88-
■	2.73-
■	3.71-15.61

e. Excessive Cold

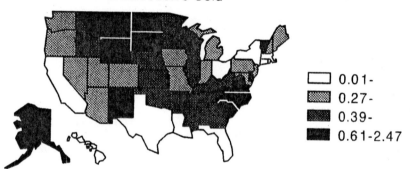

☐	0.01-
▨	0.27-
■	0.39-
■	0.61-2.47

f. Excessive Heat

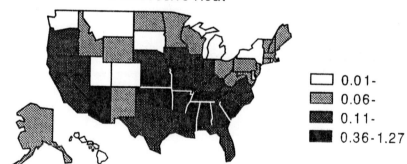

☐	0.01-
▨	0.06-
■	0.11-
■	0.36-1.27

Figure 4.12. *Continued*

57

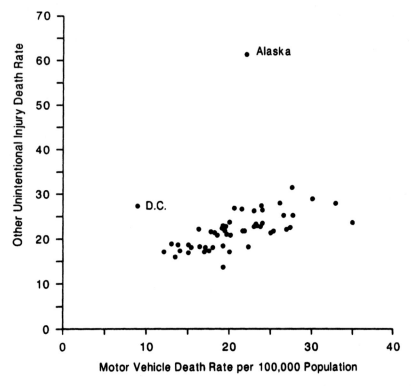

Figure 4-13.   Death Rates from Motor Vehicle Crashes versus Other Unintentional Injuries by State, 1980–1986

The death rate from all unintentional injuries is slightly higher in the summer (Figure 3-15). Ten percent of the deaths occur in July compared with 7 percent in February. The summer excess is especially prominent in drownings and deaths from lightning or electric current (Figure 4-15). In addition, motorcyclist and bicyclist deaths have very pronounced summer peaks. Deaths from housefires or clothing ignition and from unintentional poisoning by motor vehicle exhaust peak in winter. Most other types of unintentional poisonings show little monthly variation. Deaths from fatal falls are slightly more common in December and January. Long periods often elapse between fall injury and death; therefore the slight winter excess, which may be due partly to icy conditions, might be more marked if data were available for the month when the fall occurred rather than the month of death.

HISTORICAL TRENDS

From 1930 to 1986, the overall death rate from unintentional injuries declined by more than half, from 81 to 40 per 100,000 population, with a

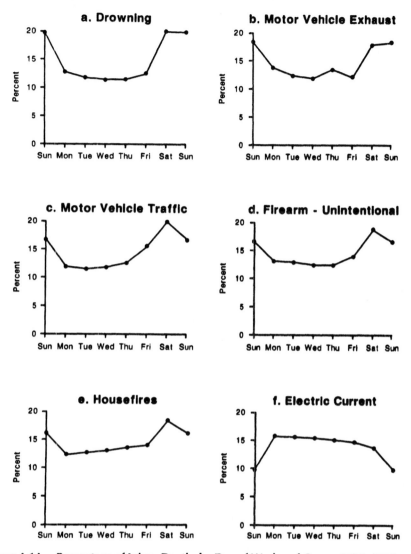

Figure 4-14. Percentage of Injury Deaths by Day of Week and Cause, 1980–1986

further decline to 35 per 100,000 in 1988. This decline, however, has been far from uniform (Figure 4-16, Table 4-4). The rates for deaths related to motor vehicles and poisoning changed relatively little. The housefire death rate increased by 6 percent over this entire period; there was a 32 percent increase from 1930 to 1980, but in more recent years there has been a 19 percent decrease (see Table 3-3).

Among all causes of unintentional injury, the greatest *absolute* drop after 1930 occurred in the death rate from falls. The greatest *proportional* decreases occurred in deaths related to nonfarm machinery, lightning, and

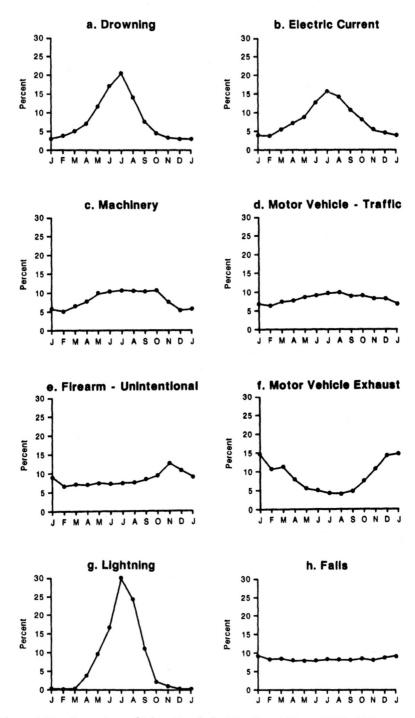

Figure 4-15. Percentage of Injury Deaths by Month and Cause, 1980–1986

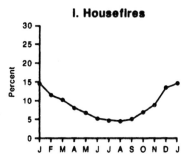

I. Housefires

Figure 4.15.   *Continued*

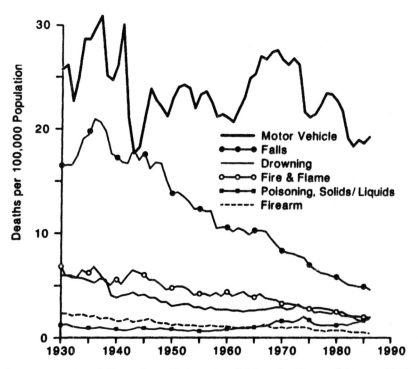

Figure 4-16.   Death Rates from Unintentional Injury by Year and Cause, 1930–
1986

Table 4-4. Percentage Change in Unintentional Injury Death Rates by Cause, 1986 compared with 1930

Cause	Death Rate per 100,000 Population 1930	1986	Percentage Change
Poisoning by solids/liquids	1.44	1.96	+36
Farm machinery	0.25	0.27	+8
Housefires and other conflagrations	1.62	1.72	+6
Aircraft	0.48	0.48	0
Motor vehicle occupants	15.44	14.66	−5
Electric current	0.80	0.35	−56
Drowning, excluding water transport	6.05	2.36	−61
Pedestrians	9.99	2.92	−71
Falls	16.27	4.75	−71
Firearms	2.53	0.60	−76
Poisoning by gases/vapors[a]	1.98	0.42	−79
Nonfarm machinery	1.40	0.23	−84
Lightning	0.29	0.03	−90
Other burns	5.30	0.34	−99
All unintentional injuries	112.89	39.50	−65

Sources: National Center for Health Statistics, published data for 1986, and Bureau of the Census, Mortality Statistics for 1930.

[a]Poisoning by gases and vapors decreased mainly because of a 96 percent decrease in the death rate between 1947 and 1980 from utility gas piped to homes; data prior to 1947 not available for utility gas.

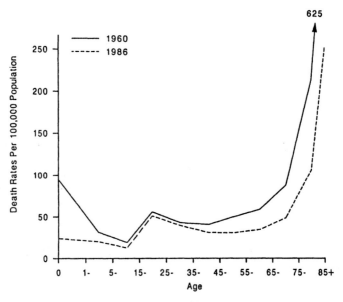

Figure 4-17. Death Rates from Unintentional Injury by Age, 1960 and 1986

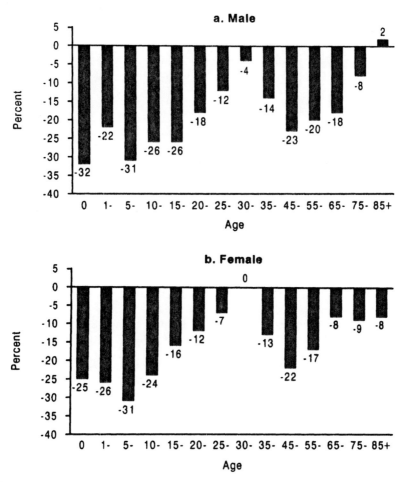

Figure 4-18.   Percentage Change in Death Rates from Unintentional Injury by Age and Sex, 1984–1986 Compared with 1977–1979

burns other than those from housefires (Table 4-4). For all of these, the rates in 1986 were one-fifth or less of the 1930 rates. Deaths attributed to suffocation and aspiration also decreased dramatically, but this may be largely an artifact caused by changes in classification of deaths from sudden infant death syndrome (SIDS, or "crib death"), many of which were formerly attributed to suffocation or aspiration of food (see Chapter 14).

Reductions in the unintentional injury death rate between 1960 and 1986 were largely due to reductions in death rates of the middle aged and elderly (Figure 4-17). For 1984–1986 compared with 1977–1979, the general trend was downward for all ages combined, with a 15 percent decline in the death rate for all unintentional injuries. During the brief interval between these two three-year periods (7 years between the midpoints), death rates from many causes of injury declined by more than 25 percent (Table 3-3). The greatest decline occurred at ages 0–19 and 45–64 (Figure 4-18), unlike the changes in the previous decade, when large decreases were seen at ages 55 and older (Baker et al. 1984).

NOTE

1. Homicide rates are highest in the first month of life and decline gradually; homicide is four times as common in the first month as in the 11th month of life.

REFERENCES

Baker, S.P. (1975). Determinants of injury and opportunities for intervention. *American Journal of Epidemiology* 101:98–102.

Baker, S.P., B. O'Neill, and R. Karpf. (1984). *The injury fact book*. Lexington, MA: Lexington Press.

Bureau of the Census (1988). Rural and rural farm population: 1987. *Current population reports—farm population* 61:11.

Devine, O.J., J.L. Annest, M.L. Kirk, P. Holmgreen, and S.S. Emrich (1991). *Injury mortality atlas of the United States 1979–1987*. Atlanta, GA: Centers for Disease Control.

Haddon, W., Jr., P. Valien, J.R. McCarroll, and C.J. Umberger (1961). A controlled investigation of the characteristics of adult pedestrians fatally injured by motor vehicles in Manhattan. *Journal of Chronic Diseases* 14:655–678.

Hogue, C.C. (1982). Injury in late life: Part I. epidemiology. *Journal of the American Geriatric Society* 30:183–90.

McKnight, R.H. (1984). *U.S. agricultural equipment fatalities 1975–1981: Implications for injury control and health education*. Unpublished doctoral dissertation, The Johns Hopkins University, Baltimore, MD.

Rivara, F.P. (1982). Epidemiology of childhood injuries. In A.B. Bergman (ed.), *Preventing childhood injuries, report of the twelfth Ross roundtable on critical approaches to common pediatric problems*. Columbus, OH: Ross Laboratories, 1982.

Rivara, F.P. (1985). Fatal and nonfatal farm injuries to children and adolescents in the United States. *Pediatrics* 76:567–573.

5

Suicide

More than 30,000 deaths in 1988 were classified as suicide, making this the eighth leading cause of death in the United States. For ages 15–34, suicide is the third leading cause, surpassed only by unintentional injury and homicide. Among white males of all ages combined, suicide is the eighth leading cause of death.

More than half of all suicidal deaths (59 percent) are caused by firearms. The next most frequent causes are hanging (15 percent), poisoning by ingestion of solids or liquids (10 percent), and carbon monoxide poisoning with motor vehicle exhaust (8 percent). Other means include jumping from high places or drowning (2 percent each) and cutting with a sharp instrument (1 percent).

Studies of nonfatal injuries that are deliberately self-inflicted indicate that drug ingestion is the most common method, accounting for at least 70 percent of such cases. Although only 1 percent of all suicides are accomplished by cutting with a sharp instrument, wrist cutting is the second most common method of attempting suicide, accounting for about 15 percent of attempts (Weissman 1974; Wexler et al. 1978). Firearm injuries are relatively uncommon among nonfatal suicide attempts because of the high fatality rate from such injuries.

Risk factors for suicide include previous suicide attempts, depression, alcoholism, divorce or separation, and firearm availability (Brent et al. 1988; Monk 1987; Moscicki et al. 1988). Alcohol use in connection with suicides has often been noted; in Alaska, there was evidence of alcohol consumption prior to the suicide in 59 percent of cases, and people with blood alcohol concentrations (BACs) of 0.10 percent or higher were more likely to have used a gun to commit suicide (Hlady and Middaugh 1987). There are few data on the effectiveness of interventions (Holinger 1990), but the importance of availability of lethal agents has been widely noted in the case of firearms (e.g., Baker 1985), as well as domestic piped gas (Hassall and Trethowan 1972), bridges (Gerberich et al. 1985), and barbiturates (Oliver and Hetzel 1973).

AGE AND SEX

Suicide is rare prior to age 10, and only 1 percent of identified suicides involve people under 15 years old. For both sexes, the suicide rate doubles each year between ages 10 and 14 and then increases more slowly to age 24 (Figure 3-3). Thereafter, the male rate is fairly constant until the late sixties, when it begins to increase again. The highest suicide rate is among elderly males. The rate for females increases until about age 50 and then declines. Overall, the female suicide rate is about one-fourth the male rate. The highest incidence of attempted suicide is at ages 20–24 (Weissman 1974), but the rate is also high for teenagers, especially among females (Trinkoff and Baker 1986).

Males and females differ substantially in their methods of committing suicide at various ages (Table 5-1). Shooting is the most common method of committing suicide for virtually all age and sex groups. Hanging is the second most common means for males of all ages, and poisoning is second for females. Among males aged 10–14, 39 percent of all suicides are by hanging. Among females aged 75 and older, hanging and poisoning are the predominant means, outranking even shooting.

The age- and sex-specific mortality pattern for all methods of suicide combined reflects the pattern for firearms (Figure 5-1) because they are used in the majority of suicides. The age- and sex-specific patterns for suicide by hanging, cutting, jumping, and drowning are roughly similar to one another. Suicide by poisoning and by drowning exhibit the smallest differences by sex. Males and females have similar death rates for suicidal poisoning by solids and liquids until age 30, after which the death rate is substantially higher among women. In the case of drownings, males have a higher rate than females for ages 15–44; at other ages the rates are similar. Peaks in female death rates occur at about age 50 for firearm suicide and for poisoning by solids and liquids, whereas female rates for suicide by hanging, drowning, and cutting increase at older ages.

RACE AND PER CAPITA INCOME

Suicide rates are highest among whites and Native Americans (13 per 100,000 population) and relatively low among Asians and blacks (6 per 100,000). The age-specific patterns for these four racial groups show major differences (Figure 5-2). Native Americans exhibit the sharpest peak at ages 20–24 and have the highest suicide rates up to age 44. After age 44, whites have the highest rates.

Racial groups differ in the methods most commonly employed to commit suicide (Figure 5-3) (Warshauer and Monk 1978). Firearms are used in only about one-fourth of suicides by Asians, compared with more than one-half of suicides by the other three groups. Hanging is the most common means among Asians and accounts for two-fifths of the suicides. It is the second most common means among Native Americans and is used in about one-fourth of their suicides (Simpson et al. 1983).

Table 5-1. Percentage of Suicides by Sex, Age, and Method, 1980–1986

Age	Firearm	Hanging	Poisoning—Solids/Liquids	Motor Vehicle Exhaust	Jumping	Drowning	Cutting	Other	Total
Males									
10–14	58.2	39.3	1.5	0.0	0.5	0.0	0.0	0.5	100.0
15–24	62.6	20.7	3.9	6.9	1.7	0.7	0.5	3.0	100.0
25–34	56.0	19.2	7.6	8.4	2.4	1.4	1.5	3.5	100.0
35–54	61.3	13.1	7.9	9.5	1.9	1.2	1.2	3.9	100.0
55–74	72.7	11.0	4.1	5.5	1.5	1.1	2.0	2.1	100.0
75+	73.2	12.8	2.7	4.1	2.4	1.9	1.5	1.4	100.0
Females									
10–14	50.0	29.6	13.0	0.0	0.0	0.0	3.7	3.7	100.0
15–24	49.6	12.8	18.7	9.4	3.0	0.8	0.8	4.9	100.0
25–34	45.9	10.7	23.9	9.1	3.5	1.7	1.0	4.2	100.0
35–54	37.5	9.4	29.5	12.4	2.3	2.6	1.4	4.9	100.0
55–74	37.5	13.0	24.1	10.3	3.4	5.2	2.7	3.8	100.0
75+	21.5	28.0	25.5	7.7	5.4	6.5	1.2	4.2	100.0

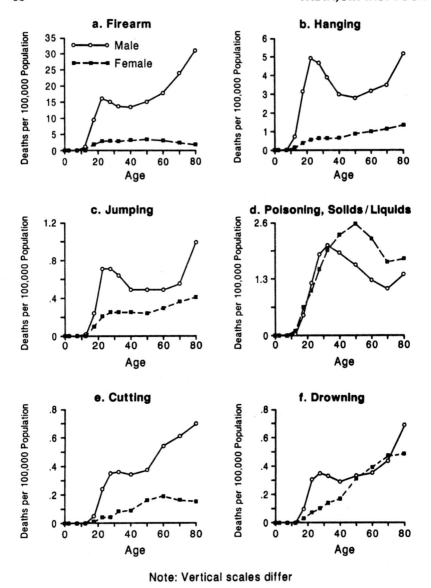

Note: Vertical scales differ

Figure 5-1.   Death Rates from Suicide by Age, Sex, and Method, 1980–1986

After age 30, age- and sex-specific suicide rates show markedly different patterns for blacks and whites (Figure 5-4). The suicide rate among black males is very high for ages 25–34 and declines dramatically thereafter. Although the downward trend reverses in black males in their sixties, the rate does not show the dramatic rise that is apparent for white males. The female suicide rate declines after age 34 for blacks and Native Americans

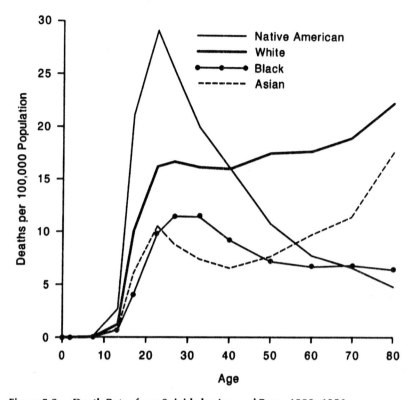

Figure 5-2.   Death Rates from Suicide by Age and Race, 1980–1986

and is highest (13 per 100,000) for Asians aged 75 and older; for white females it is highest at ages 45–54. This peak in female suicide rates at about age 50 appears to be unique among North American white females (Rockett and Smith 1989).

Overall suicide rates show little variation with per capita income of the county of residence (Figure 3-9), but specific types of suicide show strong relationships to income. Except for firearm suicide, rates for all types of suicide are lowest in low-income areas (Figure 5-5). This relationship is strongest for suicide by jumping. For suicide by firearms, however, the death rate is about twice as high in low-income areas as in high-income areas. Because firearms account for more than half of all suicides, the two trends shown in Figure 5-5 tend to offset one another, except at the upper end of the income scale.

URBAN/RURAL AND GEOGRAPHIC DIFFERENCES

The suicide rate is highest in large cities for both blacks and whites (Baker et al. 1984). Urban-rural patterns differ by type of suicide and in some cases

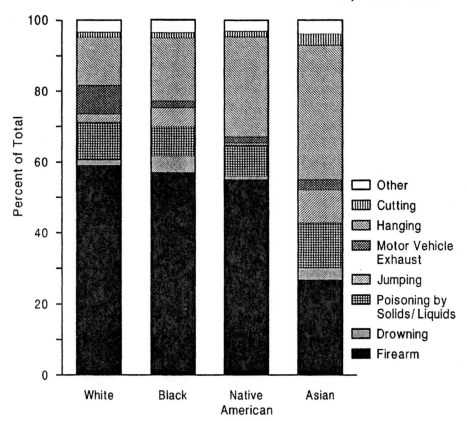

Figure 5-3. Percentage of Suicides by Race and Method, 1980–1986

reflect the availability of various methods (Figure 5-6). Large cities, where tall buildings offer a ready means of committing suicide, have especially high rates of fatal jumps. Rates of suicidal poisoning by solids and liquids are also high in large cities, whereas rates for firearm suicide are highest in rural areas, where gun ownership is most prevalent (FBI 1990). High rates of suicide by motor vehicle exhaust in areas of intermediate urbanization may reflect a greater prevalence of garages.

Suicide rates range from a low of 8 per 100,000 population in New Jersey to a high of 25 in Nevada. Although rates for all types of suicide combined are generally highest in the western states, the geographic patterns differ depending on the method (Figure 5-7). Rates for suicide by firearms are high in the mountain and southern states, where firearm ownership is generally most common (Markush and Bartolucci 1984). Even within a single state, South Carolina, firearm death rates are correlated with firearm ownership rates (Alexander et al. 1985). Suicidal poisoning by solids and liquids is especially common in Florida as well as in several western and south-

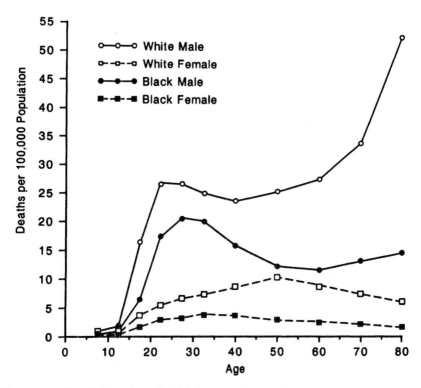

Figure 5-4. Death Rates from Suicide by Age, Race, and Sex, 1980–1986

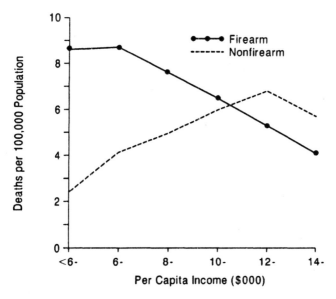

Figure 5-5. Death Rates from Firearm and Nonfirearm Suicide by per Capita Income of Area of Residence, 1980–1986

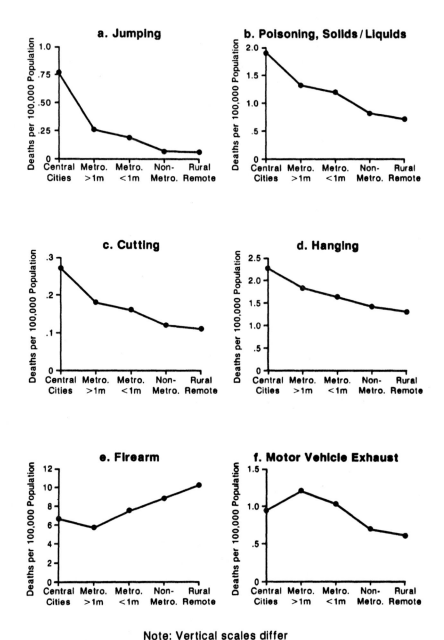

Note: Vertical scales differ

Figure 5-6.   Death Rates from Suicide by Place of Residence and Method, 1980–1986

72

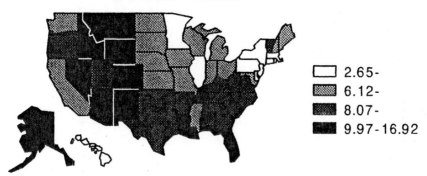

a. Suicide - Firearm

2.65-
6.12-
8.07-
9.97-16.92

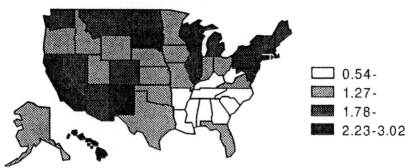

b. Suicide - Hanging

0.54-
1.27-
1.78-
2.23-3.02

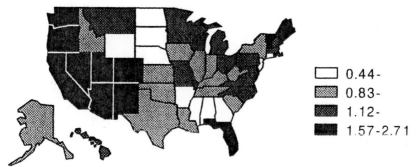

c. Suicide - Poisoning by Solids/ Liquids

0.44-
0.83-
1.12-
1.57-2.71

Figure 5-7. Death Rates from Suicide by State and Method, per 100,000 Population, 1980–1986

western states, while the highest rates for poisoning by motor vehicle exhaust are in northern states, where garages are common. The geographic patterns for both of these categories of suicidal poisoning are roughly similar to those for unintentional injury deaths from the same causes.

TEMPORAL VARIATION

Rates do not vary greatly by day of week, although more suicides are recorded on Mondays than on any other day (Figure 3-14). Seasonal fluctuations are much less marked for suicides than for unintentional injuries (Figure 3-15), but there is a slight increase in suicide in the spring and a December low in most years (the low percentage in February reflects the shorter month).

HISTORICAL TRENDS

In 1982, a 50-year decline in the suicide rate of the elderly ended; the rate has increased since then. For all ages combined, the suicide rate decreased from a high of 17 per 100,000 in 1932 to about 10 in 1943–1944, then

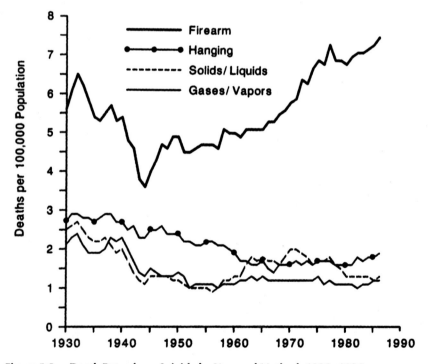

Figure 5-8.   Death Rates from Suicide by Year and Method, 1930–1986

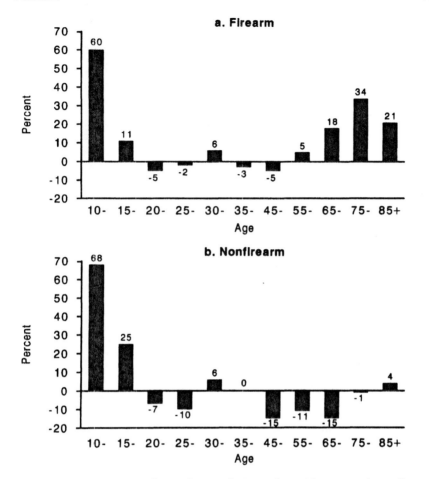

Figure 5-9. Percentage Change in Death Rates from Firearm and Nonfirearm Suicide by Age, 1984–1986 Compared with 1977–1979

increased to 13 in 1986 (Figure 5-8); in 1988 the rate was 12.4. Between 1968 and 1986 the general trend in the suicide rate was upward, with an overall increase of about 19 percent. The rate for suicide by firearms increased by 36 percent, while suicide by all other means combined remained virtually unchanged. From 1950 to 1980, suicide rates generally declined for ages 35 and older but tripled in the 15–19 age group (Carroll and Smith 1988). The increase in firearm suicide among youths coincided with dramatic increases in production and availability of firearms (Boyd and Moscicki 1986).

Comparison of the periods 1977–1979 and 1984–1986 shows increases in suicide by hanging (15 percent), motor vehicle exhaust (9 percent), and firearms (6 percent) and decreases in suicide by drowning (20 percent) and by poisoning with solids or liquids (21 percent). The largest increase was for ages 10–14, whose firearm and nonfirearm suicide rates increased by 60 percent or more (Figure 5-9). For all ages and types of suicides combined, there was a 4 percent increase in male rates and a 12 percent decrease among females in this period. The high suicide rates in young Native American males and middle-aged white females have persisted. Among black males aged 15–19, the firearm suicide rate doubled between 1982 and 1987 while the rate of suicide by other means declined (Fingerhut and Kleinman 1989).

REFERENCES

Alexander, G.R., R.M. Massey, T. Gibbs, and J. Altekruse (1985). Firearm-related fatalities: An epidemiologic assessment of violent death. *American Journal of Public Health* 75:165–168.

Baker, S.P. (1985). Without guns, do people kill people? (editorial). *American Journal of Public Health* 75:587–588.

Baker, S.P., B. O'Neill, and R. Karpf (1984). *The injury fact book*. Lexington, MA: Lexington Books.

Boyd, J.H., and E.K. Moscicki (1986). Firearms and youth suicide. *American Journal of Public Health* 76:1240–1242.

Brent, D.A., J.A. Perper, C.E. Goldstein, D.J. Kolko, M.J. Allan, C.J. Allman, and J.P. Zelenak (1988). Risk factors for adolescent suicide. *Archives of General Psychiatry* 45:581–588.

Federal Bureau of Investigation (1990). *Sourcebook of criminal justice statistics— 1989*. Washington, DC: U. S. Government Printing Office.

Fingerhut, L.A., and J.C. Kleinman (1989). Firearm mortality among children and youth. *Advance Data* 178:1–6.

Gerberich, S.G., M. Hays, J.S. Mandel, R.W. Gibson, and C.J. Van der Heide (1985). Analysis of suicide in adolescents and young adults: Implications for prevention. In U. Laaser, R. Senault, and H. Viefhues (eds.), *Primary Health Care in the Making*. Berlin: Springer-Verlag.

Griffith, E.E.H., and C.C. Bell (1989). Recent trends in suicide and homicide among blacks. *Journal of the American Medical Association* 262:2265–2269.

Hassall, C., and W.H. Trethowan (1972). Suicide in Birmingham. *British Medical Journal* 1:717–718.

Hlady, W.G., and J.P. Middaugh (1987). The epidemiology of suicide in Alaska, 1983–1984. *Alaska Medicine* 29:158–164.

Holinger, P.C. (1990). The causes, impact, and preventability of childhood injuries in the United States: Childhood suicide in the United States. *American Journal of Diseases of Children* 144:670–676.

Markush, R.E., and A.A. Bartolucci (1984). Firearms and suicide in the United States. *American Journal of Public Health* 74:123–127.

Monk, M. (1987). Epidemiology of suicide. *Epidemiologic Reviews* 9:51–69.

Moscicki, E.K., P. O'Carroll, D.S. Rae, B.Z. Locke, A. Roy, and D.A. Regier (1988). Suicide attempts in the Epidemiologic Catchment Area Study. *Yale Journal of Biology and Medicine* 61:259–268.

National Center for Health Statistics (1989). Advance report of final mortality statistics, 1987. *Monthly Vital Statistics Report* 38(5):38.

O'Carroll, P.W., and J.C. Smith (1988). Suicide and homicide. In H. M. Wallace, G. Ryan, Jr., and A.C. Oglesby (eds.), *Maternal and Child Health Practices*, 3rd ed. Oakland, CA: Third Party Publishing Company.

Oliver, R.G., and B.S. Hetzel (1973). An analysis of recent trends in suicide rates in Australia. *International Journal of Epidemiology* 2:91–101.

Rockett, I.R.H., and G.S. Smith (1989). Homicide, suicide, motor vehicle crash, and fall mortality: United States' experience in comparative perspective. *American Journal of Public Health* 79:1396–1400.

Simpson, S.G., R. Reid, S.P. Baker, and S.P. Teret (1983). Injuries among the Hopi Indians, a population-based survey. *Journal of the American Medical Association* 249:1873–1876.

Trinkoff, A.M., and S.P. Baker (1986). Poisoning hospitalizations and deaths among children and teenagers. *American Journal of Public Health* 76:657–660.

Warshauer, M.E., and M. Monk (1978). Problems in suicide statistics for whites and blacks. *American Journal of Public Health* 68:383–388.

Weissman, M.M. (1974). The epidemiology of suicide attempts, 1960 to 1971. *Archives of General Psychiatry* 30:737–746.

Wexler, L., M.M. Weissman, and S.V. Kasl (1978). Suicide attempts 1970–75: Updating a United States study and comparisons with international trends. *British Journal of Psychiatry* 132:180–185.

6

Homicide

The 22,000 deaths in 1988 due to homicide and legal intervention made this the eleventh leading cause of death for all ages combined. Homicide is the fourth leading cause of death for ages 1–14 and ranks second for ages 15–24. Among blacks aged 15–34 it is the leading cause of death. During the first year of life, homicide claims more lives than any other cause of injury (Waller et al. 1989).

Firearms are used in almost two-thirds of all homicides. Other common methods are cutting and stabbing with knives and other sharp instruments (20 percent) and strangulation (5 percent). The majority of homicides take place in the home and involve family members or other people who are known to the victim (FBI 1989). At least 600 homicides annually occur in

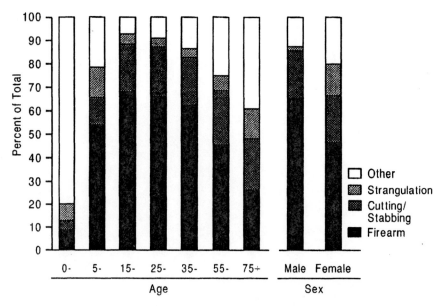

Figure 6-1. Percentage of Homicides by Age and Method, and by Sex and Method, 1980–1986

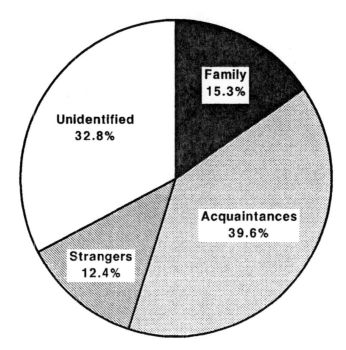

Figure 6-2. Percentage of Homicides by Victim-Offender Relationship, 1988 (*Source:* Federal Bureau of Investigation.)

connection with work, but this is no doubt an underestimate because of deficiencies in reporting such deaths as occupational (Kraus 1987). Among women, homicide is the leading cause of fatal occupational trauma, accounting for 47 percent of work injury deaths (CDC 1990).

AGE AND SEX

Among males, homicide rates are highest at ages 25–29 (Figure 3-3). Among females, the death rates peak slightly earlier, at ages 20–24. For ages 7 and older, firearms are the most common means of homicide (Figure 6-1). For young children, beatings are the most common means.

More than 15 percent of homicides are committed by family members, and nearly 40 percent are committed by acquaintances of the victims (Figure 6-2). Fatal assaults on children are usually inflicted by family members (Christoffel 1984; Jason et al. 1983). Beginning at about age 15, deaths are more often the result of assault by nonfamily acquaintances. Assaults by strangers are most important among teenagers and the elderly, but at no age do they comprise more than about one-fourth of all homicides. The higher proportion of stranger-committed homicides among people in their sixties or older is consistent with the larger proportion of homicides of older

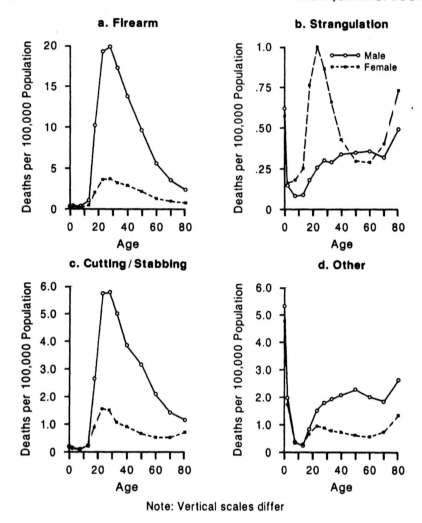

Figure 6-3.   Death Rates from Homicide by Age, Sex, and Method, 1980–1986

people committed in connection with robberies and other felonies. For ages 15–59, homicides occur primarily in connection with arguments. Because this is the age range with the highest homicide rate, arguments are a precipitating factor in almost half of all homicides (CDC 1982).

Firearms are the weapon most commonly used in fatal assaults on both males and females. Cutting and stabbing account for almost one-fifth of homicides among both sexes (Figure 6-1). Death by strangulation causes 12 percent of homicides among females but only 2 percent among males. Not only does strangulation account for a larger proportion of homicides in females, but the death *rate* is much higher than for males (Figure 6-3). The ratio of female to male death rates is especially high (4:1) at ages 15–24, when strangulation often accompanies rape (Dietz 1977).

The shape of the age- and sex-specific death rate curves for firearm homicides is virtually the same as for cutting and stabbing with knives and other sharp instruments (Figure 6-3), although the firearm rate is more than three times as high. The resemblance in the shapes of these curves is closer than for other causes of injury death, suggesting important similarities between the circumstances involved and the populations at risk of being assaulted with the two types of weapons.

Hospital data indicate that many more people are assaulted with sharp instruments than with firearms. Yet the ratio of deaths to injuries is roughly five times as great for shootings (Teret and Wintemute 1983). The evidence suggests that the primary basis for the extremely high death rate from firearms is the lethality of the weapons rather than the characteristics of the people who kill or are killed (Baker 1985).

RACE AND PER CAPITA INCOME

Homicide rates are highest for blacks (32 per 100,000 population) and lowest for whites and Asians (6 and 5 per 100,000, respectively), with Native Americans in between (14 per 100,000). The age-specific rates are highest for blacks aged 5–29, but each race has high rates at ages 20–29 (Figure 6-4).

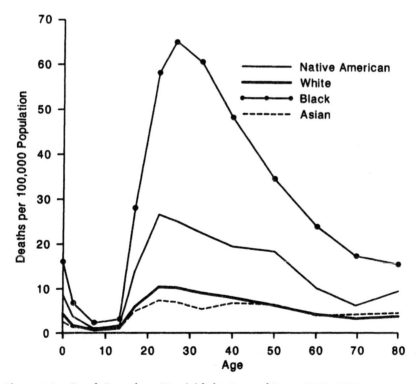

Figure 6-4.   Death Rates from Homicide by Age and Race, 1980–1986

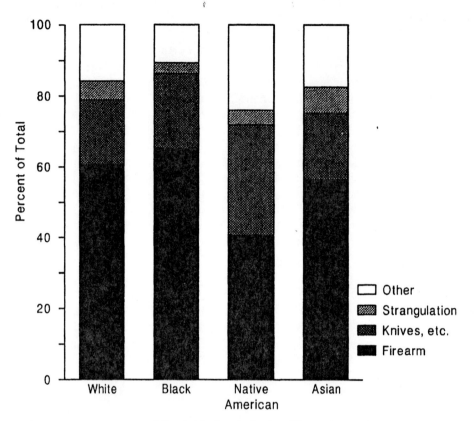

Figure 6-5.   Percentage of Homicides by Method and Race, 1980–1986

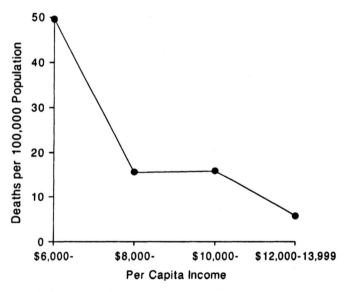

Figure 6-6.   Death Rates from Homicide in Central Cities by Per Capita Income of Area of Residence, 1980–1986

For males aged 15–24, the homicide rate for blacks is seven times that for whites (Fingerhut and Kleinman 1990).

The method of injury is roughly similar among the four racial groups, except that for Native Americans cutting and stabbing cause a larger proportion of homicides, and firearms a smaller proportion, than for the other racial groups (Figure 6-5). The preponderance of firearms among weapons used to kill Asians contrasts with the pattern seen for suicide by Asians, in which firearms are less commonly employed (see Chapter 5).

Homicide rates are two and one-half times as high in low-income areas as in high-income areas for all races combined (Figure 3-9). This difference increases to a tenfold disparity in central cities (Figure 6-6). The inverse correlation between homicide rates and income is most pronounced for firearm homicide. When socioeconomic status is controlled for, racial differences in homicide rates decrease markedly (Griffith and Bell 1989; Loftin and Hill 1974).

URBAN/RURAL AND GEOGRAPHIC DIFFERENCES

For all methods of homicide combined and for each type of homicide, the rate is about three times as high among people in central cities as among people living elsewhere (Figure 6-7).

Homicide rates range from a low of less than 2 per 100,000 population in New Hampshire and North Dakota to a high of 15 in Texas and Louisiana. The rate is substantially higher in Washington, D.C.—about 28 per 100,000. Washington is entirely urban and the central part of a much larger metropolitan area. Its high rate reflects the fact that a disproportionate number of homicides in metropolitan areas occur in inner cities.

Because firearms are used in about two-thirds of homicides, the geographic pattern for all homicides generally reflects the geographic pattern for firearm homicides, with low rates in the north central, northwest, and New England states and high rates in the South (Figures 3-13c and 6-8a).

The geographic pattern for homicides not due to firearms differs from the pattern for firearm homicides in several important respects (Figure 6-8b). In particular, New York and California have high rates of nonfirearm homicides—ranking second and third among all states, respectively—but their firearm homicide rates are not exceptionally high (17th and 21st, respectively).

Another way of looking at the relationship of firearm to nonfirearm homicides is by mapping the percentage of all homicides in which firearms are used (Figure 6-8c). Nationally, the proportion is 63 percent; state-specific rates range from 39 percent in Rhode Island to 72 percent in Kentucky. In general, the highest percentages are in the South and the lowest in the Northeast, possibly reflecting the fact that gun ownership is most common in the South and least common in the Northeast (Flanagan and Maguire 1987).

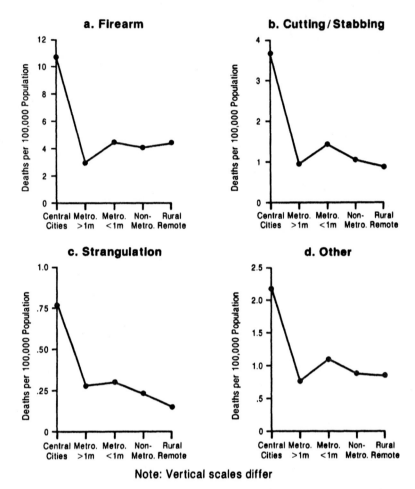

Figure 6-7. Death Rates from Homicide by Place of Residence and Method, 1980–1986

Age-adjusted homicide rates for blacks are highest in western and north central regions. For whites, they are highest in the West and South, with the top 10 states equally divided between the two regions (O'Carroll and Mercy 1989). In Seattle, age-adjusted homicide rates for blacks, Asians, and Hispanics are more than three times the rates in nearby Vancouver, which has similar rates of nonfatal assaults but much more restrictive handgun regulations (Sloan et al. 1988).

TEMPORAL VARIATION

Half of all homicides occur on Fridays, Saturdays, or Sundays, with the largest proportion (19 percent) occurring on Saturdays (Figure 3-14). As

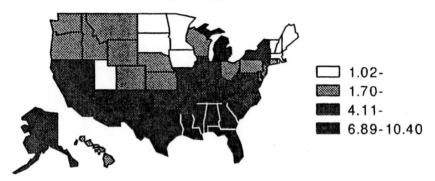

a. Firearm Homicide

☐ 1.02-
▨ 1.70-
▦ 4.11-
■ 6.89-10.40

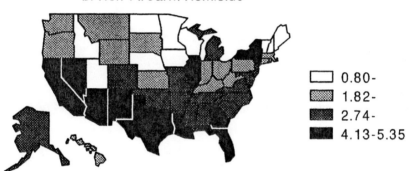

b. Non-Firearm Homicide

☐ 0.80-
▨ 1.82-
▦ 2.74-
■ 4.13-5.35

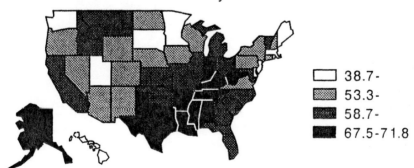

c. Percent of Homicides by Firearms

☐ 38.7-
▨ 53.3-
▦ 58.7-
■ 67.5-71.8

Figure 6-8. Death Rates from Homicide by State and Method, per 100,000 Population, 1980–1986

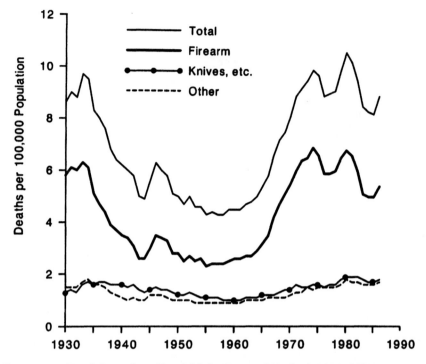

Figure 6-9.   Death Rates from Homicide by Year and Method, 1930–1986

with many unintentional injuries, the higher weekend incidence is partly
related to greater consumption of alcohol, which has been shown to be
involved in a large proportion of killings (Baker et al. 1971).

Homicide rates are highest during July and August (Figure 3-15). Compared with unintentional injury deaths, the monthly variation in homicides
is small.

HISTORICAL TRENDS

Since 1930, the homicide rate has fluctuated widely (e.g., rates per 100,000
population of 9 in 1930, 4 in 1957, 11 in 1980, and 9 in 1988), primarily
reflecting changes in the death rate from homicide by firearms (Figure 6-9).
For other types of homicides, the rates have been more stable, although the
trends have usually been in the same direction as for firearms. For example,
between 1960 and 1980 the death rate from firearm homicide increased by
160 percent (from 2.6 to 6.8 per 100,000), while the rate for all other homicides increased by 100 percent (from 1.9 to 3.8).

From 1968 to 1979, homicide rates increased in almost all age groups,
with the greatest increases among ages 1–19 and 75 or older (Baker et al.
1984). From 1977–1979 to 1984–1986, the death rate increased by 33 percent

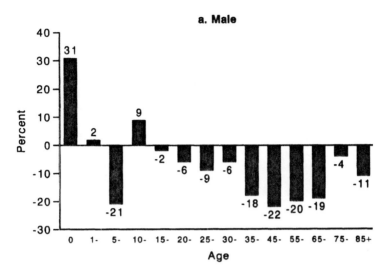

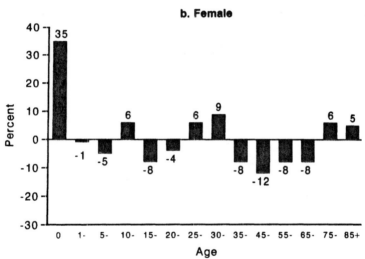

Figure 6-10. Percentage Change in Death Rates from Homicide by Age and Sex, 1984–1986 Compared with 1977–1979

in infants and decreased in most adult age groups (Figure 6-10). Among all major causes of death for children less than age 15, homicide is the only one in which the death rate has increased in recent decades (Christoffel 1984).

After reaching a peak in 1980, the trend in the homicide rate during the early 1980s was downward, especially for firearm homicide. Increases occurred for strangulation and homicide by "other" means, primarily beatings. The most recent FBI statistics (unpublished) indicate that between 1988 and 1989, firearm homicides increased by 9 percent while homicide by other means increased by less than 1 percent.

REFERENCES

Baker, S.P. (1985). Without guns, do people kill people? (editorial) *American Journal of Public Health* 75:587–588.

Baker, S.P., B. O'Neill, and R. Karpf (1984). *The injury fact book*. Lexington, MA: Lexington Books.

Baker, S.P., L.S. Robertson, and W.U. Spitz (1971). Tattoos, alcohol, and violent death. *Journal of Forensic Sciences* 16: 219–225.

Centers for Disease Control (1982). Homicide—United States. *Morbidity and Mortality Weekly Report* 31:594–602.

Centers for Disease Control (1990). Occupational homicides among women—United States, 1980–1985. *Morbidity and Mortality Weekly Report* 39:544–546.

Christoffel, K.K. (1984). Homicide in childhood: A public health problem in need of attention. *American Journal of Public Health* 74:68–70.

Dietz, P.E. (1977). Social factors in rapist behavior. In R. Rada (ed), *Clinical aspects of the rapist*. New York: Grune and Stratton.

Federal Bureau of Investigation (1989). *Uniform crime reports in the United States: 1988*. Washington, DC: U.S. Government Printing Office.

Fingerhut, L.A., and J.C. Kleinman (1990). International and interstate comparisons of homicide among young males. *Journal of the American Medical Association* 263:3292–3295.

Flanagan, T.J., and K. Maguire (eds.) (1987). *Sourcebook of criminal justice statistis*. Washington, DC: U.S. Department of Justice, Bureau of Justice Statistics.

Griffith, E.E.H., and C.C. Bell (1989). Recent trends in suicide and homicide among blacks. *Journal of the American Medical Association* 262:2265–2269.

Jason, J., L.T. Strauss, and C.W. Tyler, Jr. (1983). A comparison of primary and secondary homicides in the United States. *American Journal of Epidemiology* 117:309–319.

Kraus, J.F. (1987). Homicide while at work: Persons, industries, and occupations at high risk. *American Journal of Public Health* 77:1285–1289.

Loftin, C., and R.H. Hill (1974). Regional subculture and homicide: An examination of the Gastil-Mackney thesis. *American Sociological Review* 39:714–724.

O'Carroll, P.W., and J.A. Mercy (1989). Regional variation in homicide rates: Why is the West so violent? *Violence and Victims* 4:17–25.

Sloan, J.H., A.L. Kellermann, D.T. Reay, J.A. Ferris, T. Koepsell, F.P. Rivara, C. Rice, L. Gray, and J. LoGerfo (1988). Handgun regulations, crime, assaults, and homicide: A tale of two cities. *New England Journal of Medicine* 319:1256–1262.

Teret, S.P., and G.J. Wintemute (1983). Handgun injuries: The epidemiologic evidence for assessing legal responsibility. *Hamline Law Review* 6:341–350.

Waller, A.E., S.P. Baker, and A. Szocka (1989). Childhood injury deaths: National analysis and geographic variations. *American Journal of Public Health* 79:310–315.

7

Sports and Recreation

Sports and recreation are an important source of injuries and deaths, including the majority of drownings, many firearm fatalities, about 10 percent of all brain injuries (Kraus et al. 1984), 7 percent of spinal cord injuries (Kraus et al. 1975), and 13 percent of facial injuries treated in hospitals (Karlson 1983). Two important groups of recreational injuries, those related to swimming and bicycling, are addressed in Chapters 13 and 21, respectively. Motorcyling, which for many people is a form of recreation rather than transportation per se and which produces many injuries and deaths, is addressed in Chapter 20. For most sports, however, mortality data from the National Center for Health Statistics (NCHS) do not permit analyses that would be comparable to others in this book, including analyses by age, race, and geographic area.

This chapter includes some of the most representative statistics available. Research results on a variety of sports are incorporated to provide a comprehensive presentation of basic preventive strategies. These can be supplemented with data on many specific sports available elsewhere (Schneider et al. 1985; Waller 1985).

It is estimated that more than 6,000 deaths each year are associated with sports and recreation, not including the many thousands that occur in connection with recreational use of motor vehicles in traffic (Kraus and Conroy 1984). The ninth edition of the *International Classification of Diseases* (ICD), used since 1979 to code NCHS data, adds some detail not previously available concerning the causes of injury (WHO 1977). The ICD E-codes, however, still do not specifically identify most recreation-related injuries; Table 7-1 presents estimates of such deaths.

Three-fourths of all recreation-related deaths result from water recreation. Deaths from some sports, even those specified by E-codes, may be underestimated. For example, in 1986 the 58 recreational scuba diving deaths identifiable in NCHS data using E-codes were far fewer than the 94 reported to the National Underwater Accident Data Center (McAniff 1988). Many other sports are not identified at all, although the numbers of associated deaths may be high. Skiing, for example, is known to have caused 11 fatalities per year in Colorado and more than two per year in Vermont (Morrow et al. 1988; Colorado Department of Health 1989). Sports with very high death *rates* (more than 1 per 10,000 participants per year)

Table 7-1. Estimates of Deaths Related to Sports and Recreation, United States, 1986 (Excluding Motor Vehicles in Traffic)

ICD E-Code[a]	Circumstances of Death	Number of Deaths	Estimated Percentage Sports-Related	Estimated Number Sports-Related
910.8	Drowning in swimming pool	2322	(95)	2206
910.2	Drowning, other recreation	1178	(100)	1178
830–832(0, .1, .3, .5, .9)	Boating	945	(95)	898
910.9	Drowning, unspecified	902	(50)	451
883.0	Diving/jumping into water	46	(75)	35
830–838(.4); 910.0	Water skiing	21	(100)	21
910.1	Recreation, with diving equipment[b]	94	(100)	94
	Subtotal, water recreation			(4,847)
810–819(.6); 826.1	Bicycles	983	(75)	737
821	Off-road vehicle, excluding snow[c]	238	(50)	119
820	Off-road snow vehicle	53	(90)	48
	Subtotal, vehicles			(904)
	Airplane, personal[d]	587	(50)	294
842	Unpowered aircraft	17	(100)	17
	Subtotal, aircraft			(311)
884–888	Falls[c] <age 65	1976	(10)	198
922	Firearms, unintentional	1453	(10)	145
828.2	Animal being ridden	115	(50)	58
917.0	Struck, in sports	46	(100)	46
907	Lightning	79	(25)	20
918	Caught in/between	112	(10)	11
	Total			6,576

[a]World Health Organization (1977).
[b]*Source:* J.J. McAniff, *U.S. underwater diving fatality statistics, 1986 edition.* Washington, DC: U.S. Department of Commerce, 1988.
[c]Excluding codes unlikely to be recreation.
[d]Based on NTSB data for general aviation deaths on personal (nonbusiness) flights.

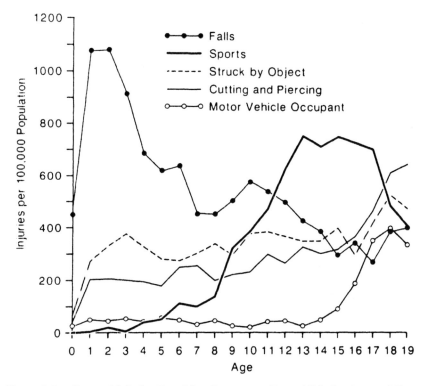

Figure 7-1. Rates of Injuries Requiring Emergency Room Visits by Age and Cause, Massachusetts, 1979–1982 (*Source:* Massachusetts Department of Public Health, Statewide Childhood Injury Prevention Program. Unpublished data.)

include hang gliding, flying home-built aircraft, sport parachuting, scuba diving, and mountain climbing (Addiss and Baker 1989; Metropolitan Life Insurance Company 1979; NSC 1988).

Sports, like falls, are even more important as a source of nonfatal injury and disability than as a cause of death. Reports from trauma centers underestimate the importance of sports and recreational injury, which are usually treated in community hospitals. For example, sports-related eye trauma in Maryland children comprises 32 percent of eye injury admissions in community-based hospitals compared with 10 percent in trauma referral centers (Strahlman et al. 1990).

A comprehensive survey of injured children aged 0–19 admitted to Massachusetts emergency rooms and hospitals revealed that sports were the leading cause of injury from age 12 to 17 (Figure 7-1). (Massachusetts SCIPP, undated). Among 13-year-olds, 30 percent of injuries were sports related. Overall, each year one child in 27 sustained a sports injury severe enough to result in hospital treatment. Almost two-thirds of all sports injuries resulted from team contact sports such as football, basketball, or soccer. Roller skating was the most common source of sports injury at ages

5–9, and football and basketball were the most common at ages 10–19. In a Washington school district, physical education and sports caused at least half of all school-related injuries in both junior and senior high students, but junior high students had rates more than twice those of senior high students and a sixfold risk of fracture (Veazie et al. 1991).

The best national estimates of nonfatal injuries from specified sports come from the Consumer Product Safety Commission (CPSC) sample of patients treated in emergency rooms, called the National Electronic Injury Surveillance System (NEISS). The NEISS data are not limited to organized sports (Table 7-2) (Rutherford et al. 1981). Reflecting their large numbers of participants, football, baseball, and basketball each result in more than 400,000 injuries annually requiring emergency room treatment.

The National Survey of Catastrophic Sports Injury compiles data on athletes participating in high school or college sports programs from many sources, including athletic organizations and a national newspaper clipping service (Mueller et al. 1989). During the six academic years from fall 1982 through spring 1988, an average of 49 catastrophic injuries were reported annually among high school participants and an average of 13 annually among college participants (Tables 7-3 and 7-4). The survey does not include injuries from informal sports or injuries of professional and Olympic ath-

Table 7-2.   Sports-Related Injuries (1980) and Deaths (1973–1980)

Sport	Estimated Number of Injuries Treated in Hospital Emergency Rooms, 1980		Number of Deaths, 1973–1980	
	All Ages	5–14	All Ages	5–14
Football	463,800	173,100	260	19
Baseball	442,900	121,700	183	40
Basketball	421,000	92,800	37	6
Soccer	94,200	37,800	11	6
Racquet sports	74,700	5,400	3	1
Volleyball	73,700	13,900	4	0
Wrestling[a]	67,500	20,000	23	2
Gymnastics	61,400	38,200	8	0
Ice hockey	36,400	10,800	10	2
Track and field	31,600	8,800	10	2
Golf[b]	18,800	4,600	28	14
Trampoline	6,100	2,900	13	6

Source: G.W. Rutherford, R.B. Miles, V.R. Brown, and B. MacDonald, *Overview of sports-related injuries to persons 5–14 years of age.* Washington, DC: U.S. Consumer Product Safety Commission, 1981.

Note: Injuries were estimated from the CPSC's NEISS. Deaths were identified from death certificates, newspaper clippings, consumer complaints, medical examiner reports, and NEISS data.

[a]Includes deaths from "roughhousing."

[b]Includes spectators and children playing with golf clubs.

Table 7-3. Reported Catastrophic Injuries from High School Sports, Mid-1982 to Mid-1988

| Sport | Fatal | | Permanent | Serious | Total | Rate/100,000 Participant Years | |
	Direct	Indirect				Male	Female
Cross country	0	5	1	0	6	0.6	0.0
Football	33	27	53	75	188	2.4	—
Soccer	1	4	0	2	7	0.5	0.2
Basketball	0	18	1	1	20	0.6	0.1
Gymnastics	1	0	3	3	7	4.8	2.3
Ice hockey	0	0	3	2	5	3.6	—
Swimming	0	2	1	3	6	0.6	0.6
Wrestling	2	8	7	6	23	1.5	—
Baseball	2	2	3	5	12	0.5	—
Lacrosse	0	1	0	0	1	1.0	—
Track	5	7	2	4	18	0.6	0.0
Tennis	0	1	0	0	1	0.1	0.0
Total	44	75	74	101	294	16.8	3.2

Source: F.O. Mueller, C.S. Blyth, and R.C. Cantu, *Sixth annual report of the National Center for Catastrophic Sports Injury Research, Fall 1982–Spring 1988.* Chapel Hill: University of North Carolina, 1989.

Table 7-4. Reported Catastrophic Injuries from College Sports, Mid-1982 to Mid-1988

| Sport | Fatal | | Permanent | Serious | Total | Rate/100,000 Participant Years | |
	Direct	Indirect				Male	Female
Cross country	0	1	0	0	1	1.7	0.0
Football	3	10	8	29	50	11.1	—
Soccer	0	0	0	1	1	1.1	0.0
Basketball	0	8	0	1	9	10.2	1.6
Gymnastics	0	0	2	1	3	31.1	8.9
Ice hockey	0	1	0	1	2	7.8	—
Swimming	0	1	1	0	2	4.1	1.1
Wrestling	0	0	0	0	0	0.0	—
Baseball	1	1	0	0	2	1.6	—
Lacrosse	0	0	1	2	3	10.3	—
Track	0	1	1	1	3	1.5	0.0
Tennis	0	2	0	0	2	2.1	2.2
Total	4	25	13	36	78	82.5	13.8

Source: F.O. Mueller, C.S. Blyth, and R.C. Cantu, *Sixth annual report of the National Center for Catastrophic Sports Injury Research, Fall 1982–Spring 1988.* Chapel Hill: University of North Carolina, 1989.

letes. Catastrophic injury includes death, permanent severe functional disability, and other severe injury such as fractured cervical vertebra without
paralysis. The majority of the deaths were not from physical trauma but
were classified as "indirect"—usually the result of cardiac failure or, less
commonly, heat exhaustion. Three-fourths of the injury deaths were associated with football.

Nonfatal injuries in this survey are likely to be underreported. Injuries
to the extremities, even when permanently disabling, are not usually included except for amputations, which are rare.

The overall rate of catastrophic injury per 100,000 person years (or player seasons) was more than four times as high for college as for high school
participants. Sports with the highest rates among high school participants were gymnastics, ice hockey, and football; among college participants, the highest were gymnastics, football, lacrosse, and basketball. The
rates were generally several times as high for males as for females participating in the corresponding sports. Other research not restricted to catastrophic
injuries indicates that injury rates per person hours of exposure for comparable intercollegiate teams are similar for men and women except in the case
of gymnastics, for which rates were higher in women (Lanese et al. 1990).

PREVENTIVE APPROACHES

Because of their importance, sports injuries will be used to illustrate approaches based on Haddon's 10 basic strategies applicable to the prevention
of injury of all types (Haddon 1980a, 1980b).

The *first strategy* is to prevent the creation of the hazard in the first
place—for example, by not manufacturing sports equipment that is apt to
cause injury. The manufacture and sale of three-wheeled all-terrain vehicles
(ATVs) was banned in 1987 because of their inherent instability and their
involvement in thousands of deaths and severe injuries (Jagger and Widome
1988). A ban on the sale of four-wheeled ATVs has also been recommended;
there is no evidence that they are safer than three-wheeled ATVs, and they
have a propensity to flip over backwards with resulting severe injuries
(Brown et al. 1989). Another illustration of the first strategy is a ban on
high-risk activities such as human pyramids, which cause catastrophic
injury to several female cheerleaders each year (Mueller et al. 1989); North
Dakota and Minnesota have instituted a ban on cheerleader pyramids.
Many medical organizations have called for a ban on boxing or drastic
modifications of the sport such as a ban on blows to the head, because of
the acute and chronic brain and eye damage associated with the sport
(Enzenauer et al. 1989).

The first strategy may also be applicable to trampolines, an important
source of spinal cord injuries. After the American Academy of Pediatrics
recommended in 1977 that school use of trampolines be banned, there was a
drop of more than 60 percent in the number of trampoline head and neck

injuries treated in hospitals participating in the CPSC's NEISS (Torg 1987; Rutherford et al. 1981). Between 1980 and 1988, the total number of hospital-treated trampoline injuries estimated by NEISS increased from 6,100 to 14,000, probably due primarily to injuries from trampolines used in non-institutional settings.

The *second strategy* is to reduce the amount of hazard that is created, for example, reducing the height from which people can fall or jump, limiting the speed capability of snowmobiles, or limiting the speed of beginning skiers by providing trails that are not too steeply sloped (Haddon et al. 1962). Mountain climbers can reduce the length of a potential fall by placing pitons at shorter intervals (Addiss and Baker 1989). Exposure can be curtailed, for example, through shorter periods of play or by permitting hunting only on certain days. In hot and humid weather, reduction of training runs and other strenuous exercise is appropriate for protecting athletes against heat stroke. Reducing the number of players who participate in a particular sport is another example, illustrated by limiting participants to a specified age group. In high school football, injury rates would be reduced by limiting contact scrimmage, contact drills, and practice games, which have more than five times the injury rates of noncontact drills and controlled scrimmage (Halpern et al. 1987). Screening prospective athletes through medical examinations might prevent some of the deaths from heart failure.

The *third strategy* involves preventing the release of a hazard, for example, by designing hunting weapons that will not discharge inadvertently. Reducing the likelihood of release of the hazard is often a more practical approach; an example is packing and grooming ski slopes to reduce hidden obstacles that might cause skiers to fall. Many behavioral strategies are relevant here, such as those related to reducing alcohol use. Alcohol was implicated in 15 of the 20 ATV-related deaths in Alaska in a two-year period (Smith and Middaugh 1986) and contributes to injuries in other sports.

The *fourth strategy* is to modify the rate or spatial distribution of release of a hazard from its source. Examples include release bindings on skis, controlled release of dammed-up water to protect boaters downstream, and the use of shorter cleats or larger numbers of cleats on football shoes so that the foot can rotate easily without transmitting a sudden force to the knee. Use of "breakaway" bases in softball games resulted in a 95 percent reduction in injuries from base sliding, compared with games played on fields with stationary bases. The sudden deceleration caused by sliding into fixed bases had previously caused 71 percent of recreational softball injuries (Janda et al. 1988).

Changes in football rules in 1976 outlawed spearing and face-tackling at the high school and college level; these techniques use the head as a primary contact point, and the abrupt forces on the head and neck are likely to exceed injury thresholds. Cervical spine injuries resulting in permanent quadriplegia decreased dramatically between 1976 and 1984: from 2.2 to 0.4

per 100,000 high school football players and from 10.7 to 0 per 100,000 college players (Torg et al. 1985). Yet, more than one-third of high school football players in Minnesota continued to use these maneuvers a year after they were banned, and one player in five reported concussion symptoms during the playing season (Gerberich et al. 1983). Head-on tackling is still causing catastrophic injuries in high school players: In 1987 there were at least three deaths, six cases of quadriplegia, and two permanent head injuries in players making tackles (Mueller et al. 1989).

The *fifth strategy* is to separate people in time or space from the hazard and its release. Starting avalanches during times when ski slopes are closed, an example of temporal separation, decreases the likelihood that avalanches will occur when skiers are on the slopes. Placing benches and other equipment farther from playing areas reduces the frequency of "out of bounds" injuries that commonly occur when players run into them (Garrick et al. 1977). Other examples of spatial separation include storing pistols used for target shooting at the shooting range rather than at home and providing paths that separate bicyclists, walkers, and joggers from motor vehicles. It has been recommended that competitive swimmers practice running starts at the deep ends of pools to reduce the chance of catastrophic injury when a swimmer's head strikes the bottom of the pool (Mueller et al. 1989).

The *sixth strategy* is to separate people from the hazard by interposing a material barrier. In many sports, the head, face, eyes, chest, or other body parts need to be protected from balls, bats, or other players. A review of sports-related injuries and deaths among players aged 5–14 revealed that 38 percent of the deaths involved baseball (Rutherford et al. 1981). Being struck on the chest by the baseball with subsequent cardiac arrest appeared to be the prominent cause, suggesting a need for chest protection for young baseball players. Eye protection devices for racquetball and squash can prevent many eye injuries, which are the most common serious injury associated with racquet sports (Karlson 1983). Facial and dental injuries among hockey and football players have been substantially reduced by face masks (Downs 1979; Rontal et al. 1977; Wilson et al. 1973). Protective helmets are needed for many sports, such as football, horseback riding, and bicycling, where head injuries are a serious problem. Often, spectators must also be protected by separation, for example, from out-of-control race cars.

The *seventh strategy* is to modify the relevant basic qualities of the hazard. Illustrations include the adoption of a softer ball in squash rather than the previously used hardball, padding the outer edge of racquets, and using balls large enough so that the bony socket of the eye affords some protection. The ends of hockey sticks, once pointed and a major source of facial injuries, are now rounded to make them less injurious. Energy-absorbing flooring materials can reduce injuries in boxers, and gymnasium walls should be designed without protrusions and either made of energy-attenuating materials or padded in areas where players might strike them. Breakaway goalposts and slalom poles that yield on impact are further examples. The boards surrounding ice hockey rinks deserve attention because of their role in head and neck injuries.

The *eighth strategy* is to make the person more resistant to damage. Conditioning of the musculoskeletal system, such as neck strengthening, is an important means of reducing injury. Exercise and therapy to reduce osteoporosis are promising approaches of special relevance to older people participating in athletic and recreational activities. The injury rate of aerobic dance students with no other fitness activity was three times the rate for students also involved in other fitness activities (Garrick et al. 1986). Grouping school athletes by skills, physical fitness, and physical maturity rather than age has reportedly reduced injury rates (Van Dusen 1981). It cannot be assumed, however, that advanced training will reduce rates of serious injury, since in some sports such as trampoline it is the most skilled participants who attempt the most hazardous maneuvers (Torg 1987).

The *ninth strategy* is to begin to counter damage already done. Athletes who may have sustained spinal cord injuries, for example, need to be carefully supported when they are moved in order to reduce the likelihood of paralysis. Football players with concussion symptoms should not be returned to play on the same day because of the potential for progressive neurological debilitation, yet one study found that most high school players who experienced loss of consciousness returned to play the same day (Gerberich et al. 1983). Communication systems and readily available emergency and hospital care are clearly important but often inadequate. Athletic trainers in high schools can help to ensure proper initial attention to injuries.

The *tenth strategy* is to stabilize, repair, and rehabilitate the injured person. Reconstructive surgery, physical and mental rehabilitation, and modification of the environment to accommodate the handicapped help to minimize adverse outcomes of serious injury.

These 10 strategies and examples of illustrative tactics suggest the wide variety of measures that can reduce the likelihood and severity of injuries, as well as the severity of the consequences of injury once it has occurred. In choosing among potentially useful preventive measures, priority should be given to the ones most likely to effectively reduce injuries. In general, these will be measures that provide built-in, automatic protection, minimizing the amount and frequency of effort required of the individuals involved (Baker 1981; Haddon 1980a; Haddon and Baker 1981; Robertson 1983).

REFERENCES

Addiss, D.G., and S.P. Baker (1989). Mountaineering and rock-climbing injuries in U.S. national parks. *Annals of Emergency Medicine* 18:975–1013.

Baker, S.P. (1981). Childhood injuries: The community approach to prevention. *Journal of Public Health Policy* 2:235–246.

Brown, B., C. Laberge-Nadeau, and A. Delisle (1989). Three- and four-wheeled all terrain vehicle-related injuries in Quebec. *Chronic Diseases in Canada* 10:10–14.

Colorado Department of Health (1989). Identifying snow-skier deaths from death certificates. *Colorado Health Statistics* 3(3):5–6.

Downs, J. (1979). Incidence of facial trauma in intercollegiate and junior hockey. *Physician and Sports Medicine* 7:88.

Enzenauer, R.W., J.S. Montrey, R.J. Enzenauer, and W.M. Mauldin (1989). Boxing-related injuries in the U.S. Army, 1980 through 1985. *Journal of the American Medical Association* 261:1463–1466.

Garrick J., G. Collins, and R. Requa (1977). Out-of-bounds in football: Player exposure to probability of football injury. *Journal of Safety Research* 9:34–38.

Garrick, J.G., D.M. Gillien, and P. Whiteside (1986). The epidemiology of aerobic dance injuries. *American Journal of Sports Medicine* 14:67–72.

Gerberich, S.G., J.D. Priest, J.R. Boen, C.P. Straub, and R.E. Maxwell (1983). Concussion incidence and severity in secondary school varsity football players. *American Journal of Public Health* 73:1370–1375.

Haddon, W., Jr. (1980a) Advances in the epidemiology of injuries as a basis for public policy. *Public Health Reports* 95:411–421.

Haddon, W., Jr. (1980b). The basic strategies for preventing damage from hazards of all kinds. *Hazard Prevention* 16:8–12.

Haddon, W., Jr., and S.P. Baker (1981). Injury control. In D. Clark and B. MacMahon (eds.), *Preventive and community medicine.* Boston: Little, Brown, pp. 109–140.

Haddon, W., Jr., A.E. Ellison, and R.E. Carroll (1962). Skiing injuries: Epidemiologic study. *Public Health Reports* 77:975–991.

Halpern, B., N. Thompson, W.W. Curl, J.R. Andrews, S.C. Hunter, and J.R. Boring (1987). High school football injuries: Identifying the risk factors. *American Journal of Sports Medicine* 15:316–320.

Jagger, J., and M.D. Widome (1988). All-terrain vehicles: Hazard in Britain. *Lancet* 2:1368–1369.

Janda, D.H., E.M. Wojtys, F.M. Hankin, and M.E. Benedict (1988). Softball sliding injuries—a prospective study comparing standard and modified bases. *Journal of the American Medical Association* 259:1848–1850.

Karlson, T.A. (1983). *The incidence of hospital-treated facial injuries.* Madison: University of Wisconsin.

Kraus, J.F., and C. Conroy (1984). Mortality and morbidity from injuries in sports and recreation. *Annual Review of Public Health* 5:163–192.

Kraus, J.F., M.A. Black, N. Hessol, P. Ley, W. Rokaw, C. Sullivan, S. Bowers, S. Knowlton, and L. Marshall (1984). The incidence of acute brain injury and serious impairment in a defined population. *American Journal of Epidemiology* 119:186–201.

Kraus, J.F., C.E. Franti, R.S. Riggins, D. Richards, and N.O. Borhani (1975). Incidence of traumatic spinal cord lesions. *Journal of Chronic Diseases* 28:471–492.

Lanese, R.R., R.H. Strauss, D.J. Leizman, and A.M. Rotondi (1990). Injury and disability in matched men's and women's intercollegiate sports. *American Journal of Public Health* 80:1459–1462.

Massachusetts Statewide Comprehensive Injury Prevention Program (SCIPP) (N.D.). Sports injuries, 1979–1982. Boston: Massachusetts Department of Health.

McAniff, J.J. (1988). *U.S. underwater diving fatality statistics, 1986 edition.* Washington, DC: U.S. Department of Commerce.

Metropolitan Life Insurance Company (1979). Sports hazards. *Statistical Bulletin* 60:2–5.

Morrow, P.L., E.N. McQuillen, L.A. Eaton, and C.J. Bernstein (1988). Downhill ski fatalities: The Vermont experience. *Journal of Trauma* 28:95–100.

Mueller, F.O., C.S. Blyth, and R.C. Cantu (1989). *Sixth annual report of the National Center for Catastrophic Sports Injury Research, Fall 1982-Spring 1988*. Chapel Hill: University of North Carolina.

National Safety Council (1988). *Accident facts, 1988 edition*. Chicago: National Safety Council.

Robertson, L.S. (1983) *Injuries: Causes, control strategies, and public policy*. Lexington, MA: Lexington Books.

Rontal, E., M. Rontal, K. Wilson, and B. Cram (1977). Facial injuries in hockey players. *Laryngoscope* 87:884–894.

Rutherford, G.W., R.B. Miles, V.R. Brown, and B. MacDonald (1981). *Overview of sports-related injuries to persons 5-14 years of age*. Washington, DC: U.S. Consumer Product Safety Commission.

Schneider, R.C., J.C. Kennedy, M.L. Plant, P.J. Fowler, J.T. Hoff, and L.S. Matthews (eds.) (1985). *Sports injuries—mechanisms, prevention, and treatment*. Baltimore, MD: Williams & Wilkins.

Smith, S.M., and J.P. Middaugh (1986). Injuries associated with three-wheeled, all-terrain vehicles, Alaska, 1983 and 1984. *Journal of the American Medical Association* 255:2454–2458.

Strahlman, E.R., M.J. Elman, E. Daub, and S.P. Baker (1990). The incidence and causes of pediatric eye injuries: A population-based study. *Archives of Ophthalmology* 108:603–606.

Torg, J.S. (1987). Trampoline-induced quadriplegia. *Clinics in Sports Medicine* 6:73–85.

Torg, J.S., J.J. Vegso, B. Sennett, and M. Das (1985). The National Football Head and Neck Injury Registry—14-year report on cervical quadriplegia, 1971 through 1984. *Journal of the American Medical Association* 254:3439–3443.

Van Dusen, K. (1981). *A model state recreational injury control program*. Atlanta, GA: U.S. Department of Health and Human Services, Public Health Service, Centers for Disease Control.

Veazie, M.A., J. Keniston-Longrie, and N. Harris (1991). *School injury surveillance in a local health department: Results and implications*. Olympia, WA: Washington State Department of Health.

Waller, J.A. (1985). *Injury control: A guide to the causes and prevention of trauma*. Lexington, MA: Lexington Books.

Wilson, K., E. Rontal, and M. Rontal (1973). Facial injuries in football. *Transactions of the American Academy of Ophthalmology and Otolaryngology* 77:434–437.

World Health Organization (1977). *Manual of the international statistical classification of diseases, injuries and causes of death*, 9th ed., Vol. 1. Geneva: World Health Organization.

8

Aviation and Rail Transportation

Motor vehicle crashes are the leading cause of injury deaths, but other forms of transportation are also significant. "Transportation" includes travel for many reasons such as recreation, the context in which the majority of transportation deaths associated with driving, flying, and boating occur. The number of deaths per person mile of travel differs markedly by mode of travel (Table 8-1). Among users of road vehicles there is a 750-fold difference between bus occupants and motorcyclists in deaths per person mile. For air travelers, the death rate in general aviation (private or business aircraft) is more than 250 times the rate in scheduled noncommuter airlines. Passengers traveling by bus or train and those on scheduled airlines have the lowest rates. Rates for boat travel are not available. About 90 percent of all "water transport" deaths are drownings related to small boats (discussed in Chapter 13).

Between 1930 and 1987, while death rates from unintentional injury that was not associated with travel decreased by two-thirds, the death rate from all forms of transportation combined declined by only one-third, from about 31 to 20 per 100,000 population. Although the death rate per mile of travel has shown a much larger decrease, it should be recognized that the human cost of traveling has changed relatively little during a period when deaths from injuries at home and in the workplace have declined substantially.

Table 8-1. Death Rates of Vehicle Occupants
per 100 Million Person Miles of Travel, by Type of Vehicle,
1986–1988

Vehicle	Deaths per 100 Million Person Miles of Travel
Motorcycle	45
General aviation	8
Car	1.23
Bus	0.06
Passenger train	0.03
Scheduled plane	0.03

Sources: National Safety Council, *Accident facts,* 1990 edition. Chicago: National Safety Council, 1990; and Aircraft Owners and Pilots Association.

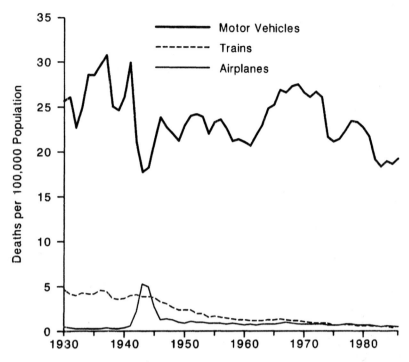

Figure 8-1.   Death Rates from Motor Vehicles, Airplanes, and Trains by Year, 1930–1986

Major shifts in mode of travel have resulted in large changes in death rates associated with specific forms of transportation. For example, since 1930 there has been an 89 percent reduction in the death rate related to trains (Figure 8-1). Dramatic changes occurred during World War II: More than 20,000 aviation deaths among military personnel occurred in the continental United States (i.e., excluding combat and other overseas military deaths) (Office of Statistical Control 1945; USMC Historical Center, undated). This increase was balanced by a comparable reduction in highway deaths during the same period, largely due to civilian gasoline rationing. Shortly after World War II, the aviation death rate was more than twice the prewar rate. In recent years the rate has declined to 1930 levels.

AVIATION

Aircraft crashes are a major cause of death, resulting in about 1,200 fatalities annually. Among white men aged 45–54, aircraft crashes are the fourth leading cause of fatal unintentional injury after motor vehicle crashes, drowning, and falls.

Aviation is also an important source of occupational injury deaths among commercial air crew, flying instructors, test pilots, crop dusters,

Table 8-2.   Aviation Deaths and Fatal Crashes per 100,000 Aircraft Hours,
1980–1988

Type of Carrier	Deaths			Fatal Crashes		
	No.	Average per year	Percentage	Crashes	No.	Rate per 100,000 Hours
Scheduled airline service	971	108	8	195	25	0.04
Nonscheduled airline service	337	37	3	30	7	0.19
Scheduled commuter service	267	30	2	224	54	0.37
On-demand air taxis	648	72	6	1,216	291	1.82
General aviation	9,339	1,038	81	26,558	4,817	1.68
Total	11,562	1,285	100	28,223	5,194	

Source: National Transportation Safety Board, *Annual report to Congress 1988.* Washington, DC: National
Transportation Safety Board, 1989.

pipeline inspectors, military pilots, and people who travel extensively by air
on business (Wiant et al. in press). From 1980 to 1985, an average of at least
220 work-related deaths each year involved aircraft; this was almost one-
fifth of all aircraft-related deaths (see Chapter 9). Bureau of Labor Statistics data indicate that commercial pilots as a whole have a death rate of 98
per 100,000 per year, which is surpassed only by loggers (Leigh 1987) (Table
9-3). One of the highest rates for any occupational subgroup is for aerial
application pilots such as crop dusters, whose rate is about 300 deaths per
100,000 (Wiant et al. in press). Death rates are not available for specific
groups of civilians such as private pilots of light aircraft, but for all licensed
pilots (most of whom are not commercial pilots) the death rate in plane
crashes exceeds 72 per 100,000 pilots annually (Baker and Lamb 1989).
Almost 60 percent of deaths of all active duty navy officers are from plane
crashes, private as well as military (Withers 1983). About 100 deaths annually occur in military aircraft crashes in the United States.

From 1980 to 1988, the number of deaths in civilian aircraft crashes
averaged about 1,300 each year (Table 8-2). Of these, 81 percent were in
general aviation crashes and only 8 percent involved scheduled airline service. The fatal crash rate per 100,000 aircraft hours was 40 times as great for
general aviation as for scheduled airlines.

Between 1980 and 1988, 267 people died in crashes of scheduled commuter flights and 648 in crashes of unscheduled air taxis in the United States
(NTSB 1989a). The rate of fatal crashes per 100,000 departures is nine times
as high for scheduled commuter flights as for scheduled airline flights (0.37
compared with 0.04). In other words, the traveler on a commuter flight is
nine times as likely to be involved in a fatal crash as the traveler on an
airliner. Factors contributing to the high rates include less experienced pilots, more demanding schedules, less sophisticated aircraft, more challeng-
ing airports, and flights at altitudes where weather, air traffic, and moun-
tainous terrain increase the hazards.

Table 8-3. General Aviation Crashes by Type of Flying, 1987

Type of flying	Crashes, Number	Fatal Crashes, Number	Deaths, Number	Deaths, Percentage	Fatal Crashes per 100,000 Hours
Personal	1,575	297	560	75.1	2.07
Business	180	46	98	13.1	
Instructional	337	30	67	9.0	0.61
Aerial application	175	11	11	1.5	0.66
Corporate/executive	19	4	10	1.3	0.12
Total[a]	2,286	388	746	100.0	

[a]Excludes crashes in which the type of flying was other or not recorded.

Source: National Transportation Safety Board, *U.S. general aviation, calendar year 1987.* Report No. NTSB/ARG-89/01. Washington, DC: National Transportation Safety Board, 1990.

Characteristics of Crashes

Three-fourths of general aviation deaths involve personal flights, and 13 percent involve noncommercial business flying such as a dental team serving rural clients (Table 8-3). Personal and business flying combined have the highest rate of fatal crashes, with 2.07 per 100,000 aircraft hours flown. Aerial application has the second highest rate (0.66) but accounts for less than 2 percent of deaths. Instructional flights are involved in 9 percent of general aviation crashes and in one-third of all midair collisions.

Fixed-wing airplanes are involved in about 90 percent of all general aviation crashes and deaths (Table 8-4). Almost one-fifth of occupants of fixed-wing airplanes that crash are killed, compared with 13 percent of helicopter occupants and 3 percent of occupants of balloons (NTSB 1990).

Pilot experience is reflected in both the total number of flight hours and the hours of experience in the type of aircraft being flown. Only 6 percent of pilots involved in general aviation crashes had fewer than 50 hours experi-

Table 8-4. Persons Aboard in Crashes by Aircraft Type and Injury Severity, General Aviation, 1987

Aircraft Type	Degree of Injury					Percentage Fatal
	Fatal	Serious	Minor	None	Total	
Fixed wing	748	371	560	2,420	4,099	18.2
Rotor craft	40	35	56	180	311	12.9
Gliders	4	7	6	37	54	7.4
Balloons	3	33	16	63	115	2.6
Total	795	446	638	2,700	4,579	17.4
Percentage	17.4	9.8	13.9	58.9	100.0	

Source: National Transportation Safety Board, *U.S. general aviation, calendar year 1987.* Report No. NTSB/ARG-89/01. Washington, DC: National Transportation Safety Board, 1990.

Table 8-5. Flying Experience of Pilots Involved in General Aviation Crashes, 1987

Flight Time (Hours)	Total Time		Time in Type	
	Number	Percentage	Number	Percentage
1–49	158	6	700	28
50–99	166	7	309	13
100–499	708	29	671	27
500–999	341	14	194	8
1000–4999	680	27	226	9
5000+	382	15	29	1
Not reported	51	2	366	14
Total	2,486	100	2,495	100

Source: National Transportation Safety Board, *U.S. general aviation, calendar year 1987.* Report No. NTSB/ARG-89/01. Washington, DC: National Transportation Safety Board, 1990.

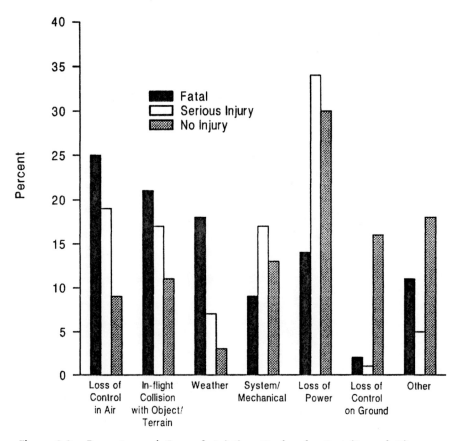

Figure 8-2. Percentage of General Aviation Crashes by Severity and Circumstances, 1986

Table 8-6. Percentage of Air Crashes by Circumstances and Type
of Operation, 1981–1986

| | Air Carrier Crashes | | | | | | General Aviation | |
| | Airlines | | Commuters | | Air Taxis | | | |
	All	Fatal	All	Fatal	All	Fatal	All	Fatal
Weather	26.0	4.5	9.0	15.6	8.1	16.8	6.0	17.9
Collision with object/terrain	14.5	27.3	22.5	34.4	26.6	35.2	20.4	27.1
Loss of power	10.7	13.6	18.8	12.5	21.0	12.1	25.8	11.9
Aircraft malfunction	12.2	4.5	12.0	15.6	7.1	3.1	4.5	5.3
Gear collapsed/ retracted	6.1	0.0	6.0	0.0	4.2	0.0	2.1	0.0
Loss of control in flight	4.5	22.7	6.0	6.3	10.9	16.8	12.4	25.5
Loss of control on ground	2.3	0.0	7.5	0.0	7.5	2.6	10.6	0.0
Fire/explosion	2.3	0.0	3.8	6.3	1.6	0.0	0.0	0.0
Midair collision	0.0	0.0	2.3	6.3	1.4	4.2	1.5	4.4
Other	21.3	27.3	11.9	3.1	11.6	9.1	16.8	8.0
Total	100.0	100.0	100.0	100.0	100.0	100.0	100.0	100.0

Sources: National Transportation Safety Board, *Annual review of aircraft accident data, U.S. air carrier operations, calendar year 1986.* Report No. NTSB/ARC-89/01. Washington, DC: National Transportation Safety Board 1989. National Transportation Safety Board, *U.S. general aviation, calendar year 1987.* Report No. NTSB/ARG-89/01. Washington, DC: National Transportation Safety Board, 1990.

ence, but 28 percent had fewer than 50 hours in the type of aircraft involved in the crashes (Table 8-5).

In the majority of fatal general aviation crashes, the first event leading to the crash, as cited by the National Transportation Safety Board (NTSB), was either loss of control in air, in-flight collision with terrain or objects (such as trees or power lines), or bad weather or turbulence. Weather-related general aviation crashes have a very high fatality rate; bad weather was cited as the first event in 18 percent of fatal crashes compared with 3 percent of no-injury crashes (Figure 8-2). In contrast, for airline crashes, encounters with bad weather were the first event for less than 5 percent of fatal crashes but for 26 percent of all crashes (Table 8-6).

Age, Sex, and Race

In the general population, overall aviation death rates are highest for ages 25–54 (Figure 4-2) and are five times as high for males as for females. Whites and Native Americans have the highest rates (0.68 and 0.52 per

100,000 population, respectively), compared with 0.08 and 0.19 for blacks and Asians, respectively.

Among general aviation pilots involved in crashes, only 8 percent are less than 25 years of age (NTSB 1990). When exposure is taken into account, female pilots have general aviation crash rates that are less than half the rates for males (Booze 1977).

Geographic Factors

Aviation deaths are strongly associated with geographic factors. The patterns are determined primarily by the general aviation component of aviation mortality rather than by commercial aviation. Mortality is highest among residents of remote rural areas and increases with income (Figure 8-3). Death rates are highest in the western half of the United States (Figure 8-4), in part because of the greater use of private aircraft in rural areas. Death rates are especially high in the Rocky Mountains, where bad weather, hostile terrain, and poor aircraft performance at high altitude create lethal situations (Baker and Lamb 1989). Even when adjusted for exposure, most

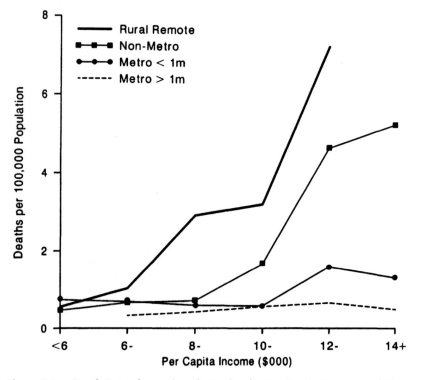

Figure 8-3.   Death Rates from Aircraft Crashes by Per Capita Income and Place of Residence, 1980–1986

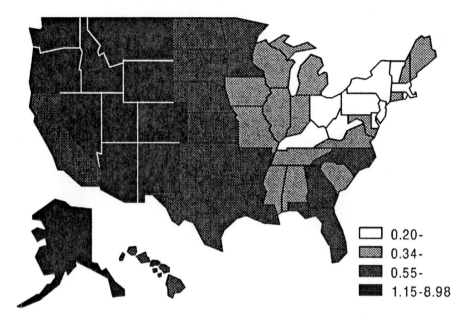

☐	0.20-
▦	0.34-
▨	0.55-
■	1.15-8.98

Figure 8-4. Death Rates from Aircraft Crashes by State, per 100,000 Population, 1980–1986

of these states have crash rates that are at least twice the expected values (Booze 1977).

Aviation-related mortality is exceptionally high in Alaska (Middaugh 1986), where the death rate of 9 per 100,000 population is almost 4 times the rate in the next highest state (Nevada) and 15 times the average for the United States. Of all unintentional injury deaths in Alaska, 11 percent result from airplane crashes, compared with 1 percent nationally. In part, the high rates in Alaska reflect the fact that a large proportion of all travel is by air because of the lack of roads in many areas. Frequent adverse weather conditions and very short periods of daylight for much of the year contribute to the high aviation death rates in Alaska. The remoteness of many small Alaskan communities influences death rates from all types of injuries through lack of speedy access to medical treatment.

Season, Day, and Time

More than half of all aviation deaths occur on Friday, Saturday, and Sunday. July and August are the peak months when almost one-third of the deaths occur, due in part to greater air travel in the summer months. In addition, high temperature adversely affects the performance capability (especially the climb performance) of low-powered aircraft; as a result, crashes caused by the inability of airplanes to climb above mountain terrain are especially common in the summer (Baker and Lamb 1989).

Information on commercial air travel by time of day has been obtained from the FAA for major airports where most scheduled flights arrive or depart. These data have been used to calculate crash rates per million operations (arrivals and departures) for air carriers (Figure 8-5). Although the largest numbers of crashes occur in the daytime, the rates increase after 10 P.M and are highest during the night, especially from 2 to 4 A.M. Fatigue and unadjusted circadian rhythms probably contribute to the high rates at night.

Time Trends and Preventive Measures

The number of deaths related to air transportation decreased from 1,919 in 1978 to 1,160 in 1988, a 40 percent change (Table 8-7). Impressive decreases also occurred in fatalities from unscheduled ("on-demand") air taxis, commuter flights, and general aviation, which dropped by 63 percent, 56 percent, and 49 percent, respectively. The number of deaths in major airline crashes fluctuated dramatically, since a single crash sometimes results in several hundred deaths.

Many recent efforts to improve airline pilot performance have emphasized fatigue (Graeber 1988) and crew interaction and coordination (Foushee and Helmreich 1988). Human factors in general aviation, including design-induced errors, have received less attention (Snyder 1981b).

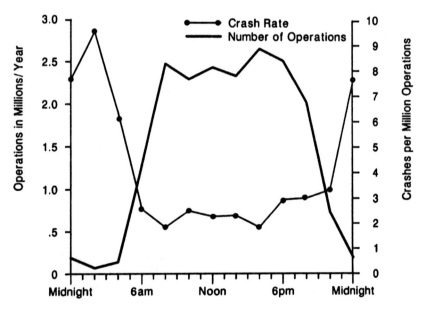

Figure 8-5.   Crash Rates and Number of Operations of Scheduled Carriers by Hour of Day, 1980–1988

Table 8-7. Number of Aviation Deaths by Type of Operation and Year, United States, 1978–1988

	Airlines	Commuters	Air Taxis	General Aviation	Total
1978	160	48	155	1556	1919
1979	354	66	77	1221	1718
1980	1	37	105	1239	1382
1981	4	34	94	1282	1414
1982	234	14	72	1187	1507
1983	15	11	62	1064	1152
1984	4	48	52	1039	1143
1985	526	37	76	950	1589
1986	4	4	65	965	1038
1987	232	61	64	817	1174
1988	285	21	58	796	1160

Source: National Transportation Safety Board, *Annual report to Congress 1988.* Washington, DC: National Transportation Safety Board, 1989.

Alcohol use by pilots has not been implicated in airline crashes (Modell and Mountz 1990), but has been established in about one-tenth of fatal general aviation crashes (Ross and Ross 1985) and has been shown to adversely affect pilot performance as long as 14 hours after ingestion (Yesavage and Leirer 1986). The correlation between pilot alcohol intoxication and a history of arrest for driving while intoxicated suggests the potential usefulness of the National Driver Register to identify pilots with chronic alcohol problems (Hricko 1970).

Most efforts to reduce aviation deaths have focused on preventing crashes. Comparable attention should be given to preventing injuries when crashes occur; contrary to popular opinion, most airplane crashes need not produce forces on their occupants in excess of injury thresholds. Such crashes would therefore be survivable in well-designed aircraft (Snyder 1981a; Snyder and Armstrong 1979).

A substantial portion of serious injuries and deaths in general aviation as well as in scheduled airline service could be prevented through application of available knowledge and technology to seat designs and other structural components. Crashworthy fuel systems in Army helicopters virtually eliminated deaths from postcrash fires, previously a major cause of death (Springate et al. 1989). Similarly, more crashworthy fuel systems should be incorporated into all powered aircraft (U.S. Army 1980). Fire-retardant cabin furnishings that do not emit toxic gases and better means of egress would further reduce the large number of preventable deaths in postcrash fires (NTSB 1980; Snyder 1983a, 1983b).

RAILROADS

Half of the 1,100 deaths related to trains each year involve occupants of motor vehicles, and 42 percent are people on foot who are struck by trains. About 50 railroad employees are killed each year (NSC 1990). Freight train conductors, brakemen, and flagmen have the highest on-duty death rates among railroad employees (Metropolitan Life Insurance Company 1981). Passengers represent less than 1 percent of all deaths related to rail transport. Their death rate per 100 million person miles of travel is estimated to be about one-fortieth of the rate for passenger car occupants (Table 8-1).

Death rates of occupants of motor vehicles struck by trains are especially high in whites and Native Americans and among residents of low-income and rural counties. Collisions between trains and motor vehicles are further discussed in Chapter 17, because virtually all of the deaths and injuries in such collisions are to motor vehicle occupants.

Age, Sex, and Race

People unprotected by vehicles, such as pedestrians and motorcyclists, are at extremely high risk of death when struck by trains. Pedestrians killed by trains, who number almost 500 annually, are predominantly adult males. The rate for Native Americans is almost three times the rate for blacks and five times the rate for whites. Death rates are highest from age 15 to 24 among whites and from age 20 to 54 for blacks and Native Americans.

Among Native Americans, the pedestrian-train death rate per 100,000 population is highest in remote rural areas, while among whites the rate is highest in the central cities (Baker et al. 1984). Since the rates described are population based, the differences cannot be explained by the fact that Native Americans are more likely than whites to live in remote areas. Collection and analysis of state- or county-specific data on the characteristics of those killed (including the role of acute and chronic alcoholism), as well as the circumstances of death, amount of train mileage, and ways of separating pedestrians from train tracks might explain some of the demographic differences in death rates and suggest ways to reduce the rates.

Season

Unlike other motor vehicle occupant deaths, motor vehicle–train fatalities are most common in December and January (Figure 8-6), perhaps because of the longer periods of darkness. In contrast, pedestrian–train fatalities are most common in the summer—the number in July and August is twice the number in January and February. It is likely that the winter peak in deaths from motor vehicle–train collisions is related to weather conditions and increased hours of darkness, reducing the ability of drivers to make timely and appropriate decisions. The summertime peak in pedestrian deaths may reflect greater outdoor activity in warm months.

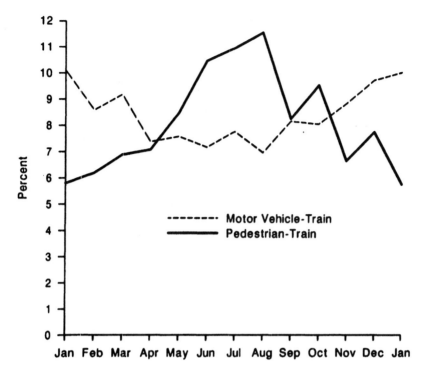

Figure 8-6. Percentage of Deaths from Motor Vehicle-Train and Pedestrian-Train Collisions by Month, 1980–1986

Historical Trends and Preventive Measures

Pedestrian–train fatality rates for 1984–1986 compared with 1977–1979 showed an increase of about 40 percent for ages 20–34 and a decline for most other ages, with a decrease of 22 percent for all ages combined. During the same period, death rates from motor vehicle collisions with trains declined for all ages, with an overall decrease of 40 percent. The tremendous forces involved when trains strike people on foot make it essential to reduce the potential for such events. Where trains or light rail vehicles pass through communities or other high-risk areas, physical barriers, vertical separation, and easy means of crossing the tracks safely are needed to protect pedestrians. Rapid rail systems that allow passengers to wait for and get on or off trains without risk of falling onto the track illustrate effective means of separation.

REFERENCES

Baker, S.P., and M.W. Lamb (1989). Hazards of mountain flying: Crashes in the Colorado Rockies. *Aviation, Space, and Environmental Medicine* 60:531–536.

Baker, S.P., B. O'Neill, and R. Karpf (1984). *The injury fact book*. Lexington, MA: Lexington Books.

Booze, C.F., Jr. (1977). Epidemiologic investigation of occupation, age, and exposure in general aviation accidents. *Aviation, Space, and Environmental Medicine* 48:1081–1091.

Foushee, H.C., and R.L. Helmreich (1988). Group interaction and flight crew performance. In E.L. Wiener and D.C. Nagel (eds.), *Human factors in aviation*. San Diego, CA: Academic Press.

Graeber, R.C. (1988). Aircrew fatigue and circadian rhythmicity. In E.L. Wiener and D.C. Nagel (eds.), *Human factors in aviation*. San Diego, CA: Academic Press.

Hricko, A.R. (1970). Alcohol has menacing role in flight safety as on highways. Reprinted from *National Underwriter*, August 7 and 14, 1970, by the Insurance Institute for Highway Safety, Washington, DC.

Leigh, J.P (1987). Estimates of the probability of job-related death in 347 occupations. *Journal of Occupational Medicine* 29:510–519.

Metropolitan Life Insurance Company (1981). Railroad accident fatalities. *Statistical Bulletin* 62 (July-September):4–7.

Middaugh, J.P. (1986). *The epidemiology of involuntary injuries associated with general aviation in Alaska, 1963–1981*. Anchorage: Alaska Division of Public Health.

Modell, J.G., and J.M. Mountz (1990). Drinking and flying—the problem of alcohol use by pilots. *New England Journal of Medicine* 223:455–461.

National Safety Council (1990). *Accident facts, 1990 edition*. Chicago: National Safety Council.

National Transportation Safety Board (1980). *Safety report—the status of general aviation aircraft crashworthiness*. Washington, DC: National Transportation Safety Board.

National Transportation Safety Board (1989a). *Annual report to Congress 1988*. Washington, DC: National Transportation Safety Board.

National Transportation Safety Board (1989b). *Annual review of aircraft accident data, U.S. air carrier operations, calendar year 1986*. Report No. NTSB/ARC-89/01. Washington, DC: National Transportation Safety Board.

National Transportation Safety Board (1991). *U.S. general aviation, calendar year 1988*. Report No. NTSB/ARG-91/01. Washington, DC: National Transportation Safety Board.

Office of Statistical Control (1945). *Army Air Forces statistical digest—World War II*. Washington, DC: U.S. Army.

Ross, L.E., and S.M. Ross (1985). Alcohol and drug use in aviation. *Alcohol and Research World*. Summer: 34–41.

Snyder R.G. (1981a). General aviation aircraft crashworthiness: An evaluation of FAA safety standards for protection of occupants in crashes. Frederick, MD: Aircraft Owners and Pilots Association.

Snyder, R.G. (1981b). Human factors—the missing link in general aviation accident investigation. In *Proceedings of the Fifth Human Factors Workshop on Aviation: Biomedical and behavioral factors in aviation*. Oklahoma City, OK: Federal Aviation Administration, U.S. Department of Transportation.

Snyder, R.G. (1983a). Comparison of automobile and airplane crashes: Implications for preventing injuries. In *Proceedings of th American Medical Association*

Conference on Prevention of Disabling Injuries. Chicago: American Medical Association.

Snyder, R.G. (1983b). Survival in airplane crashes. *The UMTRI Research Review* 13:1–11.

Snyder, R.G., and T.J. Armstrong (1979). *Crashworthiness analysis of field investigation of business aircraft accidents.* Society of Automotive Engineers Paper No. 790587. Warrendale, PA: Society of Automotive Engineers.

Springate, C.S., R.R. McMeekin, and C.J. Ruehle (1989). Fire deaths in aircraft without the crashworthy fuel system. *Aviation, Space, and Environmental Medicine* 60: (10, Suppl.) B 35–38.

United States Army (1980). *Aircraft crash survival design guide. Vols. 1–5.* Report No. USARTL-TR-79-22a. Fort Eustis, VA: Applied Technology Laboratories.

United States Marine Corps Historical Center (N.D.). Reference Files. Subject: Marine Corp casualties during World War II.

Wiant, C.J., S.P. Baker, W. Marine, R. Vancil, and S.M. Keefer (in press). Work-related aviation fatalities in Colorado, 1982–1987. *Aviation, Space, and Environmental Medicine.*

Withers, B. (1983). Raison d'être. *Society of U.S. Naval Flight Surgeons Newsletter.* 7(4)4.

Yesavage, J.A., and V.O. Leirer (1986). Hangover effects on aircraft pilots 14 hours after alcohol ingestion: A preliminary report. *American Journal of Psychiatry* 143:1546–1550.

9

Occupational Injury

Among people aged 20 to 64, one-third of all injuries (NCHS 1985) and one-sixth of all injury deaths occur on the job. Occupational hazards and their resulting injuries have changed markedly in recent decades as job characteristics have altered and increased protection has been provided. In some industries, injury rates have been reduced as more hazardous tasks have been mechanized and the number of clerical staff has increased, so that a smaller proportion of the work force is at risk of severe trauma. In other industries, risks may have increased, for example, because a larger proportion of jobs entail driving trucks, cars, and other highway vehicles. Estimates of occupational deaths related to motor vehicles range as high as 37 percent of all occupational injury deaths (NSC 1989).

Other changes reflect better reporting and inclusion of injuries that formerly were not considered to be work related. Homicide, for example, long unrecognized as a category of occupational death (Baker et al. 1982; Davis 1987; Kraus 1987), surpasses falls as a cause of fatal occupational injury (Table 9-1). Even for fatalities, however, occupational injury data are still incomplete. Estimates of the annual number of deaths range from about 3,000 (BLS 1990) to 10,600 (NSC 1989). The Bureau of Labor Statistics (BLS) estimates exclude many groups of workers, such as government and railroad workers, members of the military, miners, the self-employed, and workers in places with fewer than 11 nonfamily employees. As a result, the majority of deaths of farmers and many other workers in hazardous jobs are not included in BLS estimates.

The most detailed census of occupational injury deaths is the National Traumatic Occupational Fatality (NTOF) file. Compiled by the National Institute of Occupational Safety and Health (NIOSH), NTOF data include all cases of persons aged 16 or older for whom the death certificate indicates that a fatal injury occurred at work (Bell et al. 1990; DSR 1990). Because of incomplete death certificate identification of injury at work, NTOF data underestimate the actual number of deaths, especially in certain categories. In California, a new system to identify work-related fatalities revealed that 83 percent of such deaths among people aged 65 or older are missed by the usual "reporting system" of checking "injury at work" on the death certificate (Kraus et al. 1990).

The most serious underreporting involves injury from road vehicles, since often it is not obvious to someone filling out a death certificate that a

Table 9-1.   Deaths and Death Rates from Occupational Injuries by Cause and Sex, 1980–1985

	Male		Female		Total	
Cause	Deaths	Rate	Deaths	Rate	Deaths	Rate
Motor vehicle traffic	6,809	1.99	493	0.19	7,302	1.20
Motor vehicle nontraffic	768	0.22	31	0.01	799	0.13
Aviation	1,480	0.43	78	0.03	1,558	0.26
Railway	262	0.08	4	0.00	266	0.04
Water transport	583	0.17	11	0.00	594	0.10
Drowning/suffocation	1,202	0.35	38	0.01	1,240	0.20
Poisoning	493	0.14	7	0.00	500	0.08
Falls	3,378	0.99	113	0.04	3,491	0.57
Fires and flames	627	0.18	55	0.02	682	0.11
Firearm	181	0.05	12	0.00	193	0.03
Natural/environmental factor	394	0.12	30	0.01	424	0.07
Falling object	2,342	0.68	19	0.01	2,361	0.39
Struck against	531	0.16	10	0.00	541	0.09
Caught in/between	333	0.10	9	0.00	342	0.06
Machinery	4,950	1.45	93	0.03	5,043	0.83
Explosive material	770	0.22	44	0.02	814	0.13
Explosion of pressure vessel	212	0.06	5	0.00	217	0.04
Electric current	2,695	0.79	15	0.01	2,710	0.45
Suicide	1,017	0.30	113	0.04	1,130	0.19
Homicide	3,586	1.05	861	0.32	4,447	0.73
Other and unspecified	1,445	0.42	111	0.04	1,556	0.26
Total	34,058	9.94	2,152	0.81	36,210	5.95

Source: National Institute of Occupational Safety and Health.

motor vehicle death is job related. Further underestimation occurs because NTOF data from areas employing almost 10 percent of the U.S. workforce (Louisiana, Nebraska, New York City, and Oklahoma) do not include homicide and suicide at work.

An average of more than 6,000 deaths annually were identified by NTOF in 1980–1985 as work related (Table 9-1). The five leading causes were motor vehicles in traffic, machinery, homicide, falls, and electric current (Figure 9-1).

This chapter reports death rates per 100,000 workers based on NTOF data and death rates per 100,000 population based on NCHS data. For the NCHS data, four causes especially likely to be identified on death certificates as "injury at work" are emphasized: machinery, electric current, explosion, and deaths caused by falling objects. In each of these categories NTOF data include about half of all deaths in the NCHS mortality file; the highest proportion (62 percent) is for electrocutions.

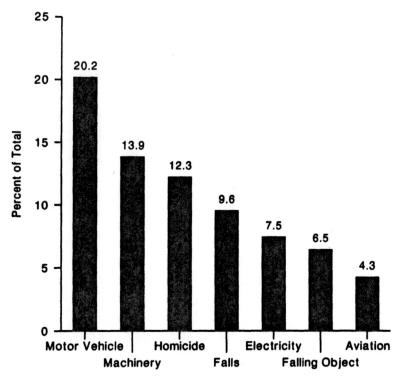

Figure 9-1. Leading Causes of Occupational Injury Death, United States, 1980–1985 (*Source:* National Institute of Occupational Safety and Health, unpublished data.)

NONFATAL INJURY

Data for nonfatal occupational injury are poor at the national level and almost nonexistent at the state level (Kraus 1985). Work relatedness of hospitalized trauma is rarely coded, and underreporting of injury by employers is a major problem.

For many groups of workers, motor vehicles play a major role in nonfatal as well as fatal injuries. One study of 30,000 municipal employees found that motor vehicles accounted for 16 percent of all injury costs; each year about one out of every 50 workers had motor vehicle-related injuries, including injuries not related to crashes (Runyan and Baker 1988).

In a study that deserves replication in other places and for other types of injuries, residents of San Diego County were found to have work-related hospitalized brain injury rates of 20 per 100,000 workers. The rate was 37 per 100,000 for the military, with more than one-half related to transportation, and 15 per 100,000 for civilian workers, with more than one-half due to falls (Kraus and Fife 1985).

Back injuries are the most common compensable nonfatal injury and account for the greatest total cost (Klein et al. 1984): These injuries occur in about one out of 50 workers each year (Snook 1982). Among all occupations, laborers and sanitation workers have the highest rates with 12.3 and 11.1 back injuries per 100 workers per year, respectively (Klein et al. 1984). Contributing factors include prolonged postural stress or vibration, prolonged sitting or standing, and overexertion (Baker et al. 1990). For example, the rate of back injuries in concrete reinforcement work, which requires stooped posture and heavy lifting, is more than 10 times the rate among house painters (Wickstrom et al. 1985).

AGE AND SEX

Rates of nonfatal injury have often been found to be highest for young workers (Mueller et al. 1987; Rossignol et al. 1986). Fatal injury rates, however, are highest in the elderly for all occupational injuries combined (Table 9-2). Workers aged 65 and older comprise less than 3 percent of all workers but sustain 7 percent of the deaths. They have the highest death

Table 9-2. Death Rates from Occupational Injuries by Cause and Age, 1980–1985

Cause	16–19	20–24	25–34	35–44	45–54	55–64	65+
Motor vehicle traffic	0.94	1.22	1.16	1.10	1.25	1.34	1.94
Motor vehicle nontraffic	0.13	0.16	0.09	0.11	0.12	0.17	0.50
Aviation	0.06	0.24	0.35	0.30	0.20	0.18	0.13
Railway	0.02	0.02	0.04	0.03	0.06	0.08	0.02
Water transport	0.10	0.16	0.09	0.08	0.09	0.09	0.08
Drowning/suffocation	0.27	0.28	0.20	0.15	0.17	0.21	0.33
Poisoning	0.11	0.12	0.09	0.07	0.07	0.05	0.09
Falls	0.30	0.48	0.47	0.42	0.66	0.96	1.80
Fires and flames	0.06	0.09	0.10	0.09	0.12	0.16	0.37
Firearm	0.05	0.03	0.03	0.03	0.02	0.03	0.05
Natural/environmental	0.06	0.05	0.05	0.06	0.07	0.09	0.39
Falling object	0.27	0.35	0.33	0.37	0.44	0.48	0.87
Struck against	0.06	0.11	0.08	0.08	0.09	0.11	0.19
Caught in/between	0.05	0.07	0.05	0.05	0.06	0.06	0.10
Machinery	0.76	0.77	0.61	0.57	0.79	1.24	4.05
Explosive material	0.06	0.14	0.15	0.15	0.13	0.12	0.11
Explosion of pressure vessel	0.04	0.04	0.03	0.03	0.04	0.03	0.06
Electric current	0.55	0.70	0.52	0.38	0.31	0.24	0.26
Homicide	0.39	0.63	0.66	0.69	0.76	0.90	2.14
Suicide	0.12	0.17	0.13	0.16	0.23	0.30	0.39
Other and unspecified	0.17	0.24	0.22	0.19	0.25	0.40	0.88
Total	4.57	6.07	5.45	5.11	5.93	7.24	14.75

Source: National Institute of Occupational Safety and Health.

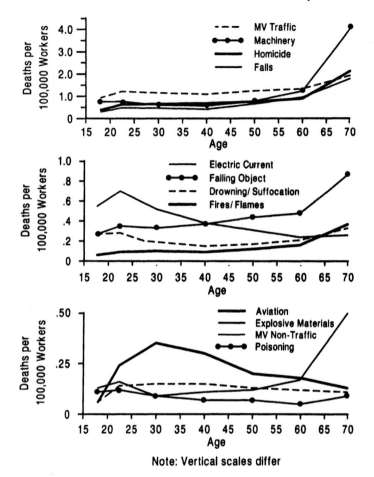

Figure 9-2. Death Rates from Occupational Injury by Cause and Age, per 100,000 Workers, 1980–1985 (*Source:* National Institute of Occupational Safety and Health, unpublished data.)

rates from many specific causes, including falls, homicide, motor vehicles, fire/flames, machinery, and falling objects (Figure 9-2). In workers aged 65 or older in California, 46 percent of the work injury deaths occurred among self-employed persons, 27 percent resulted from homicide, and 10 percent involved tractor overturns (Kraus et al. 1990).

Workers aged 25–44 have especially high death rates from airplane crashes (Figure 9-2). The highest rates from electric current, poisoning, water transport, and drowning or suffocation are found in workers younger than 25. Many causes for which death rates are highest in the elderly, such as those related to motor vehicles, also show a peak at ages 20–24.

Using NCHS data, death rates in Figure 9-3 are calculated separately for farm and nonfarm machinery. For nonfarm machinery, the death rate is

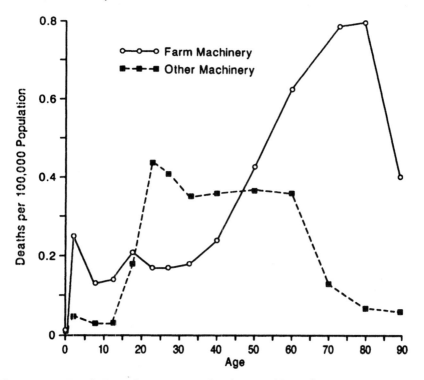

Figure 9-3.   Death Rates from Farm and Other Machinery by Age, per 100,000
Population, 1980–1986

high from age 20 to 64; however, farm machinery death rates increase
sharply after age 40 and are highest for ages 65–84. Children aged 1–4, who
often are carried on tractors or play near farm machinery, also have high
death rates. Two-thirds of such childhood deaths are caused by falling from
and/or being run over by tractors (McKnight 1984).

Six percent of all people killed at work are females (Table 9-1). When
adjustment is made for the number of workers of each sex, the overall
occupational injury death rate for males is 12 times the female rate (9.9
versus 0.8 per 100,000 workers). The male to female ratio of death rates
ranges from about 3 to 1 for homicide to 80 to 1 for electric current. Among
females, homicide is the most common cause of fatal injury at work, and
motor vehicle-related death is the second most common, accounting for 40
percent and 23 percent, respectively, of all female deaths from injury at
work.

Figure 9-4 presents death rates based on NCHS data for injuries due to
explosions and electric current, which are typically work related. For
females, whose deaths from these causes probably are not as likely to be
work related as deaths of males, death rates do not show the sharp rise in the
adolescent and young adult years that characterizes the rates for males.

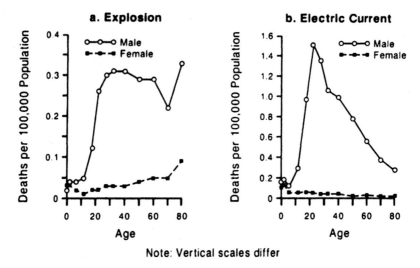

Figure 9-4.   Death Rates from Explosion and Electric Current by Age and Sex, per 100,000 Population, 1980–1986

The rates shown in Figure 9-4 are based on the entire population and include deaths that are not work related. Some occupational injury rates adjusted for the numbers of workers and days of work have revealed high rates of nonfatal injury among workers in their thirties and forties (Robertson and Keeve 1983). A study of work-related injury deaths in Maryland indicated that when the number of workers was taken into account, males aged 25–44 were at greatest risk of fatal, on-the-job injury (Baker et al. 1982). NTOF data, however, indicate that workers 65 or older have the highest rate (Table 9-2).

PER CAPITA INCOME AND RACE

Low-income counties have very high rates of death for causes that are typically work related. The rates are 10 times as high in the lowest-income versus the highest-income counties for deaths from machinery and four times as high for falling objects, electric current, and explosions (Figure 3-12).

Prominent racial differences are seen in death rates from machinery and electric current, for which rates per 100,000 population are almost twice as high for whites as for blacks. Native Americans have the highest death rates from explosions and falling objects. Asians have very low rates for all four causes (see Appendix). Per 100,000 workers, death rates from all occupational injuries combined are about 12 percent higher for nonwhites than for whites (DSR 1990).

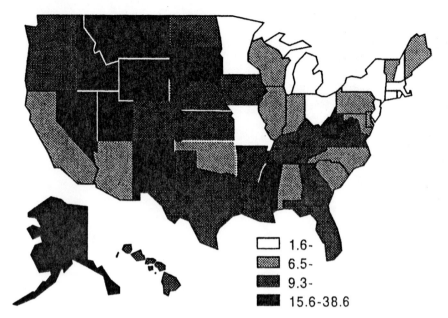

Figure 9-5.   Death Rates from Occupational Injury by State, per 100,000 Workers, 1980–1985

GEOGRAPHIC DIFFERENCES

Occupational injury death rates per 100,000 workers range from 1.6 in Connecticut to 33.3 in Wyoming and 38.6 in Alaska. In general, the highest rates based on NTOF data are in the mountain states and the lowest are in the northeastern states (Figure 9-5). States vary in the degree to which injury at work is reported on death certificates, and underreporting may be the reason for low rates in some states.

Population-based death rates for causes of death that typically occur in connection with work are mapped in Figure 9-6. Death rates from explosions and electric current generally are higher in western and southern states. Death rates from nonfarm machinery tend to be high in the mountain states, while rates associated with farm machinery are high in the north central states.

Death rates from work-related injury are generally high in states where much of the population lives in rural areas. Moreover, within individual states, the highest death rates tend to be in the most rural areas. In Colorado, 47 percent of all work injury deaths occur in rural areas where only 17 percent of the workforce is employed (Marine et al. 1990). Nationally, when examined by urban/rural characteristics of the counties, the death rates from machinery, falling objects, electric current, and explosion all increase in the most rural areas, where they are 3 to 10 times the rates in central cities (Figure 9-7).

a. Machinery

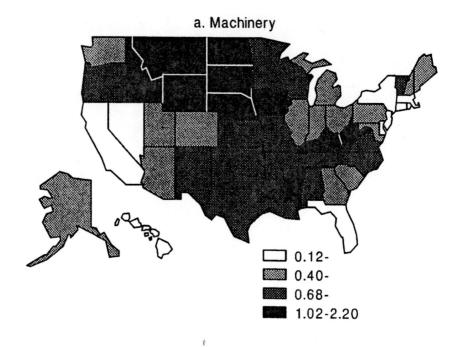

☐	0.12-
▨	0.40-
▦	0.68-
■	1.02-2.20

b. Explosion

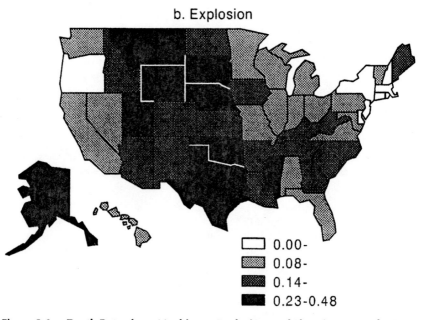

☐	0.00-
▨	0.08-
▦	0.14-
■	0.23-0.48

Figure 9-6.   Death Rates from Machinery, Explosion, and Electric Current by State, per 100,000 Population, 1980–1986

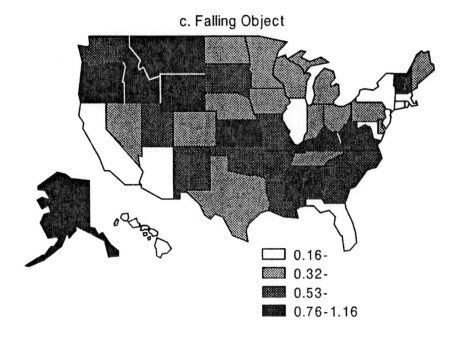

c. Falling Object

- ☐ 0.16-
- ▨ 0.32-
- ▦ 0.53-
- ■ 0.76-1.16

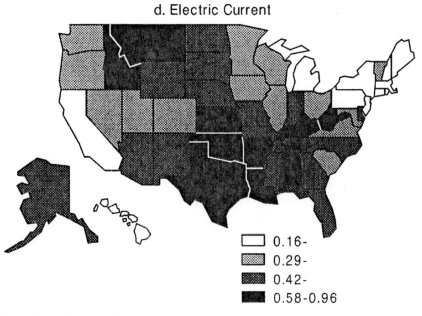

d. Electric Current

- ☐ 0.16-
- ▨ 0.29-
- ▦ 0.42-
- ■ 0.58-0.96

Figure 9-6. *Continued*

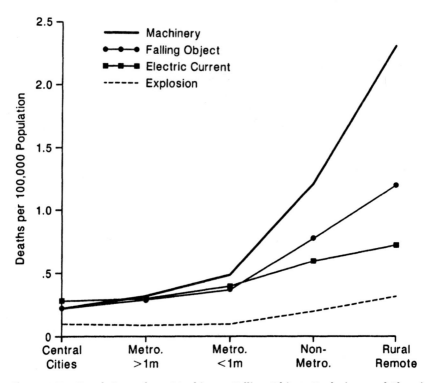

Figure 9-7. Death Rates from Machinery, Falling Object, Explosion, and Electric Current, by Place of Residence, per 100,000 Population, 1980–1986

TEMPORAL VARIATION

Unlike injury deaths in general, which are most frequent on weekends, deaths from machinery, falling objects, electric current, and explosions are least common on Saturday and Sunday, especially the latter. Summer, when greater exposure to some hazards may occur, is the season of highest frequency for all four causes (Figure 9-8). Especially prominent is the July–August peak for electric current deaths, which may be partly related to seasonal patterns in construction work, since many electrocutions involve contact with overhead wires by cranes or other equipment. The summer peak may also be related to farm electrocutions, which sometimes occur when long sections of irrigation pipe touch overhead wires while being repositioned (Helgerson and Milham 1985). Other factors that may contribute to summertime electrocutions include greater use of poorly grounded outdoor electrical equipment and a tendency for people to perspire, which markedly lowers the skin's resistance to electric current. In addition, rainfall and moist earth in late spring and summer may increase electrical hazards.

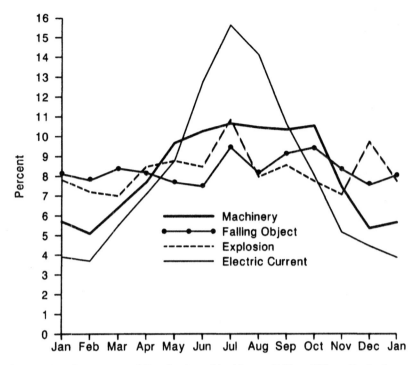

Figure 9-8. Percentage of Deaths from Machinery, Falling Object, Explosion, and Electric Current by Month, 1980–1986

OCCUPATION AND INDUSTRY

The preceding death rates in this chapter are for all occupational groups and industries combined. Death rates for various groups of workers differ greatly. Transport workers and farmers, for example, are more than 30 times as likely as clerical workers to be fatally injured on the job (Figure 9-9). Separation into more specific occupations reveals even greater differences, with the highest rates for loggers and pilots (Table 9-3; Leigh 1987).

Among industries, the highest rates are experienced by workers in mining, construction, transportation and agriculture (Table 9-4). The rate for agriculture is more than five times that for manufacturing, which is the fifth most hazardous industry (DSR 1990). Estimates of nonfatal injury rates for major industry groups tend to obscure the great differences among subgroups (NSC 1989). For example, in transportation and public utilities, the overall rate of lost workdays is relatively low (3.5 per 100 workers per year) because the large numbers of workers in low-risk subgroups such as communications mask the very high rates for smaller high-risk subgroups such as trucking (Table 9-5).

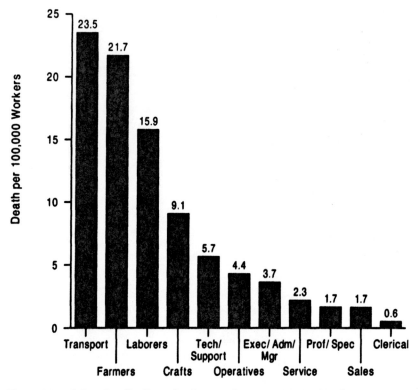

Figure 9-9.   Injury Fatality Rates by Occupation, per 100,000 Workers, 1980–1985 (*Source:* National Institute of Occupational Safety and Health.)

HISTORICAL TRENDS AND PREVENTIVE MEASURES

Overall death rates from work-related injury have declined in recent years; from 1980 to 1985, there was a 23 percent decrease (Bell et al. 1990). In California, the rate of occupational injury fatalities declined by an average of 7 percent annually from 1972 to 1983 (Goldberg et al. 1989). In some industries, however, substantial increases have been reported. Among mobile offshore drilling units, the death rate per 100,000 workers secondary to major mishaps (i.e., exclusive of deaths in routine operations) increased sharply in the 1970s, due in part to high fatality rates involving jack-up rigs (Clemmer and Diem 1985). Similarly, death rates of offshore fishermen were 39 percent higher in 1971–1980 than in the prior decade (Reilly 1985). Trends in rates of reported nonfatal work injuries have been mixed; amputations decreased dramatically from 23.3 per 100 million hours worked in 1953 to 4.7 in 1985, while fractures decreased until 1980 and then increased (Robinson 1988). Occupational Safety and Health Administration (OSHA) inspections have been credited with some of the decrease in nonfatal rates (Robertson and Keeve 1983).

Table 9-3. Occupations with Highest Job-Related Death Rates, 11 States, 1977–1980

Occupation	Estimated Deaths Annually per 100,000 Workers
Timber cutters/loggers	129
Pilots	98
Asbestos/insulation workers	79
Structural metal workers	72
Electric line installers/repairers	51
Firefighters	49
Garbage collectors	40
Truck drivers	40
Bulldozer operators	39
Earth drillers	39
Specified craft apprentices	38
Mine operatives	38
Boilermakers	35
Taxi drivers/chauffeurs	34
Construction laborers	34

Source: J.P. Leigh, Estimates of the probability of job-related death in 347 occupations. *Journal of Occupational Medicine* 29 (1987):510–519.

Table 9-4. Occupational Injury Fatality Rates by Industrial Division, 1980–1985

Industrial Division	Fatality Rate per 100,000 Workers
Mining	27.9
Construction	21.9
Transportation, communication, and public utility	21.4
Agriculture, forestry, and fishing	18.7
Finance, insurance, and real estate	11.5
Manufacturing	4.0
Services	2.4
Wholesale trade	0.9
Retail trade	0.4

Source: National Institute of Occupational Safety and Health.

Table 9-5.   Lost Workday Rates in the Transportation
and Public Utilities Industry, 1987

Industry Area	Lost Workday Cases per 100 Employees
Industry rate	3.5
Local and long distance trucking	17.6
Local and interurban passenger transit	8.4
Railroad transportation	5.5
Water transportation	3.7
Air transportation	2.8
Electric/gas/sanitary services	2.6
Communication	0.8

Source: National Safety Council, 1989.

Severe injury and death from fixed machinery in factories and mills, once major problems, have been greatly reduced by incorporation of machine guards, fail-safe devices, and other types of automatic protection. By 1986, only 14 percent of all deaths from occupational injuries were attributed to machinery and only 2 percent of all deaths from machinery were due to power presses, saws, or other woodworking and metalworking machines—that is, the machines that now commonly incorporate a variety of automatic protection devices (Table 9-6).

Between 1980 and 1986, death rates from both farm and nonfarm machinery decreased by about one-fifth. During the previous 50 years, however, markedly different trends characterized deaths from farm and nonfarm machinery. Between 1930 and 1980, the farm machinery death rate per 100,000 population increased by 44 percent, while the death rate from all other machinery dropped by 79 percent (Figure 9-10). The latter decrease involved not only deaths from fixed machinery but also those from elevators, which in 1930 surpassed deaths from farm machinery (348 versus 314 deaths, respectively). Although the number of elevators increased markedly, elevator-related deaths became rare as stringent codes were developed and

Table 9-6.   Deaths from Machinery, 1988

Type of Machinery	Number	Percentage
Agricultural machines	599	51.0
Cranes, forklifts, lifting machines	180	15.3
Earth-moving machines	115	9.8
Mining and earth-drilling machines	45	3.8
Metalworking and woodworking machines	32	2.7
Other or unspecified	205	17.4
Total	1,176	100.0

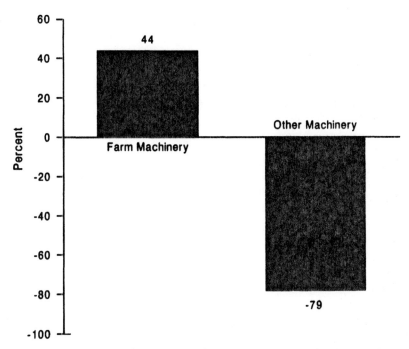

Figure 9-10.   Percentage Change in Death Rates from Farm and Other Machinery, per 100,000 Population, 1980 versus 1930

enforced.[1] Unlike road vehicles, home appliances, and most other consumer products sold in the United States, farm machinery is not covered by federal product safety standards. Employers of more than 10 farm workers must provide employees with equipment that meets OSHA requirements, but the great majority of farm workers are not covered under OSHA because they are family members or work on small farms (Baker et al. 1982; Karlson and Noren 1979).

Of some 1,200 annual machinery-related deaths, more than one-half involve farm equipment. In Georgia, the rate of tractor-related deaths in 1971–1981 among male farm residents was 24 per 100,000, exceeding the overall national death rate for injuries from road vehicles (Goodman et al. 1985). Detailed analysis of death certificate information on 4,500 farm machinery fatalities in the United States during 1975–1981 revealed that about three-fourths involved tractors (McKnight 1984). The major problems were tractor overturns, falling from and/or being run over by tractors, and entanglement by the power take-off shaft. Corn pickers, augers, and combines also caused substantial numbers of deaths. Farm machinery operating on public roads was involved in about 200 deaths annually, including occupants of other vehicles.

Cranes were the most common type of nonroad land vehicle involved in deaths of Maryland workers (Baker et al. 1982). As in the case of tractors, deaths from cranes, forklifts, and bulldozers often involve overturns. In addition, electrocution is an important contributor to fatalities related to cranes and augers.

At work sites that are out of doors and at remote locations, prevention of deaths and injuries from machinery—for example, in the fishing industry and among farmers and loggers—presents a special challenge. In addition to the hazards of unguarded machines lacking automatic protection, injured people may be working alone, often under difficult conditions and time pressures created by maturing crops and changes in the weather. Access to emergency services and skilled trauma care is often inadequate.

Despite improvements in machinery in recent years, further design changes are needed to provide automatic protection from death or severe injury under a wide variety of predictable circumstances. For example, not only is it necessary to separate workers from cutting and grinding mechanisms, but also means are needed to clear machinery that is jammed by cornstalks or other material, so that workers will not have to intervene while machinery is running. Old tractors need to be retrofitted with rollover protection devices, and power take-offs should have integrated guards that cannot be removed. Along with forklifts and other vehicles that are apt to overturn, tractors need improved design to prevent backward and sideward overturns.

Countermeasures for electrical injuries and deaths include burying transmission lines or otherwise placing them out of reach and designing irrigation pipes that fold or separate into pieces that are too short to reach power lines. Improving insulation on crane booms and other equipment likely to be used near electrical wires, using electronic sensors that preclude contact with dangerous electrical fields or conductors, reducing the voltage, and installing ground fault interrupters are a few more examples of approaches that would reduce exposure to lethal doses of electricity. The need to protect electrical workers against postdisaster electrical hazards has recently been recognized (CDC 1989).

Increased use of personal protective devices and advances in equipment design are essential. Use of well-designed helmets by loggers and jockeys, for example, would substantially reduce head injuries, which are the most frequent source of disability or death in these occupations (Boglioli et al. 1987; Holman et al. 1987). Being stuck by a syringe or other needled device, which is the most common injury sustained by health care workers, could be largely prevented by designs for these items that virtually eliminate the potential for such injuries and consequent exposure to blood-borne diseases (Jagger et al. 1988).

Road vehicles cause the greatest number of occupational deaths, yet they have been largely ignored as a contributor to occupational death and injury (Baker et al. 1982; Runyan and Baker 1988). The crashworthiness of trucks and their aggressiveness in crashes could be greatly improved using current technology. Occupational injuries and deaths could be reduced by improving and implementing federal motor vehicle safety standards and by providing air bag-equipped vehicles to workers who drive on the job (IIHS 1985). Heavy truck safety is discussed in more detail in Chapter 18.

Detailed examination of the circumstances of worker deaths and injuries can help to identify hazards and focus preventive efforts. For example, review of confined-space fatalities revealed that two-thirds of the jobs were related to water, wastewater, or sewerage systems (Manwaring and Conroy 1990). Although established procedures can potentially prevent some deaths, only 4 percent of the workers killed in confined spaces had received relevant training. Fully one-third worked for companies with 10 or fewer employees and most of the remainder for companies with 11 to 100 employees. Unfortunately, small companies, which tend to have higher-than-average injury rates, are less likely than larger firms to have comprehensive safety programs.

Despite the importance of workplace design and automatic protection of the worker, emphasis is often on training (Olson and Gerberich 1986) and on identifying high-risk workers. The concept of "accident proneness" in the workplace, as in other settings, has been discredited, and it has been shown that removing workers with an excessive number of injuries would not appreciably reduce injuries in the succeeding time period (Mohr and Clemmer 1988).

The possible role of alcohol and drug abuse in workplace injuries has often prompted speculation, but there are few data to support such an association (Smith and Kraus 1988). Several studies have reported that 11 to 13 percent of fatally injured workers had measurable BACs and that 7 to 9 percent had BACs of 0.10 percent or higher (Lewis and Cooper 1989; Sniezek and Horiagon 1989). In Maryland and Texas, high BACs were rare among fatally injured workers except those killed in motor vehicle crashes or shootings (Baker et al. 1982; Lewis and Cooper 1989). Alcohol and prescription drugs are detected far more frequently than illicit drugs in postmortem toxicology screens of workers (Lewis and Cooper 1989).

NOTE

1. Elevator deaths are now so uncommon that they are not separately coded; they are combined with the far more numerous deaths from forklifts and cranes.

REFERENCES

Baker, S.P., A.H. Myers, G.S. Smith (1990). Injury prevention in the workplace. In *Proceedings of The Johns Hopkins University Conference on Research in Work, Health, and Productivity*. New York: Oxford University Press.

Baker, S.P., J.S. Samkoff, R.S. Fisher, and C.B. Van Buren (1982). Fatal occupational injuries. *Journal of the American Medical Association* 248:692–697.

Bell, C.A., N.A. Stout, T.R. Bender, C.S. Conroy, and W.E. Crouse (1990). Fatal occupational injuries in the United States, 1980 through 1985. *Journal of the American Medical Association* 263:3047-3050.

Boglioli, L.R., M.L. Taff, and L.I. Lukash (1987). Harness racing injuries and deaths. Report of a fatal accident and review of 178 cases. *American Journal of Forensic Medicine and Pathology* 8:185-207.

Bureau of Labor Statistics (1990). *Occupational injury and illness in the United States by industry, 1988. Bulletin 2366.* Washington, DC: U.S. Department of Labor.

Centers for Disease Control (1989). Update: Work-related electrocutions associated with hurricane Hugo, Puerto Rico. *Morbidity and Mortality Weekly Report* 38:718-720, 725.

Clemmer, D.I., and J.E. Diem (1985). Major mishaps among mobile offshore drilling units. *International Journal of Epidemiology* 14:106-112.

Davis, H. (1987). Workplace homicides of Texas males. *American Journal of Public Health* 77:1290-1293.

Division of Safety Research (1990). National traumatic occupational fatalities: 1980-1985. Cincinnati, OH: National Institute for Occupational Safety and Health.

Goldberg, R.L., L. Bernstein, D.H. Garabrant, and J.M. Peters (1989). Fatal occupational injuries in California, 1971-1983. *American Journal of Industrial Medicine* 15:177-185.

Goodman, R.A., J.D. Smith, R.K. Sikes, D.L. Rogers, and J.L. Mickey (1985). Fatalities associated with farm tractor injuries: An epidemiologic study. *Public Health Reports* 100:329-333.

Helgerson, S.D., and S. Milham (1985). Farm workers electrocuted when irrigation pipes contact powerlines. *Public Health Reports* 100:325-328.

Holman, R.G., A. Olszewski, and R.V. Maier (1987). The epidemiology of logging injuries in the Northwest. *Journal of Trauma* 27:1044-1050

Insurance Institute for Highway Safety (1985). Fleet buyers get latest facts and figures. *Status Report* 20(15):1-4.

Jagger, J., E.H. Hunt, J. Brand-Elnaggar, and R.D. Pearson (1988). Rates of needlestick injury caused by various devices in a university hospital. *New England Journal of Medicine* 319:284-288.

Karlson, T.A., and J. Noren (1979). Farm tractor fatalities: The failure of voluntary safety standards. *American Journal of Public Health* 69:146-149.

Klein, B.P., R.C. Jensen, and L.M. Sanderson (1984). Assessment of workers' compensation claims for back strains/sprains. *Journal of Occupational Medicine* 26:443-448.

Kraus, J.F. (1985). Fatal and nonfatal injuries in occupational settings: A review. *Annual Review of Public Health* 6:403-418.

Kraus, J.F. (1987). Homicide while at work: Persons, industries, and occupations at high risk. *American Journal of Public Health* 77:1285-1289.

Kraus, J.F., and D. Fife (1985). Incidence, external causes, and outcomes of work-related brain injuries in males. *Journal of Occupational Medicine* 27:757-760.

Kraus, J.F., J. Macurda, J. Sahl, and C. Anderson (1990). Work-related fatal injuries in older California workers, 1979-1985. *Journal of Occupational Accidents* 12:223-235.

Leigh, J.P. (1987). Estimates of the probability of job-related death in 347 occupations. *Journal of Occupational Medicine* 29:510–519.

Lewis, R.J., and S.P. Cooper (1989). Alcohol, other drugs, and fatal work-related injuries. *Journal of Occupational Medicine* 31:23–28.

Manwaring, J.C., and C. Conroy (1990). Occupational confined space-related fatalities: Surveillance and prevention. *Journal of Safety Research* 21:157–164.

Marine, W.M., C. Garrett, S.M. Keefer, R. Vancil, R. Hoffman, and L. McKenzie (1990). *Occupational injury deaths in Colorado 1982–1987*. Denver: Colorado Department of Health.

McKnight, R.H. (1984). *U.S. agricultural equipment fatalities 1975–1981: Implications for injury control and health education*. Unpublished doctoral dissertation, The Johns Hopkins University, Baltimore.

Mohr, D.L., and D.I. Clemmer (1988). The "accident prone" worker: An example from heavy industry. *Accident Analysis and Prevention* 20:123–127.

Mueller, B.A., D.L. Mohr, J.C. Rice, and D.I. Clemmer (1987). Factors affecting individual injury experience among petroleum drilling workers. *Journal of Occupational Medicine* 29:126–131.

National Center for Health Statistics (1985). Persons injured and disability days due to injuries. United States, 1980–1981. *Vital and Health Statistics* 10(149).

National Safety Council (1989). *Accident Facts 1989*. Chicago: National Safety Council.

Olson, D.K., and S.G. Gerberich (1986). Traumatic amputations in the workplace. *Journal of Occupational Medicine* 28:480–485.

Reilly, M.S. (1985). Mortality from occupational accidents to United Kingdom fishermen 1961–1980. *British Journal of Industrial Medicine* 42:806–814.

Robertson, L.S., and J.P. Keeve (1983). Worker injuries: The effects of workers' compensation and OSHA inspections. *Journal of Health Politics, Policy and Law* 8:581–597.

Robinson, J.C. (1988). The rising long-term trend in occupational injury rates. *American Journal of Public Health* 78:276–281.

Rossignol, A.M., J.A. Locke, C.M. Boyle, and J.F. Burke (1986). Epidemiology of work-related burn injuries in Massachusetts requiring hospitalization. *Journal of Trauma* 26:1097–1101.

Runyan, C.W., and S.P. Baker (1988). Occupational motor vehicle injury morbidity among municipal workers. *Journal of Occupational Medicine* 30:883–886.

Smith, G.S., and J.F. Kraus (1988). Alcohol and residential, recreational, and occupational injuries: A review of the epidemiologic evidence. *Annual Review of Public Health* 9:99–121.

Snook, S.H. (1982). Low back pain in industry. In A.A. White and S.L. Gordon (Eds.), *Symposium on idiopathic low back pain*. St. Louis, MO: Mosby, pp. 23–28.

Sniezek, J.E., and T.M. Horiagon (1989). Medical-examiner-reported fatal occupational injuries, North Carolina, 1979–1984. *American Journal of Industrial Medicine* 15:669–678.

Wickstrom, G., T. Niskanen, and H. Riihimak (1985). Strain on the back in concrete reinforcement work. *British Journal of Industrial Medicine* 42:233–239.

10

Falls

Falls, the second leading cause of unintentional injury death, are the most common cause of injuries and of hospital admissions for trauma. The source of 87 percent of all fractures in the elderly (Fife and Barancik 1985), they are also the second leading cause of both spinal cord and brain injury, accounting for about one-fifth of these injuries (Kraus et al. 1984; Kraus et al. 1975). Each year one person in 20 receives emergency room treatment because of a fall (Barancik et al. 1983). The total lifetime cost of fall injuries sustained in 1985 was about $37 billion, an amount only slightly less than the cost of motor vehicle-related injury (Rice et al. 1989).

Hip fractures result in more hospital admissions than any other injury and were the primary cause of 254,000 hospital admissions in 1988. Fracture of the hip typically occurs as the result of a fall and only rarely precedes a fall (Cummings et al. 1990). Incidence is especially influenced by age, with people 65 years or older sustaining 85 percent of all hip fractures. On average, hip fractures in this age group require 13.5 days of hospitalization in a short-stay hospital, compared with an average stay of 8.9 days for all causes of hospital admission in this group (Graves 1990). About three million hospital days are required annually to treat hip fractures in the population age 65 or older. These figures exclude the many days of nursing home care and do not convey the tragic changes in life style and loss of independence that commonly ensue.

In addition to producing substantial morbidity and disability, falls are a major cause of unintentional injury death, surpassed only by motor vehicles. In recent years more than 11,000 deaths annually have been attributed to falls. In an even greater number of cases a fall initiates or contributes to the sequence of events leading to death but is not coded as the underlying cause of death, even though it is mentioned on the death certificate (Fife 1987). Only falls listed as the underlying cause of death are included in the following mortality analyses.

Injuries from falls result from an abrupt dissipation of mechanical energy. As in motor vehicle crashes, the intensity of the forces exerted on a person who falls depends in part on the person's velocity at the moment of impact. In turn, the velocity is determined primarily by the height from which the person has fallen and whether the fall has been interrupted, for example, by grasping a handrail or landing on shrubbery. The impact velocity may also be increased by other aspects of the dynamics of a fall, as when a person slips on ice and spins backward.

When a person falls, the likelihood of injury decreases as the decelerative, or stopping, distance increases. This stopping distance depends on several things, including the energy-absorbing qualities of the structure that a person falls onto or against, the thickness and energy-absorbing qualities of clothing, and the yield or compressibility of the part of the body on which the forces operate.

Spreading the forces of a fall over a larger area of the body is also an important means of reducing injuries from falls. Falling against a narrow, sharp, or pointed structure focuses the forces and increases the chance of injury, whereas a wider contact area distributes the forces less harmfully over a larger portion of the body, with less likelihood of injury.

The implications of these basic determinants of fall injuries are often unrecognized, despite the pioneering work of Hugh DeHaven (DeHaven 1942; Haddon 1980; Haddon et al. 1964). His classic study of people who survived falls from great heights showed that injury severity in falls is largely determined by the characteristics of the environment, including the impact surface and what is beneath it. The study also demonstrated that under appropriate conditions the human body can withstand very high deceleration forces without significant injury. Subsequent work by Snyder identified survival of falls of up to 70 meters (Snyder 1963). Such cases often involve landing on snow or other energy-attenuating surfaces. When concrete and other rigid surfaces are involved, injury can occur in falls from low heights. Free-fall investigations and simulations revealed that, although children are generally injured less severely than adults under similar fall circumstances, headfirst falls onto rigid surfaces from a height of 2 meters can cause serious injury to children (Foust et al. 1977; Mohan et al. 1979).

The biomechanics of falls also influences outcome. Hip fracture is much more likely when an elderly person lands on the hip or side of the leg rather than on the buttocks or other part of the body, and when the local soft tissues do not absorb enough of the energy to prevent a fracture (Cummings and Nevitt 1989; Hayes et al. 1990). The fragility of bones, as often manifested in osteoporosis, is a major determinant of fracture likelihood.

PLACE OF INJURY

The place where injury occurred is specified for about two-thirds of all fatal falls (Table 10-1). In the majority of cases specified, the injury occurs at home; the proportion that occurs in the home is highest among young children and the elderly.

NIOSH identifies about 800 work-related fatal falls annually. Although the numbers are underestimates, only road vehicles, machinery, and homicide cause more deaths at work (see Chapter 9). Except for about 300 falls per year in which the death certificate mentions industrial sites and mines, it

Table 10-1. Percentage of Fall Deaths by Circumstances and Place of Injury, 1980–1986

Place of Injury	Circumstances						
	Stairs	Ladder /Scaffold	Building /Structure	Different Level	Same Level	Other /Unspecified	All Falls
Home	77.2	44.5	37.3	27.2	50.0	35.3	39.7
Resident institution	2.3	1.0	3.1	21.9	15.6	12.9	11.8
Public building	5.4	8.7	8.7	3.3	4.0	2.0	3.1
Recreation/sport	0.2	0.3	0.9	4.3	2.6	0.4	0.8
Farm	0.1	1.9	2.1	1.4	0.4	0.2	0.4
Industrial/mine	0.4	19.0	13.0	4.8	0.9	0.9	2.4
Other	4.7	11.6	22.5	22.4	14.2	6.6	9.1
Unspecified	9.7	13.0	12.4	14.7	12.3	41.7	32.7
Total	100.0	100.0	100.0	100.0	100.0	100.0	100.0

is not yet possible to identify work-related falls in the NCHS mortality files. A review of all fatal occupational injuries in Maryland found that 9 percent were due to falls, a proportion surpassed only by vehicle-related and firearm deaths (Baker et al. 1982). More than 1,400 fatal falls are known to occur each year in residential institutions such as nursing homes. Studies conducted in such facilities for the elderly reveal high rates of falls and fall injuries, including hip fractures (Gryfe et al. 1977). The preponderance of falls, however, occur in the home, where they are often associated with tripping (Blake et al. 1988).

AGE AND SEX

Almost one-third (32 percent) of all deaths from falls occur among people aged 85 or older, although this age group makes up only 1 percent of the population. Fifty-nine percent of all fall deaths involve people 75 or older, who comprise about 5 percent of the population. The importance of the problem is illustrated by comparing fall deaths among the elderly with motor vehicle occupant deaths among teenage males, who are well known to be at high risk of death in motor vehicle crashes. There are more deaths from falls among people 85 or older than there are motor vehicle occupant deaths among males aged 18–19 (3,700 versus 2,900), and the death rate per 100,000 population is about three times as high. The elderly have high death rates from falls because of several concomitants of advanced age: greater likelihood of falling due to various medical problems and impairment of vision, gait, and balance; increased fragility of certain bones caused by osteoporosis, a loss of bone mass that is greater in females and increases with age (Engh et al. 1968; Johnson and Specht 1981); and greater susceptibility to fatal complications following injury.

The circumstances of fatal falls vary with age. During childhood the majority of fatal falls are from buildings or other structures or are coded on the death certificate as falls "from another level." Fatal falls from buildings, ladders, and scaffolds are prominent during the working years. Falls on stairs become relatively important after about age 45. Among the elderly, who have the highest death rates from *all* types of falls, the circumstances are not specified for about 80 percent of falls. The age and sex pattern of unspecified falls closely resembles the pattern for falls on the same level (Figure 10-1) suggesting that most of the unspecified falls occur on one level.

The male to female ratio of death rates for all ages and for all types of falls combined is 1.2 to 1. The ratio varies, however, by type of fall, ranging from 29 to 1 for falls from ladders and scaffolds to about 1 to 1 for falls on one level. These sex ratios, like others in this book, are not adjusted for age. At each age, the male death rate for each category of fall exceeds the female rate. If death rates were age adjusted, the male to female ratio for falls on

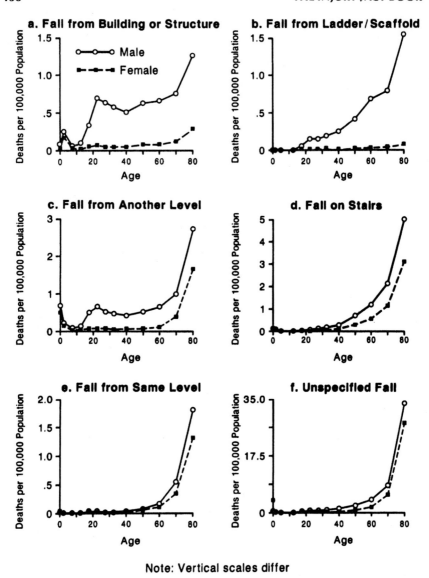

Note: Vertical scales differ

Figure 10-1.   Death Rates from Falls by Age, Sex, and Circumstances, 1980–1986

one level would be slightly greater than 1. However, the larger proportion of elderly women in the total female population causes the unadjusted death rate for females to be similar to the rate for males in the case of falls on one level and to exceed it in the case of unspecified falls. The higher age-specific death rates among males contrast with their lower age-specific fracture rates (Table 10-2). Case fatality rates in white men hospitalized for hip fractures are substantially higher than rates for white women, even when controlled for age, circumstances of fall, other injuries, and serious concomitant

Table 10-2.   Hip Fracture Incidence in the Elderly by Age, Race,
and Sex, 1984–1987

	Women		Men	
	Number [4 years]	(Annual Rate per 100,000)	Number [4 years]	(Annual Rate per 100,000)
Whites				
65–74	103,150	(27)	40,323	(13)
75–84	233,140	(103)	64,344	(48)
85+	287,810	(260)	47,205	(150)
Blacks				
65–74	3,424	(10)	2,697	(11)
75–84	6,819	(38)	3,063	(29)
85+	6,900	(119)	2,049	(76)

Sources: Based on incidence data from S.J. Jacobsen, J. Goldberg, T.P. Miles, J.A. Brody, W. Stiers, and A.A. Rimm, Hip fracture incidence among the old and very old: A population-based study of 745,435 cases. *American Journal of Public Health* 80(1990):871–873; and Bureau of the Census population estimates for 1986.

illnesses (Myers et al. 1991). Differences between the sexes in use of alcohol may contribute to higher death rates in men, because severe injuries are more likely to involve alcohol than are minor injuries. At least among pedestrians, falls resulting in head injuries are frequently associated with alcohol but other falls are not (Merrild and Bak 1983). In addition to increasing the likelihood of a fall, alcohol has been shown to be associated with a loss of bone density, which would contribute to the likelihood of fracture when a fall occurs (Felson et al. 1988).

The age-associated increase in fracture rates is especially pronounced for fractures of the hip (Figure 3-7). After age 75, hip fractures in both sexes outnumber all other fractures combined as a cause of hospitalization. Among white women, the rate of hip fractures at age 85 and older is almost 10 times the rate at ages 65–74 (Table 10-2). Although white men have lower hip fracture rates, they show as great a rate of increase with age. For both sexes, the hospitalization rate for all fractures excluding those of the hip is about three times as high for ages 85 and older as for ages 65–74. Although fractures are a significant problem among elderly males as well as females, most scientific attention has been given to fractures among elderly women, who outnumber elderly men and also have higher fracture rates.

For both sexes, advanced age substantially increases the likelihood of hospital admission following minor fractures. However, age does not greatly influence the probability of admission following hip fractures, almost all of which result in hospitalization.

Children are also at high risk of fall injury, but their death rate is low. Based on Massachusetts data, about one-tenth of all children aged 1–3 require emergency room treatment each year for falls, with the highest incidence at age 1. Falls on stairs account for one-eighth of the childhood falls

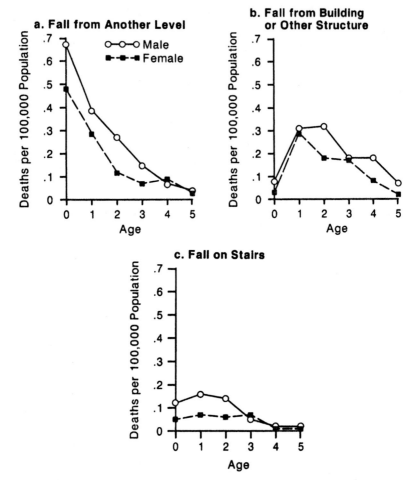

Figure 10-2.   Death Rates from Falls by Age, Sex, and Circumstances, for Ages 0–5, 1980–1986

treated in emergency rooms and one-fourth of the hospital admissions. Reflecting the greater impact forces in falls from heights, most hospital admissions for falls among children involve falls from another level, such as a roof, porch, stairs, or dressing table (Finison 1983; Gallagher et al. 1982).

In 1986, 117 children younger than 5 years old were killed in falls, primarily from buildings or other structures, on stairs, or other falls from another level (Figure 10-2). Falls on stairs of children in walkers are especially likely to result in serious injury. During childhood, fatal falls from buildings and on stairs are most common at ages 1–2, whereas other fatal falls from a different level (a bed or chair) are most common during the first year of life for both sexes (Figure 10-2). These differences may reflect differing developmental patterns of childhood activity and suggest the need for research on the relationships among age, sex, degree of supervision, and the role of the physical environment in childhood injury.

RACE AND PER CAPITA INCOME

Racial patterns of fall mortality differ substantially from racial patterns of other injury deaths. For falls among all ages combined, the death rate among whites is about 50 percent higher than among blacks and Native Americans and more than three times the rate for Asians. In children and for ages 25–64, however, the death rate from falls is higher among blacks than whites (Figures 10-3 and 10-4). Native Americans have the highest rates among infants and at ages 5–44. Asian children have high rates at ages 1–4, a pattern also noted in China (Li and Baker, 1991). The higher rate among elderly whites is consistent with the greater prevalence of osteoporosis and the higher rate of fracture of the hip for whites (Engh et al. 1968; Jacobsen et al. 1990; Trotter et al. 1960).

The racial pattern varies with the type of fall. For falls on one level, which predominantly involve the elderly, the death rate is three times as high

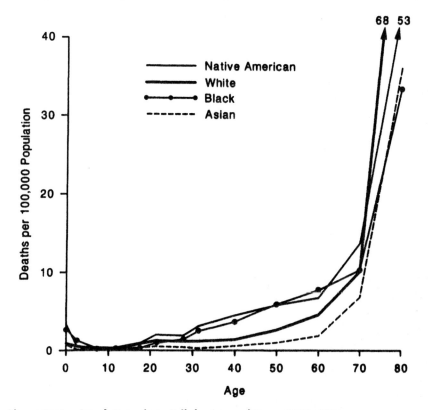

Figure 10-3.   Death Rates from Falls by Age and Race, 1980–1986

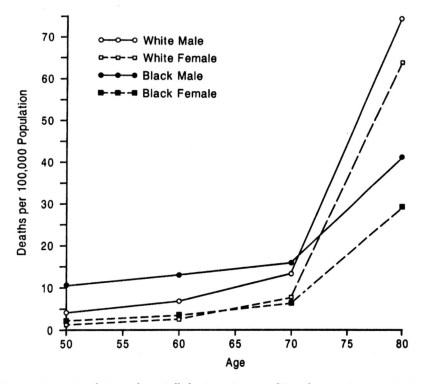

Figure 10-4.   Death Rates from Falls by Age, Race, and Sex, for Age Groups 45–54 and Older, 1980–1986

among whites as blacks. For falls from buildings or other structures, the death rate is 43 percent higher among blacks than whites. In considering such comparisons, it must be remembered that the circumstances are not specified for a large proportion of falls.

Compared with rates for other injuries, death rates for all types of falls combined show the least relationship to per capita income of the area of residence (Figure 4-10). Although this pattern holds for both whites and blacks, the death rates among Native Americans and Asians in low-income areas are about twice the rates in high-income areas (Baker et al. 1984).

URBAN/RURAL AND GEOGRAPHIC DIFFERENCES

For all falls combined, death rates are highest in central cities and rural areas. Patterns vary among specific kinds of falls (Figure 10-5). Falls from buildings or other structures have especially high rates in large cities.

There is considerable geographic variation in death rates from falls, with northern states generally having higher death rates than southern states (Figure 4-12). This is true in summer as well as winter, suggesting that the phenomenon is not explained by the longer and icier northern winters. Rates

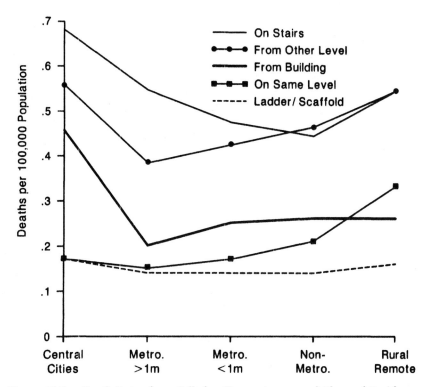

Figure 10-5.   Death Rates from Falls by Circumstances and Place of Residence, 1980–1986

of hospitalization for hip fractures also vary geographically; they are highest for both sexes in the west north central states, where the rate for white females is 50 percent greater than the overall rate for the United States (Bacon et al. 1989). The generally higher rates in the northern half of the country appear not to be explained by the age mix of the 65-and-older population, because even age-adjusted rates for this age group are high in northern states (Iskrant and Joliet 1968).

Given the seriousness of the problem of falls among the elderly, further exploration of the geographic differences would be worthwhile. Some of the differences could be due to variations in describing and coding deaths, so such research should include comparisons of state practices regarding the certification of the cause and manner of death from late complications of injury.

HISTORICAL TRENDS

The trend in death rates from falls has been downward in recent years. Although the overall death rate decreased by about 18 percent (from 6.0 in 1977–1979 to 4.9 in 1984–1986), this decrease was not uniform across age

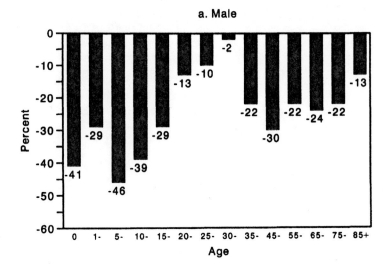

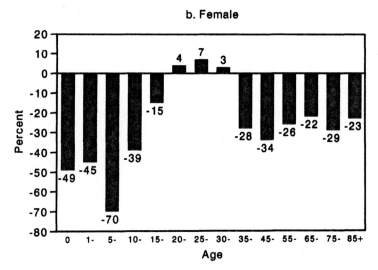

Figure 10-6.   Percentage Change in Death Rates from Falls by Age and Sex, 1984–1986 Compared with 1977–1979

groups (Figure 10-6). The least change occurred among ages 20–34, for which there was a slight decrease for men and an increase for women. This increase in young women was related primarily to falls from different levels, including from buildings and structures. The greatest decrease, about 40 percent, was among children less than 15 years old.

During the past three decades, there has been an important shift in the sex ratio for fall deaths among elderly whites. In 1960, the female rate was about 20 percent higher than the male rate for ages 75 and older (Iskrant and Joliet 1968). By 1980–1986, it was 25 percent lower than the male rate.

This shift occurred because the death rate from falls in the elderly declined more for women than for men. From 1977–1979 to 1984–1986, the decrease for ages 85 and older was 23 percent for women and 13 percent for men.

The shift in the sex ratio for fall mortality may result from an improved ability of the medical care system to prevent fatal complications following injury. Consistent with this hypothesis is the fact that among the elderly who die following falls, a greater proportion of males have fallen on stairs or from heights and thus would be expected to have sustained more severe injuries, on average, than females. Reductions in injury mortality probably have been greatest for less severe injuries because they are not immediately fatal, providing an opportunity for successful surgical and medical treatment. Specific studies are needed, however, to explore the complex relationships among age, sex, height of fall, severity of injury, and survival patterns.

PREVENTIVE MEASURES

In general, preventive efforts have emphasized the behavioral aspects of falls, despite the difficulty of changing relevant behaviors such as hurrying, shuffling, or thrill seeking. Largely ignored has been the potential benefit from modifying the environment. Particular attention needs to be given to the design of private homes, where most fall injuries occur; nursing homes and other facilities for the elderly where the population is at especially high risk of fall injury; and playgrounds, for which guidelines are available for equipment and surfaces (CPSC 1981a, 1981b). In these and many other places, falls should be anticipated and the potential for serious injury reduced or eliminated. In cities where many families live in high apartment buildings, children appear to be at special risk of being killed in falls from buildings. In recognition of this problem, the New York City Board of Health requires landlords to provide window guards for apartments in which children aged 10 or younger are living (Spiegel and Lindaman 1977).

Good lighting and visual clues, walking surfaces that provide adequate friction and are free of irregularities, and appropriate railings and other structures are among the means of preventing falls. Even when falls occur, the likelihood of injury can be greatly reduced by reducing the height of falls (with playground slides built into hillsides, for example) or by placing energy-attenuating surfaces under playground equipment, on the floors of nursing homes, below windows, and in other high-risk areas. One of the most ignored opportunities to prevent injuries is the rounding of likely contact points such as table edges, cabinet corners, and stair edges to spread impact forces. Body padding, ranging from knee pads for hockey players to hip pads for the elderly, can also attenuate impact forces. To reduce injuries in the elderly, exercise programs are recommended to improve gait and balance and increase bone density and muscle strength (Tinetti and Speechley 1989) and estrogen therapy is proposed to reduce hip fractures (Cummings et al. 1990).

In view of the advanced age and imperfect health of many residents of nursing homes and other facilities for the elderly, a large number of falls with serious sequelae should be anticipated in these institutions. Because of the prolonged disability and the high cost of falls to the individual, the family, and society, much could be gained from measures to reduce both the incidence and severity of fall injuries in such institutions. These measures include not only structural changes but also exercise programs and monitoring of medications, which often contribute to falls (Sorock 1988). Attention is also needed to the designs of wheelchairs and other assistive devices that contribute to falls.

REFERENCES

Bacon, E.W., G.S. Smith, and S.P. Baker (1989). Geographic variation in the occurrence of hip fractures among the elderly white U.S. population. *American Journal of Public Health* 79:1556–1558.

Baker, S.P., B. O'Neill, and R. Karpf. (1984). *The injury fact book.* Lexington, MA: Lexington Books.

Baker, S.P., J.S. Samkoff, R.S. Fisher, and C.B. Van Buren (1982). Fatal occupational injuries. *Journal of the American Medical Association* 248:692–697.

Barancik, J.I., B.F. Chatterjee, Y.C. Greene, E.M. Michenzi, and D. Fife (1983). Northeastern Ohio Trauma Study: I. Magnitude of the problem. *American Journal of Public Health* 73:746–751.

Blake, A.J., K. Morgan, M.J. Bendall, M. Dallosso, S.B.J. Ebrahim, T.H.D. Arie, P.H. Fentem, and E.J. Bassey (1988). Falls by elderly people at home: Prevalence and associated factors. *Age and Ageing* 17:365–372.

Consumer Product Safety Commission (1981a). *A handbook for public playground safety. Vol. 1: General guidelines for new and existing playgrounds.* Washington, DC: Consumer Product Safety Commission.

Consumer Product Safety Commission (1981b). *A handbook for public playground safety. Vol. 2: Technical guidelines for equipment and surfacing.* Washington, DC: U.S. Consumer Product Safety Commission.

Cummings, S.R., and M.C. Nevitt (1989). A hypothesis: The causes of hip fractures. *Journal of Gerontology* 44:M107–111.

Cummings, S.R., S.M. Rubin, and D. Black (1990). The future of hip fractures in the United States: Numbers, costs, and potential effects of postmenopausal estrogen. *Clinical Orthopedics and Related Research* 252:163–166.

DeHaven, H. (1942). Mechanical analysis of survival in falls from heights of fifty to one hundred and fifty feet. *War Medicine* 2:539–546.

Engh, G., A.J. Bollet, G. Hardin, and W. Parson (1968). Epidemiology of osteoporosis II. Incidence of hip fractures in mental institutions. *Journal of Bone and Joint Surgery* 50A:557–562.

Felson, D.T., D.P. Kiel, J.J. Anderson, and W.B. Kannel (1988). Alcohol consumption and hip fractures: The Framingham study. *American Journal of Epidemiology* 128:1102–1110.

Fife, D. (1987). Injuries and deaths among elderly persons. *American Journal of Epidemiology* 126:936–941.

Fife, D., and J.I. Barancik (1985). Northeastern Ohio Trauma Study III: Incidence of fractures. *Annals of Emergency Medicine* 14:244–248.

Finison, K. (1983). Target injuries to young children. *SCIPP Reports* (Massachusetts Department of Public Health) 4(1):1–5.

Foust, D.R., B.M. Bowan, and R.G. Snyder (1977). Study of human impact tolerance using investigations and simulations of free-falls. In *Proceedings of the Twenty-First Stapp Car Crash Conference*, pp. 3–59.

Gallagher, S.S., B. Guyer, M. Kotelchuck, J. Bass, F.H. Lovejoy, Jr., E. McLoughlin, and K. Mehta (1982). A strategy for the reduction of childhood injuries in Massachusetts: SCIPP *New England Journal of Medicine* 307: 1015-1019.

Graves, E.J. (1990). 1988 Summary: National Hospital Discharge Survey. *Advance Data* 185:1–12.

Gryfe, C.I., A. Amies, and M.J. Ashley (1977). A longitudinal study of falls in an elderly population: I. Incidence and morbidity. *Age and Ageing* 6:201-210.

Haddon, W., Jr. (1980). Advances in the epidemiology of injuries as a basis for public policy. *Public Health Reports* 95:411–421.

Haddon, W., Jr., E.A. Suchman, and D. Klein (1964). *Accident research: Methods and approaches*. New York: Harper & Row.

Hayes, W.C., N.M. Resnick, L.A. Maitland, E.R. Myers, L.A. Lipsitz, and S.L. Greenspan (1990). Fall biomechanics—a better determinant than bone density of hip fracture in elderly women. Boston, MA: Departments of Medicine and Orthopedics, Beth Israel Hospital.

Iskrant, A.P., and P.V. Joliet (1968). *Accidents and homicide*. Cambridge, MA: Harvard University Press.

Jacobsen, S.J., J. Goldberg, T.P. Miles, J.A. Brody, W. Stiers, and A.A. Rimm (1990). Hip fracture incidence among the old and very old: A population-based study of 745,435 cases. *American Journal of Public Health* 80:871–873.

Johnson, R.E., and E.E. Specht (1981). The risk of hip fracture in postmenopausal females with and without estrogen drug exposure. *American Journal of Public Health* 71:138–144.

Kraus, J.F., C.E. Franti, R.S. Riggins, D. Richards, and N.O. Borhani (1975). Incidence of traumatic spinal cord lesions. *Journal of Chronic Diseases* 28:471–492.

Kraus, J.F., M.A. Black, N. Hessol, P. Ley, W. Rokaw, C. Sullivan, S. Bowers, S. Knowlton, and L. Marshall (1984). The incidence of acute brain injury and serious impairment in a defined population. *American Journal of Epidemiology* 119:186–201.

Li, G., and S.P. Baker (1991). A comparison of injury death rates in China and the United States, 1986. *American Journal of Public Health*, 81:605–609.

Merrild, U., and S. Bak (1983). An excess of pedestrian injuries in icy conditions: A high-risk fracture group—elderly women. *Accident Analysis and Prevention* 15:41–48.

Mohan, D., B.M. Bowman, R.G. Snyder, and D.R. Foust (1979). A biomechanical analysis of head impact injuries to children. *Journal of Biomechanical Engineering* 101:250–260.

Myers, A.H., S.P. Baker, E.G. Robinson, and K. Collins (1991). Hip fractures among the elderly: Factors associated with mortality in 27,370 hospitalizations. Baltimore, MD: Johns Hopkins Injury Prevention Center.

Rice, D.P., E.J. MacKenzie, and associates (1989). *Cost of injury in the United States: A report to Congress.* San Francisco: Institute for Health and Aging, University of California and Injury Prevention Center, The Johns Hopkins University.

Snyder, R.G. (1963). Human tolerance to extreme impacts in free-fall. *Aerospace Medicine* 34:695–709.

Sorock, G.S. (1988). Falls among the elderly: Epidemiology and prevention. *American Journal of Preventive Medicine* 4:282–288.

Spiegel, C.N., and F.C. Lindaman (1977). Children can't fly: A program to prevent childhood morbidity and mortality from window falls. *American Journal of Public Health* 67:1143–1147.

Tinetti, M.E., and M. Speechley (1989). Prevention of falls among the elderly. *New England Journal of Medicine* 320:1055–1059.

Trotter, M., G.E. Broman, and R.R. Peterson (1960). Densities of bones of white and Negro skeletons. *Journal of Bone and Joint Surgery* 42A:50–58.

11

Firearms

Firearm deaths are usually analyzed separately as unintentional, suicidal, or homicidal. Often, however, it is appropriate to consider them as a whole in order to clarify the magnitude of the problem and to identify preventive measures that may be effective regardless of the intent and circumstances of injury (Christoffel 1985; Wintemute et al. 1987). This chapter presents data for unintentional firearm injury and for firearm deaths as a whole; in addition, some of the similarities and differences between rates of intentional and unintentional firearm deaths will be pointed out. Additional details on firearm suicide can be found in Chapter 5 and on homicide in Chapter 6.

Firearms are the eighth leading cause of death in the United States and the leading cause for black males aged 15–34. The 17,000 firearm deaths in 1988 among Americans aged 1–34 represented 15 percent of deaths from all causes in that age group (Fingerhut et al. 1991).

Firearms account for one-fifth of all injury deaths and are second only to motor vehicles as a cause of fatal injury. In 1988, shootings caused 34,000 deaths (Table 11-1). Among all causes of fatal unintentional injuries at ages 10–19, shootings are surpassed only by motor vehicles and drowning. Three out of five homicides and suicides are caused by firearms, as are almost all deaths from legal intervention (see Chapter 6). Also an important source of work-related fatalities, firearms are an especially serious hazard to law enforcement agents as well as taxi drivers, storekeepers, and others whose jobs make them likely targets for armed robberies (Baker et al. 1982).

It is estimated that there were 236,000 nonfatal firearm injuries in 1985 of which 65,000 resulted in hospitalization, with a lifetime cost exceeding

Table 11-1. Firearm Deaths as a Percentage of All Injury Deaths, by Intent, 1988

Intent	Firearm Deaths	All Injury Deaths	Percent Firearm
Unintentional	1,501	97,100	2
Suicide	18,181	30,407	60
Homicide	13,666	21,784	63
Legal intervention	232	248	94
Undetermined and other	443	3,033	15
Total	34,023	152,572	22

$14 billion (Rice et al. 1989). A population-based study in northern California found that only motor vehicle crashes and falls surpassed shootings as a cause of spinal cord injury (Kraus et al. 1975). Reflecting the severity of firearm-related injury, the death rate among patients hospitalized because of head injuries is many times higher for gunshot wounds than for any other type of injury (Jagger et al. 1984).

AGE AND SEX

The death rate from unintentional shootings is highest for males aged 14–18 (Figure 4-5). Among females, the highest rates are seen at ages 19–23. For all ages combined, the male death rate is 6.5 times the female rate. For homicide and suicide by firearm, the male to female ratios are 4.8 to 1 and 5.7 to 1, respectively (Figure 3-4).

For all firearm deaths combined, regardless of intent, death rates are highest for ages 20–29. The relative contribution of suicide, homicide, and

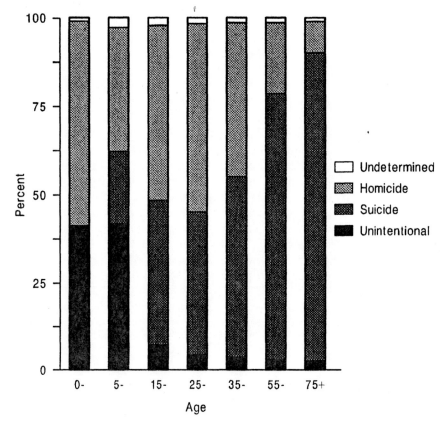

Figure 11-1.   Percentage of All Firearm Injury Deaths by Intent and Age, 1980–1986

unintentional shooting varies dramatically with age; suicide is the most important above age 45 and homicide the most important for younger age groups except ages 5–14, among whom unintentional firearm injury is most prominent (Figure 11-1). The absolute number of firearm deaths is substantial at all ages except during early childhood. In 1986, for example, 1,300 children and teenagers aged 10–19 used guns to commit suicide (Webster 1991).

RACE AND PER CAPITA INCOME

Death rates from unintentional shootings are highest among Native Americans: 2.3 per 100,000, compared with 0.9 per 100,000 for blacks, 0.7 per 100,00 for whites, and 0.2 per 100,000 for Asians. The rate peaks among whites in the 15–19-year age group, whereas among blacks the rate is highest for ages 20–34, and in Native Americans the rate is extremely high at ages 20–29 (Figure 11-2).

When all firearm injuries are combined without regard to intent, the rates are highest among blacks (Figure 11-3). Exceptions are the higher rates

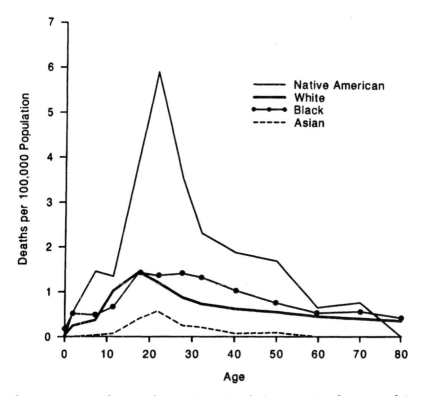

Figure 11-2.   Death Rates from Unintentional Firearm Injury by Age and Race, 1980–1986

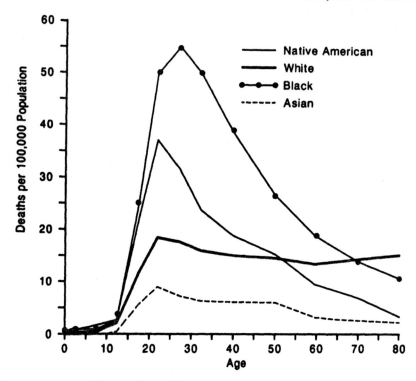

Figure 11-3.   Death Rates from All Firearm Injury by Age and Race, 1980–1986

for Native Americans at ages 5–14, because of high death rates from unintentional shootings, and for whites aged 65 and older, because of high firearm suicide rates.

For each major category of firearm fatality, death rates vary inversely with the per capita income of the area of residence (Figure 11-4). Rates from unintentional shootings in low income areas are almost identical among whites and blacks. Among whites, the rate for unintentional firearm deaths is about 10 times as high in areas of low per capita income as in high-income areas (Baker et al. 1984). For the population as a whole, the association between high death rates and low per capita income is extremely strong, with a rate seven times as high in low-income as in high-income areas. In very rural areas, however, the death rate is highest for high-income counties, many of which are in Alaska.

For firearm suicide, the rate is twice as high in low-income as in high-income areas, and for firearm homicide there is a threefold difference with income (Figure 11-4).

URBAN/RURAL AND GEOGRAPHIC DIFFERENCES

The death rate in remote rural areas from unintentional shootings is four times the rate in central cities (Figure 11-5). For firearm suicide, the rate is

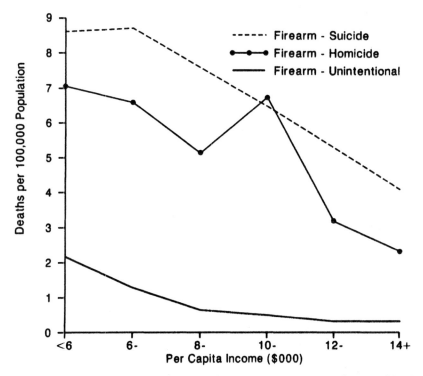

Figure 11-4. Death Rates from Firearms by Per Capita Income of Area of Residence for Unintentional Injury, Suicide, and Homicide, 1980–1986

one and a half times as high in rural areas; however, for homicide the rate in central cities is more than twice the rate in other areas. Consistent with the high death rates from unintentional shootings in rural areas, the regions with the highest rates are generally the northern mountain and southern states (Figure 11-6). This pattern generally resembles the geographic pattern for firearm suicides (Figure 5-7). Death rates from firearm homicide are also high in the South but relatively low in some of the northern mountain states (Figure 6-8), where death rates from unintentional shootings are high. In 1987, the proportion of respondents who reported having one or more guns in the home was 55 percent in the South, 47 percent in the West, 46 percent in the Midwest, and 31 percent in the Northeast (Flanagan and Maguire 1987).

SEASON AND TYPE OF WEAPON

Unintentional firearm deaths exhibit a pronounced seasonal pattern, with almost one-fourth occurring in November and December, the primary hunting season in most areas (Figure 4-15). Unfortunately, ICD codes do not distinguish deaths that occur in connection with hunting.

The best information on the type of weapon involved in homicides

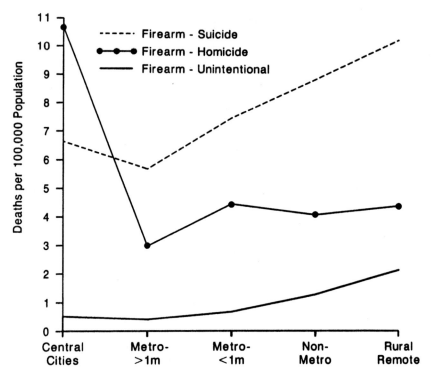

Figure 11-5.   Death Rates from Firearms by Place of Residence for Unintentional
Injury, Suicide, and Homicide, 1980–1986

comes from police investigations. According to the Federal Bureau of Investigation (FBI), 75 percent of firearm homicides are by handguns (Figure 11-7; FBI 1989). Comparable police data are not available for suicides and unintentional shootings, but local studies suggest that handguns are involved in about two-thirds of firearm suicides (Stone 1987; Wintemute et al. 1988).

The specific type of firearm is not recorded on the death certificate in four out of five firearm homicides and two out of three firearm suicides and unintentional shootings. A bias toward recording long guns, but leaving the weapon unspecified in the case of handguns, is suggested by the fact that among the relatively few firearms specified on homicide death certificates, the number of shotguns exceeds the number of handguns even though the more complete FBI data show that three-fourths of homicides are by handguns. The discrepancy indicates that currently available national death certificate data should not be used to estimate the contribution of specific types of weapons to deaths from firearms.

HISTORICAL TRENDS

From 1930 to 1986, the death rate from unintentional firearm injury decreased by almost three-fourths. Firearm suicide and homicide rates de-

a. Firearm - Unintentional

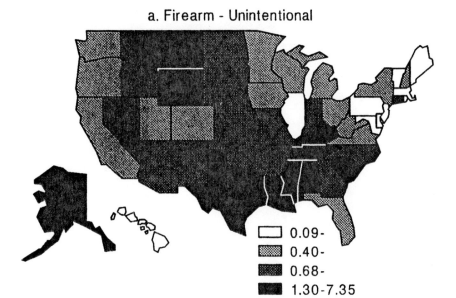

0.09-
0.40-
0.68-
1.30-7.35

b. Firearm - Legal Intervention

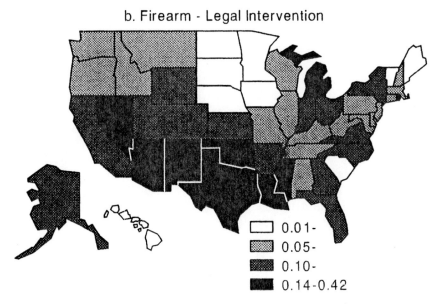

0.01-
0.05-
0.10-
0.14-0.42

Figure 11-6.   Death rates from Unintentional Firearm Injury and Legal Intervention by State, per 100,000 Population, 1980–1986

creased substantially during World War II and then increased, so there was little net change (Figures 5-8 and 6-9). During the 1960s, a substantial increase in firearms produced in the United States was paralleled by increases in firearm homicide and suicide. From 1946 to 1985, there was a high correlation (with coefficients exceeding 0.91) between the number of

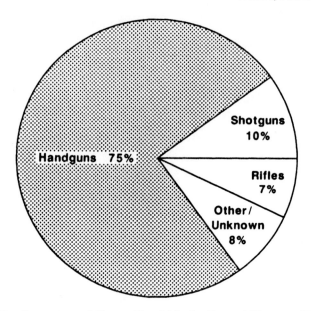

Figure 11-7.   Percentage of Fiream Homicides by Type of Weapon, 1988 (*Source:* Federal Bureau of Investigation, 1989.)

domestically produced handguns and both homicide and suicide by firearm (Wintemute 1988).

Unintentional firearm death rates declined by 21 percent for the period 1984–1986 compared with 1977–1979, with a larger decrease among children (Figure 11-8). For the same period, death rates from firearm suicides increased by 6 percent overall; the largest increases occurred for young adolescents (a 60 percent jump) and the elderly. For firearm homicides, there was a 15 percent decrease overall, with rates declining for all ages except 0–4 and 10–14. Recent FBI data indicate that for all ages combined there was a 9 percent increase in firearm homicides from 1987 to 1988.

The decline in unintentional shooting deaths over the past half-century has been greater than the decrease for unintentional injury deaths as a whole, 74 percent versus 45 percent. This may reflect increasing urbanization and general improvements in the economic status of the population. The very high rural to urban ratio of death rates from firearms and the exceptionally strong correlation with low per capita income are consistent with such speculation. In addition, improved classification of firearm suicides has probably contributed to a decrease in deaths previously classified as unintentional.

For all firearm deaths combined, the rate doubled between the late 1950s and the early 1970s. One of the most striking changes in recent decades has been the emergence of teenagers and young adults as a high-risk group (Wintemute 1987). Between 1984 and 1988, the firearm death rate for black males aged 15–19 more than doubled, to 80 per 100,000—2.8 times their rate for all natural causes of death (Fingerhut et al, 1991).

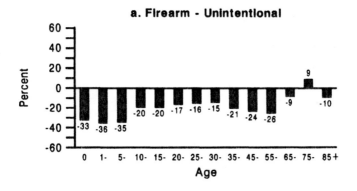

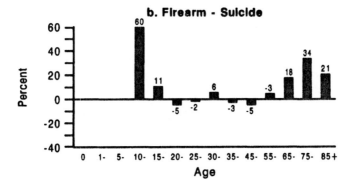

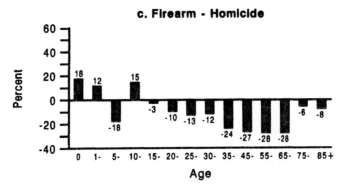

Figure 11-8. Percentage Change in Death Rates from Firearms by Age for Unintentional Injury, Suicide, and Homicide, 1984–1986 Compared with 1977–1979

PREVENTIVE MEASURES

Many firearm injuries and deaths, intentional as well as unintentional, may be prevented through application of a broad spectrum of approaches. Educational efforts emphasizing safer use of firearms have not led to a significant reduction in deaths (AMA Council on Scientific Affairs 1989); however, a better understanding of this complex problem on the part of decision makers (legislators, educators, the media, etc.) is essential if it is to be reduced and better protection of the public is to be provided.

Potentially effective measures include reducing availability of weapons and ammunition through limitations on production or importation. Efforts to keep guns from young children and to prevent handgun possession by criminals are likely to have only limited success if widespread ownership by the general public is permitted. The common tendency to focus on gun purchases by potential criminals ignores the difficulty of regulating the sale and distribution of a widely available commodity, as well as the facts that most homicides are committed by relatives and acquaintances and that suicides are not related to criminal activity. Although home protection is the major reason given for handgun ownership, one study found that for every case in which a person was killed by a handgun in the home as an act of self-protection, handguns were used in the home for 1.3 fatal unintentional shootings, 5 homicides, and 37 suicides (Kellermann and Reay 1986).

The motives and circumstances of many shootings suggest possible benefit from altering the incentives (e.g., placing cash where it will be unavailable to robbers) and disincentives (e.g., brightly illuminating convenience stores and other likely targets). Other preventive possibilities include providing high-risk employees with bullet-proof barriers or clothing and altering the characteristics of ammunition and weapons (Baker and Dietz 1979; Baker et al. 1980; Robertson 1983; Teret and Wintemute 1983). An example of needed weapon alteration is making guns more difficult for young children to fire. Shootings by children cause almost two-thirds of all unintentional firearm deaths of California children (Wintemute et al. 1987).

The type of firearm involved in shooting deaths is relevant to injury-prevention policy. Handguns are readily concealed, a characteristic that makes them easier to use to kill people intentionally but is not essential to their usefulness in target practice, hunting, or even home protection. It was noted earlier that the trend over time in homicides has been largely determined by firearm homicides (Figure 6-9). In fact, the shape of the homicide curve since about 1970 has been dictated by *handgun* homicides alone, with relatively little change in death rates from rifles and shotguns (Teret and Wintemute 1983). Between 1973 and 1987, while reported ownership (i.e., having a gun in the home) of all types of firearms decreased slightly, reported handgun ownership increased by 25 percent (Flanagan and Maguire 1987). Handgun ownership in male nonurban adolescents has been found to be three times as common among school dropouts as among enrollees (Sadowski et al. 1989). Because some handguns have virtually no legitimate utility, the Maryland legislature recently gave a specially designated handgun board the authority to identify the handguns that cannot legally be sold in Maryland (Teret, Alexander, and Bailey 1990).

For suicide, handguns appear to be used more commonly than would be expected based on their proportion of total firearms available. In California, handguns were used for 69 percent of firearm suicides, although only 35 percent of the firearms owned by households in the region were reported to be handguns (Wintemute et al. 1988).

BB guns and other nonpowder firearms that use compressed air to propel projectiles are the source of more than 20,000 injuries each year. Children predominate among those injured. These products are not regulated by any federal product safety standards. About a dozen states restrict the sale or use of nonpowder firearms, for example, by prohibiting sales to minors (Christoffel and Christoffel 1987).

REFERENCES

American Medical Association Council on Scientific Affairs (1989). Firearms injuries and deaths: A critical public health issue. *Public Health Reports* 104: 111–120.

Baker, S.P., and P.E. Dietz (1979). The epidemiology and prevention of injuries. In G.D. Zuidema, R.B. Rutherford, and W.G. Ballinger II (Eds.), *The Management of trauma*. Philadelphia: Saunders.

Baker, S.P., B. O'Neill, and R. Karpf (1984). *The injury fact book*. Lexington, MA: Lexington Books.

Baker, S.P., S.P. Teret, and P.E. Dietz (1980). Firearms and the public health. *Journal of Public Health Policy* 1:224–229.

Baker, S.P., J.S. Samkoff, R.S. Fisher, and C.B. Van Buren (1982). Fatal occupational injuries. *Journal of the American Medical Association* 248:692–697.

Christoffel, K.K. (1985). American as apple pie: Guns in the lives of U.S. children and youth. *Pediatrician* 12:46–51

Christoffel, T., and K. Christoffel (1987). Nonpowder firearm injuries: Whose job is it to protect children? *American Journal of Public Health* 77:735–738.

Federal Bureau of Investigation (1989). *Uniform crime reports for 1988*. Washington, DC: U.S. Government Printing Office.

Fingerhut, L.A., J.C. Kleinman, E. Godfrey, and H. Rosenberg (1991). Firearm mortality among children, youth, and young adults 1–34 years of age, trends and current status: United States, 1979–88. *Monthly Vital Statistics Report* 39(11 Supp):1–14.

Flanagan, T.J., and K. Maguire (Eds.) (1987). *Sourcebook of criminal justice statistics*. Washington, DC: U.S. Department of Justice, Bureau of Justice Statistics.

Jagger, J., J.I. Levine, J.A. Jane, and R.W. Rimel (1984). Epidemiologic features of head injury in a predominately rural population. *Journal of Trauma* 24:40–44.

Kellermann, A.L., and D.T. Reay (1986). Protection or peril? An analysis of firearm-related deaths in the home. *New England Journal of Medicine* 314:1557–1560.

Kraus, J.F., C.E. Franti, R.S. Riggins, D. Richards, and N.O. Borhani (1975). Incidence of traumatic spinal cord lesions. *Journal of Chronic Diseases* 28:471–492.

Rice, D.P., E.J. MacKenzie, and associates. (1989). *Cost of injury in the United States: A report to Congress*. San Francisco: Institute for Health and Aging, University of California and Injury Prevention Center, The Johns Hopkins University.

Robertson, L.S. (1983). *Injuries: Causes, control strategies, and public policy*. Lexington, MA: Lexington Books.

Sadowski, L.S., R.B. Cairns, and J.A. Earp (1989). Firearm ownership among nonurban adolescents. *American Journal of Diseases of Children* 143:1410–1413.

Stone, I.C., Jr. (1987). Observations and statistics relating to suicide weapons. *Journal of Forensic Sciences* 32:711–716.

Teret, S.P., and G.J. Wintemute (1983). Handgun injuries: The epidemiologic evidence for assessing legal responsibility. *Hamline Law Review* 6:341–350.

Teret, S.P., G.R. Alexander, and L.A. Bailey (1990). The passage of Maryland's gun law: Data and advocacy for injury prevention. *Journal of Public Health Policy* 11:26–38.

Webster, D.W. (1991). Determinants of pediatricians' firearm injury prevention counseling practices. Baltimore, MD: The Johns Hopkins University.

Wintemute, G.J. (1987). Firearms as a cause of death in the United States, 1920–1982. *Journal of Trauma* 27:532–536.

Wintemute, G.J. (1988). Handgun availability and firearm mortality. *Lancet* II:1136–1137.

Wintemute, G.J., S.P. Teret, and J.F. Kraus (1987). The epidemiology of firearm deaths among residents of California. *Western Journal of Medicine* 146:374–377.

Wintemute, G.J., S.P. Teret, J.F. Kraus, and M.W. Wright (1988). The choice of weapons in firearm suicides. *American Journal of Public Health* 78:824–826.

Wintemute, G.J., S.P. Teret, J.F. Kraus, M.A. Wright, and G. Bradfield (1987). When children shoot children: 88 unintended deaths in California. *Journal of the American Medical Association* 257:3107–3109.

12

Fires, Burns, and Lightning

Burns and fires are surpassed only by motor vehicle crashes, falls and drownings as a cause of unintentional injury death. In recent years, they have caused about 5,000 deaths annually. This figure does not include deaths related to arson or suspicious circumstances, estimated at about 300 annually, and about 150 burn deaths of suicidal intent (Table 12-1). Deaths associated with postcrash fires are counted among deaths from motor vehicle and airplane crashes.

Burns and fires result in 1.4 million injuries each year. Of these, more than 54,000 are admitted to hospitals. The lifetime cost of all fire and burn injuries sustained in 1985 was estimated at $3.8 billion (Rice et al. 1989). For severely burned patients such as those who need skin grafting, lengthy hospitalizations and multiple admissions are often necessary. Disability, disfigurement, and emotional problems are common sequelae.

Burns are usually caused by thermal energy. They may also result from exposure to chemicals, electricity, ultraviolet radiation, and ionizing radia-

Table 12-1. Causes of Fire and Burn Deaths, 1988

Cause	Number	Percentage of Total
Housefire (conflagration)	4,088	72.7
Conflagration, other building	118	2.1
Other uncontrolled fire	74	1.3
Controlled fire	54	1.0
Ignition of clothing	205	3.7
Ignition of highly flammable material	75	1.3
Hot liquid or steam	98	1.7
Suicide	155	2.8
Arson	277	4.9
Undetermined intent	124	2.2
Other or unspecified fire or hot substance	353	6.3
Total	5,621	100.0

tion. This chapter focuses on thermal energy burns, which occur when heat reaches the body in amounts or at rates that exceed the body's ability to dissipate the heat. Included among deaths attributed to fires are those resulting from exposure to the toxic byproducts of combustion. In housefires and other conflagrations, the great majority of deaths are actually due to carbon monoxide poisoning. In 1988, of all deaths from fires in private dwellings, 76 percent were attributed to smoke and fumes, 20 percent to burns, and 4 percent to falls, building collapse, or unspecified causes.

HOUSEFIRES

Among deaths from fires and burns, housefires cause 73 percent of all deaths and 80 percent of unintentional deaths (Table 12-1). Death rates are highest among young children and the elderly (Figure 12-1), in part because of their difficulty in escaping from burning buildings. In addition, children and the elderly have higher case-fatality rates than people of intermediate ages with burn injuries of comparable extent and severity (Bull 1971). However, the relationship between age and ability to survive injury is less important for housefires than for other burns, because housefire deaths usually involve either carbon monoxide poisoning or incineration, a lethal event at any age.

The male to female ratio for housefire deaths is 1.6 to 1, less than for most injury deaths (Figure 3-4). Among children, the greatest sex difference is at ages 2–4 (Figure 4-6); boys at these ages also have the highest rates for nonfatal burns from playing with matches (CPSC 1976). About 10 percent of residential fire deaths are attributed to children playing with matches, cigarette lighters, or other ignition sources (U. S. Fire Administration, no date).

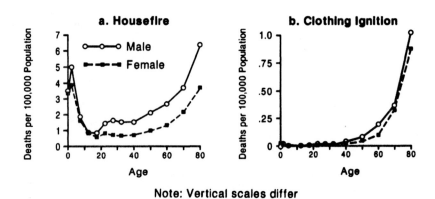

Figure 12-1.   Death Rates from Housefires and Clothing Ignition by Age and Sex, 1980–1986

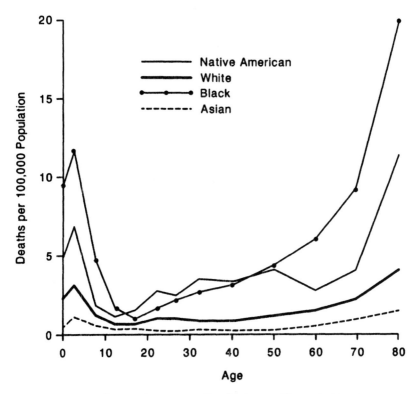

Figure 12-2. Death Rates from Housefires by Age and Race, 1980–1986

Cigarettes, cited in 28 percent of the deaths, are the leading cause of fatal housefires, which are often started by smoldering cigarettes that ignite upholstered furniture or mattresses (Birky et al. 1979; McLoughlin and McGuire 1990). Other major causes are heating equipment (15 percent) and arson or suspicious fires (16 percent) (U. S. Fire Administration, no date).

Among both blacks and Native Americans, housefire death rates are more than twice the rate for whites. In these groups, the rates are high among young children and also increase throughout the adult years (Figure 12-2). The racial differences in housefire death rates diminish in higher-income areas (Baker et al. 1984; Mierley and Baker 1983).

For all races combined, housefire death rates are almost five times as high in areas of low per capita income as in high-income areas (Figure 4-10). Ignition sources vary with income. A Baltimore study found that although cigarettes were the primary ignition source at all income levels, the proportion of fires ignited by faulty heating or electrical systems was greatest in low-income areas (Mierley and Baker 1983).

Housefire death rates for whites show little variation with place of residence; however, for blacks the rates are about twice as high in rural areas as in other areas. These urban-rural differences probably reflect not only economic disparities but also differences in housing materials and heating

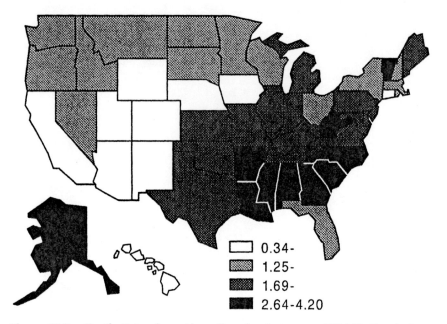

Figure 12-3. Death Rates from Housefires by State, per 100,000 Population, 1980–1986

methods, the likelihood of fires being detected, and, especially in remote areas, the availability and response time of fire equipment.

There is a pronounced geographic pattern in housefire deaths, with high death rates in the East, especially the Southeast, and low rates in the western half of the United States (Figure 12-3). These geographic patterns are generally similar for all racial groups. Although the high death rate in the southeastern states has not been thoroughly researched, kerosene heaters and other noncentral heating equipment may be a more common ignition source in fatal fires in these states than in the rest of the United States. The availability and use of wood for building materials and fuel also probably plays a role in regional differences.

The majority of housefire deaths occur during December through March, when the weather is cold, the hours of darkness long, and heating and lighting systems most utilized. Deaths are three times as common in January as in July (Figure 4-15). Weekends are disproportionately represented (Figure 4-14), which is consistent with evidence of high blood alcohol concentrations in about half the adults who die in housefires (Halpin et al. 1977; Mierley and Baker 1983). Fires ignited by cigarettes are more likely than other fires to involve alcohol (Howland and Hingson 1987). The association between cigarettes and alcohol use is important because intoxication increases the likelihood that a lighted cigarette will fall unnoticed onto a chair or bed and remain undetected. After smoldering, often for several hours, fire may erupt and spread very rapidly. Typically, deaths from cigarette-initiated housefires occur between midnight and 6:00 A.M.

Injuries from housefires and other conflagrations, although the major cause of fire- or burn-related death, account for only a small fraction of hospital admissions for burns—about 4 percent of all burn admissions in New York State (Feck et al. 1979). The fatality rate among patients hospitalized for burns from conflagrations is higher than for burns from other causes; almost 12 percent of patients admitted with burns from conflagrations died during their first hospitalization compared with 3 percent of other burn patients (Table 12-2). Because deaths prior to admission are often not included, the true ratio of deaths to admissions for housefires would be many times greater.

Compared with 1977–1979, the housefire death rate for 1984–1986 decreased by 19 percent. From 1930 to 1980, there had been a 32 percent increase in the housefire death rate in the United States, but the rate from burns from other causes had decreased by more than 85 percent (Figure 12-4). A major factor in the difference between the two trends may have been advances in the medical care of burned patients; most deaths related to housefires occur before medical treatment can be given, while deaths from other burns generally occur days or weeks later. In addition, there may have been greater reductions in the incidence of clothing ignitions than of housefires because of the standard for flame-retardant children's sleepwear and other changes in clothing and ignition sources (McLoughlin et al. 1977; Young and Baker 1978).

Further improvement in housefire death and injury rates would result from reducing the ignition potential of cigarettes and other important ignition sources such as heating and electrical equipment in low-income housing. Cigarettes are especially important because not only are they the most common ignition source in fatal housefires, they are also the ignition source

Table 12-2. Leading Causes of Hospital Admissions for Burns, New York State, 1974–1975

Cause	Number of First Admissions	Percentage of Total	Deaths per 100 Admissions
Hot liquids	1,654	29	1.2
Clothing ignition	583	10	10.6
Gasoline	367	6	2.7
Automotive	354	6	0.6
Chemicals	342	6	1.5
Grease	305	5	0.3
Conflagrations	213	4	11.7
Stoves	192	3	2.6
Other	1,781	31	2.6
Total	5,791	100	3.0

Source: G.A. Feck, M.S. Baptiste, and C.L. Tate, Jr., *An epidemiologic study of burn injuries and strategies for prevention.* Atlanta, GA: U.S. Department of Health and Human Services, Public Health Service, Centers for Disease Control, 1978.

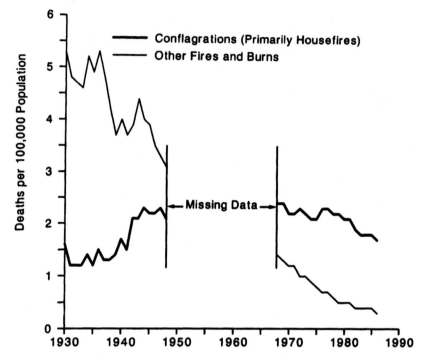

Figure 12-4. Death Rates from Conflagrations and from Other Fires and Burns by Year, 1930–1986

in 44 percent of fires from ignited bedding and 68 percent of fires that begin in upholstered furniture (CPSC 1980). Most brands of cigarettes can smolder and ignite furniture and bedding. However, experimental cigarettes produced by cigarette manufacturers and tested by the federal government are significantly less apt to ignite fires (McLoughlin and McGuire 1990; Technical Study Group 1987).

Much can be done to reduce the flammability of materials and the toxicity of their combustion products. Also important are building designs that inhibit the spread of fires and provide adequate escape routes. The value of smoke detectors is widely recognized, and they are especially prevalent where required by housing regulations (McLoughlin et al. 1985); however, unless wired to a home's electrical circuit, they often are not in working condition. Five out of six homes in the United States had smoke detectors by 1988, but one-third of the detectors lacked working batteries (Hall 1988).

Sprinkler systems that automatically extinguish fires could reduce deaths in homes as well as those in hotels, offices, airplanes, and other settings. Smoke detectors alone give insufficient protection, in part because the majority of people killed in housefires are elderly or intoxicated or very young and therefore may not be able to escape from a fire. The American Medical Association has recommended legislation that would require the installation of automatic sprinkler systems in all new residential and commercial buildings and in all existing high-rise buildings (AMA Council on Scientific Affairs 1987).

CLOTHING IGNITION

Clothing ignition is the cause of about 200 deaths annually, or about 3 percent of all deaths related to fires and burns. More than three-fourths of these deaths occur among people aged 65 or older. There is little sex difference in clothing ignition deaths, which now are rare among children (Figure 12-1; Young and Baker 1978). Death rates from clothing ignition are extremely low among Asians: 0.01 per 100,000, compared with 0.10 among whites and Native Americans and 0.20 among blacks. The death rate is five times as high in low-income areas as in high-income areas. These findings for fatal burns are consistent with clothing burn injury rates, which one study found to be highest in low-income census tracts (Barancik and Shapiro 1976). The relationship between burn rates and per capita income was most pronounced for clothing burns related to appliances and equipment.

Until the 1960s, clothing-related burns were an important cause of death among young girls, whose nightgowns and bouffant dresses were easily ignited by matches, fires, space heaters, or other sources (Oglesbay 1969). Although clothing ignition deaths were combined with other fire deaths in national statistics until 1968, they were so common among young girls that the death rate from all flame burns and fires (including housefires) was substantially higher for girls than for boys.

Figure 12-5 illustrates the sex difference prior to the mid-1960s in burn death rates of children aged 5–9 and the subsequent changes in the sex ratio. During the 1960s, dresses and nightgowns became less bouffant (thus reducing the ease with which they could be ignited), pants and other tight-fitting clothing became popular among girls and women, the use of some highly flammable materials for clothing decreased, and burn survival rates improved (Bull 1971; Young and Baker 1978). During the same decade, the preponderance of females among total burn deaths disappeared. In 1968, the first year for which national mortality data specific to clothing ignition burns became available, 40 girls and 11 boys aged 5–9 died following ignition of clothing. In 1986 there were no deaths at this age of either boys or girls. In fact, the only deaths before age 20 were in 1- to 4-year-old children, two boys and one girl. For all ages combined, the death rate from clothing ignition was 40 percent lower in 1984–1986 than in 1977–1979.

By 1975, children's sleepwear standards required a flame test for sleepwear sizes 0–6X; by 1975–1978, the proportion of clothing ignitions that involved sleepwear dropped from 55 percent to 27 percent among ages 0–12 but did not change for older age groups (CPSC 1980). Nonfatal burns resulting from clothing ignition are still a matter of concern because they are often severe and potentially disfiguring. Cases admitted to hospitals have a

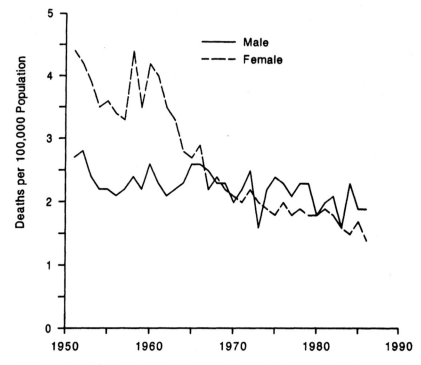

Figure 12-5. Death Rates from All Fires and Burns by Year and Sex, for Ages 5–9, 1951–1986

fatality rate surpassed only by housefires (Table 12-2). Because some fabrics used in clothing may actually melt and stick to the skin, clothing-related burns tend to be deeper and more extensive than nonfatal burns from many other sources (Barancik and Shapiro 1976).

SCALDS AND OTHER BURNS

Burns other than those from housefires are associated with extensive morbidity. In Massachusetts, the average hospital stay was 29 days for ages 65 and over and 12 days for other patients (Rossignol et al. 1985). Although the elderly did not have a higher incidence of burns, their death rates were high, reflecting high case-fatality rates (six times the rate for younger patients).

Burns from scalds and other contacts with hot substances result in about 100 deaths each year. More than 80 percent are caused by hot liquids or steam. Caustic or corrosive substances and hot objects cause the remainder. Deaths from scalds are uncommon between ages 5 and 64. Death rates and rates of hospitalized burn injuries are three times as high for blacks as for whites (Rossignol 1986a).

Although the case-fatality rate is low, scalds are a major source of burn morbidity and associated costs. Scalds from hot liquids caused 29 percent of all hospital admissions for burns in New York State (Table 12-2). Children aged 0–4 accounted for 45 percent of all admissions for hot liquid scalds in New York State (Baptiste and Feck 1980). Hot beverages, notably coffee, are a major cause of scalds to young children. For all ages combined, hot water, including tap water in bathtubs and showers, is the leading cause of scalds and of all hospital admissions for burns. Based on NEISS data, an estimated 3,500 people with scald burns from showers and bathtubs received emergency treatment in 1988; one-fourth were admitted to the hospital, and more than two-thirds were children less than five years old.

The relative importance of various burn sources changes with age. Hot liquids are the most important cause of hospitalized burns among children and the elderly. Clothing ignition is the second leading cause of burns resulting in hospital admission. In the 15- to 24-year-old age group, the largest numbers of burn admissions in New York State were related to automobiles. Crashes caused more than one-fourth of such burns. Steam from radiators was also a frequent cause. The low ratio of deaths to injuries shown in Table 12-2 for automotive burns is partly because most deaths from postcrash fires occur at the scene of the fire; these and other cases that did not involve hospitalization were not included in the study (Feck et al. 1978).

Work-related burns cause more than 100 deaths annually (Chapter 9) and account for 60 percent of hospitalized burn injuries among employed males in Massachusetts (Rossignol et al. 1986b). In the 15–24-year-old age group in Ohio, the majority of hospital-treated burns occur on the job; this age group has the highest rate of occupational burns, which occur primarily in eating places (Chatterjee et al. 1986).

Substantial decreases have occurred in deaths from scalds and other burns by hot substances. From 1968 to 1979, death rates from scalds decreased by about three-fourths for ages 0–19 and by almost half for all ages combined. By 1984–1986, the death rate was only 0.07 per 100,000 compared with 0.09 in 1977–1979.

Probably the greatest potential for preventing tap water scalds lies in modifying hot water systems either by adjusting temperature settings on the heater or by installing mixing valves or temperature-sensitive valves at the faucet. A Wisconsin program that included distribution of thermometers resulted in lowered temperatures in about 20,000 water heaters (Katcher 1987). It is not uncommon for the temperature of tap water in homes and public buildings to be 160° F (71° C) or more, although first degree burns can result from about 30 seconds of exposure to water above 130° F (54° C) (Moritz and Henriques 1947). More severe burns result from longer exposures or from higher temperatures. Consequently, all water heaters and systems should be designed or modified so that water is not discharged at temperatures above 120° F. This is especially important in bathtubs and showers, where large areas of the skin are exposed to water (Baptiste and Feck 1980; Feck et al. 1978, 1979; Feck and Baptiste 1979).

NEISS estimates of hospital-treated injuries in 1986 included 17,800 from gasoline and 12,600 from fireworks. Firecrackers, bottle rockets, and sparklers cause the greatest numbers of hospitalized injuries from fireworks (Berger et al. 1985). States in which a wide variety of fireworks can legally be sold had a sevenfold risk of injuries when compared with states that strictly limit the availability of fireworks.

Burns associated with gasoline are a serious problem in young boys. At one burn center, 62 percent of admissions of children aged 10–15 involved gasoline. These burns, deeper and more extensive than most other burns treated at the center, typically resulted from gasoline being thrown on a fire or ignited by a match (Cole et al. 1986).

LIGHTNING

Lightning kills about 80 people each year in the United States, more than the average annual number of deaths attributable to all types of natural disasters. As with other injury-producing events, being struck by lightning is most common in certain high-risk groups. The rate of deaths from lightning is highest at ages 10–19, and it is seven times as high among males as females (Figure 12-6). Death rates are highest in southern and mountain states (Figure 12-7). There have been no deaths in Alaska for at least 30 years, and

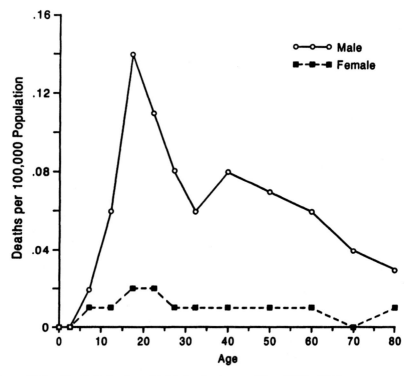

Figure 12-6.   Death Rates from Lightning by Age and Sex, 1980–1986

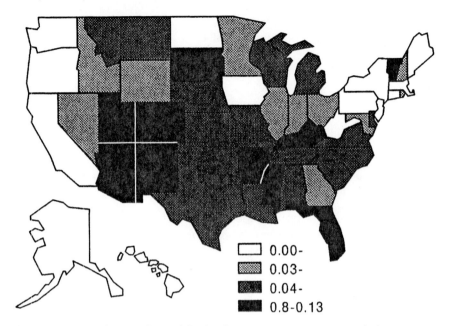

Figure 12-7   Death Rates from Lightning by State, per 100,000 Population, 1980–1986

rates are very low in other Pacific states (Duclos and Sanderson 1990). Because of small numbers of cases, state-specific rates are unstable. Wyoming, for example, had one of the three highest rates for the entire period 1968–1985 (Duclos and Sanderson 1990) but was near the national average for 1980–1986.

Deaths are most common during the summer, when people are likely to be outdoors and thunderstorms are most common. Seventy-one percent of all deaths occur in June, July, and August (Figure 4-15). Most involve people who are in open fields or on the water and/or are touching metal equipment, such as antennae. Between one-fifth and one-third of fatal lightning strikes involve a worker, typically at a farm, construction site, or other outdoor workplace (Duclos and Sanderson 1990). One death in six is related to recreation; such deaths are apt to involve golfers, fishermen, and campers (Weigel 1976).

During the past 50 years, the death rate from lightning has shown one of the largest decreases of all injuries (see Table 4-2). While part of the reported decrease is because deaths from fires ignited by lightning are no longer included with lightning deaths, the number of all lightning-related deaths is now small. Probably much of the decrease reflects improvements in electrical systems and decreases in the farm population. Between 1979 and 1986, the proportion of lightning deaths that occurred on farms decreased from 17 percent to 9 percent. Respiratory arrest subsequent to a lightning strike can often be reversed by cardiopulmonary resuscitation; it is possible that improved emergency response and knowledge of CPR has contributed to the reduction in the death rate.

REFERENCES

American Medical Association Council on Scientific Affairs (1987). Preventing death and injury from fires with automatic sprinklers and smoke detectors. *Journal of the American Medical Association* 257:1618-1620.

Baker, S.P., B. O'Neill, and R. Karpf (1984). *The injury fact book*. Lexington, MA: Lexington Books.

Baptiste, M.S., and G. Feck (1980). Preventing tap water burns. *American Journal of Public Health* 70:727-729.

Barancik, J.I., and M.A. Shapiro (1976). *Pittsburgh Burn Study. Pittsburgh and Allegheny County, Pennsylvania, 1 June 1970-15 April 1971*. Washington, DC: U.S. Consumer Product Safety Commission.

Berger, L.R., S. Kalishman, and F.P. Rivara (1985). Injuries from fireworks. *Pediatrics* 75:877-882.

Birky, M.M., B.M. Halpin, Y.H. Caplan, R.S. Fisher, J.M. McAllister, and A.M. Dixon (1979). Fire fatality study. *Fire and Materials* 4:211-217.

Bull, J.P. (1971). Revised analysis of mortality due to burns. *Lancet* 2:1133-1134.

Chatterjee, B.F., J.I. Barancik, R.B. Fratianne, R.C. Waltz, and D. Fife (1986). Northeastern Ohio Trauma Study: V. Burn injury. *Journal of Trauma* 26: 844-847.

Cole, M., D.N. Herndon, M.H. Desai, and S. Abston (1986). Gasoline explosions, gasoline sniffing; an epidemic in young adolescents. *Journal of Burn Care Rehabilitation* 7:532-534.

Consumer Product Safety Commission, Bureau of Epidemiology (1976). *Annual report of flammable fabric data, fiscal year 1975*. Washington, DC: U.S. Consumer Product Safety Commission.

Consumer Product Safety Commission (1980). *Eighth annual flammable fabrics report*. Washington, DC: U.S. Consumer Product Safety Commission.

Duclos, P.J., and L.M. Sanderson (1990). An epidemiological description of lightning-related deaths in the United States. *International Journal of Epidemiology* 19:673-678.

Feck, G.A., and M.S. Baptiste (1979). The epidemiology of burn injury in New York. *Public Health Reports* 94:312-318.

Feck, G.A., M.S. Baptiste, and C.L. Tate, Jr. (1978). *An epidemiologic study of burn injuries and strategies for prevention*. Atlanta, GA: U.S. Department of Health and Human Services, Public Health Service, Centers for Disease Control.

Feck, G.A., M.S. Baptiste, and C.L. Tate, Jr. (1979). Burn injuries: Epidemiology and prevention. *Accident Analysis and Prevention* 11:129-136.

Hall, J.R., Jr. (1988). *U.S. experience with smoke detectors*. Quincy, MA: National Fire Protection Association.

Halpin, B.M., J.J. Dinan, and O.J. Deters (1977). *Fire problems program—assessment of the potential impact of fire protection systems on actual fire incidents*. Laurel, MD: The Johns Hopkins University Applied Physics Laboratory.

Howland, J., and R. Hingson (1987). Alcohol as a risk factor for injuries or death due to fires and burns: Review of the literature. *Public Health Reports* 102: 475–483.

Katcher, M.L. (1987). Prevention of tap water scald burns: Evaluation of a multi-media injury control program. *American Journal of Public Health* 77:1195–1197.

McLoughlin, E., and A. McGuire (1990). The causes, cost, and prevention of childhood burn injuries. *American Journal of Diseases of Children* 144:677–683.

McLoughlin, E., N. Clarke, K. Stahl, and J.D. Crawford (1977). One pediatric burn unit's experience with sleepwear-related injuries. *Pediatrics* 60:405–409.

McLoughlin, E., M. Marchone, L. Hanger, P.S. German, and S.P. Baker (1985). Smoke detector legislation: Its effect on owner-occupied homes. *American Journal of Public Health* 75:858–862.

Mierley, M.C., and S.P. Baker (1983). Fatal house fires in an urban population. *Journal of the American Medical Association* 249:1466–1468.

Moritz, A.R., and F.C. Henriques, Jr. (1947). Studies of thermal injury: II. The relative importance of time and surface temperature in the causation of cutaneous burns. *American Journal of Pathology* 23:695–720.

Oglesbay, F. B. (1969). The flammable fabrics problem. *Pediatrics* 44 (Supp.):827–832.

Rice, D.P., E.J. MacKenzie, and associates (1989). *Cost of injury in the United States: A report to Congress.* San Francisco: Institute for Health and Aging, University of California and Injury Prevention Center, The Johns Hopkins University.

Rossignol, A.M., J.A. Locke, C.M. Boyle, and J.F. Burke (1985). Consumer products and hospitalized burn injuries among elderly Massachusetts residents. *Journal of the American Geriatrics Society* 33:768–772.

Rossignol, A.M., C.M. Boyle, J.A. Locke, and J.F. Burke (1986a). Hospitalized burn injuries in Massachusetts: An assessment of incidence and product involvement. *American Journal of Public Health* 76:1341–1343.

Rossignol, A.M., J.A. Locke, C.M. Boyle, and J.F. Burke (1986b). Epidemiology of work-related burn injuries in Massachusetts requiring hospitalization. *Journal of Trauma* 26:1097–1101.

Technical Study Group (October 1987). *Toward a less fireprone cigarette: Final report of the Technical Study Group on Cigarette and Little Cigar Fire Safety.* Gaithersburg, MD: Center for Fire Research.

U.S. Fire Administration (n.d.). *Fire in the United States 1983–1987.* Emmitsburg, MD: U.S. Fire Administration.

Weigel, E.P. (1976). Lightning: The underrated killer. *National Oceanic and Atmospheric Administration Magazine* p. 6.

Young, G.S., and S.P. Baker (1978). Recent trends in childhood burn deaths. Presented at the Annual Meeting of the American Public Health Association, Los Angeles, CA.

13

Drowning

Drowning is the third most common cause of unintentional injury death for all ages and ranks second for ages 5–44. Among Native Americans and Asians, only motor vehicles exceed drownings as a cause of fatal unintentional injury. In 10 states (Alaska, Arizona, California, Florida, Hawaii, Montana, Nevada, Oregon, Utah, and Washington), drowning surpasses all other causes of death in children less than 15 years old (Waller et al. 1989). In addition to the 5,000 drownings annually, there are many cases of extreme, permanent disability resulting from near-drowning. It is estimated that for every 10 children who drown, 36 are admitted to hospitals and 140 are treated in emergency rooms (Wintemute 1990).

Drowning is classified into two major groups. The larger group, numbering about 4,200 deaths in 1988, includes drownings not related to boats. The smaller group, about 1,000 annually, involves boats, primarily small recreational craft. Because drownings related to boats are categorized as "water transport" deaths, they are often excluded from drowning statistics. Although some boating deaths related to water transport are due to falls, burns, crushing, or other mechanisms, 84 percent result from drowning and can be clearly identified in NCHS data.

An additional group of drownings, about 350 each year, is included with motor vehicle-related deaths and not separately identified in NCHS mortality statistics. Suicidal or homicidal drownings and drownings of undetermined intent add another 900 deaths annually to the toll.

National data detailing the circumstances of nonboat drownings are limited. A survey of news reports that identified three-fourths of all nonboat drownings in 1971 indicated that one-fourth were swimmers; four out of five who drowned while swimming were not at designated swimming areas. About one-third, including about 500 children under age 5, were people who fell into water. Drownings from scuba diving, skin diving, and surfing together accounted for less than 2 percent of the total (Metropolitan Life Insurance Company 1977a). A complete census of the 133 Maryland drownings in the same year revealed that although sailing and ocean swimming are common sports in the state, only one person drowned while sailing and one while swimming in the ocean (Dietz and Baker 1974). Lakes and rivers were the most common drowning sites in Maryland and in King

County, Washington (Quan et al. 1989). Circumstances vary geographically as well as by age: In Los Angeles, the most common sites of drowning for young children and the elderly were swimming pools and bathtubs, and for young adults the most common sites were swimming pools and the ocean (O'Carroll et al. 1988). Nationally, about 350 drownings occur annually in bathtubs (Budnick and Ross 1985).

Details on recreational (noncommercial) boating deaths are available from the U.S. Coast Guard (USCG). In 1987, recreational boats were involved in 1,036 fatalities, including some from causes other than drowning. The majority of boats were open motorboats (Table 13-1), and half were less than 16 feet long. Capsizing or falling overboard caused 60 percent of the deaths (Table 13-1). In more than 20 percent of all deaths, the boats had too few personal flotation devices or none at all. In contrast, only 2 percent of all boats involved in incidents reported to the Coast Guard had insufficient personal flotation devices (USCG 1988).

Table 13-1. Recreational Boat Fatalities by Type of Boat and Event, 1987

	Number	Percentage
Type of Boat		
Open motorboat	546	53
Canoe/kayak	78	7
Rowboat	103	10
Sailboat	21	2
Cabin motorboat	84	8
Other	92	9
Unknown	112	11
Total	1,036	100
Event		
Capsizing	361	35
Falling overboard	272	26
Collision		
other vessel	80	8
fixed object	58	5
floating object	17	2
Swamping/flooding/sinking	122	12
Struck by boat or propeller	12	1
Fire/explosion	8	1
Other	45	4
Unknown	61	6
Total	1,036	100

AGE AND SEX

The overall death rate from drowning is highest at ages 1 and 18. For drownings not related to boats, the rate is highest among children aged 1 and 2 (Figure 13-1); this fact is not well known because rates are usually calculated for broader age groups rather than by single year of age. In the 1–4 age group, about 85 percent of drownings in 1977 resulted from falling into water; baths and playing in water accounted for about 5 percent each (Metropolitan Life Insurance Company 1977a). In some geographic areas, the majority of drownings in children 1 to 4 years old occur in home swimming pools (Wintemute 1990). In 1983, an estimated 235 children less than 5 years old drowned in residential pools. Two-thirds were being supervised by one or both parents, and only 30 percent were wearing swimwear (Present 1987).

The male to female ratio of drowning rates is about 14 to 1 for drowning related to boats and 5 to 1 for others. The male drowning rate peaks at age 2, declines until age 10, and then sharply rises to the maximum at age 18 (Figure 13-2). Among females, the death rate is highest at age 1; it then decreases sharply and does not rise again. The contrast between male and

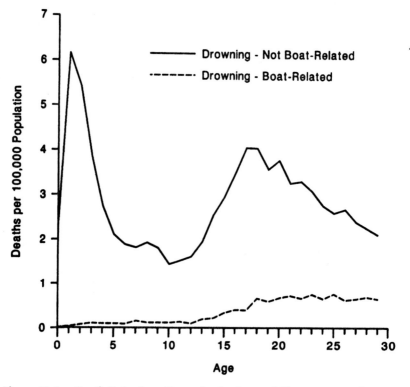

Figure 13-1.   Death Rates from Drowning by Age and Circumstances, for Ages 0–29, 1980–1986

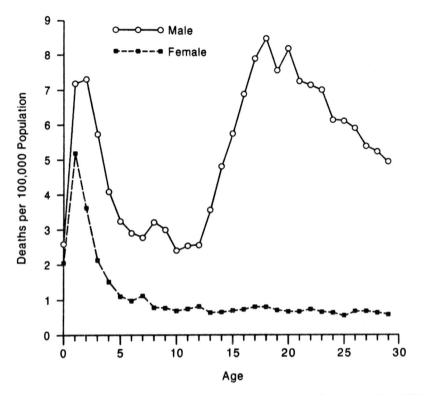

Figure 13-2.   Death Rates from Drowning by Age and Sex, for Ages 0–29, 1980–1986

female drowning rates after age 10 is a striking example of the effect of likely differences between the sexes in exposure, supervision, cultural expectations, biological makeup, and other factors such as alcohol use that influence death rates from potentially hazardous activities.

RACE AND PER CAPITA INCOME

Drowning rates are highest for Native Americans (6.9 per 100,000) and lowest among Asians and whites (2.1 and 2.3 per 100,000, respectively) (Figure 13-3). Some Native Americans who live in areas where swimming is uncommon may have few opportunities to learn to swim. Others may be exposed to occupational risks of drowning or extremely low water temperatures, as in Alaska.

For all ages combined, the drowning rate for blacks (4.2) is almost twice that for whites (2.3). Among children aged 1–4, the pattern is reversed, with that for whites almost twice that for blacks. This difference, which in Maryland is associated with more swimming pool drownings among white

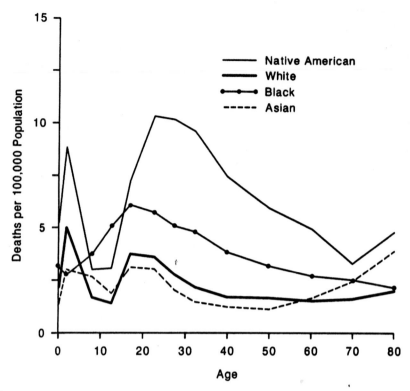

Figure 13-3.   Death Rates from Drowning by Age and Race, 1980–1986

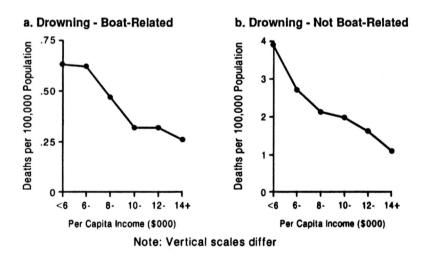

Note: Vertical scales differ

Figure 13-4.   Death Rates from Drowning by Per Capita Income of Area of Residence and Circumstances, 1980–1986

children (Dietz and Baker 1974), is an additional example of the influence of the physical environment on racial differences in injury death rates.

Drowning rates vary inversely with the per capita income of the area of residence, decreasing from 4.5 to 1.4 as the per capita income increases. Similar effects occur for both boat-related and nonboat-related drowning (Figure 13-4). Because pool ownership increases with socioeconomic status (Wintemute 1990), it is likely that this component of drownings increases with income.

URBAN/RURAL AND GEOGRAPHIC DIFFERENCES

Drowning rates are highest among residents of rural areas, especially among blacks. Differences among states and regions reflect many other factors, including climate (Figure 13-5). Rates for drownings that do not involve boats are generally highest in southern and mountain states. Alaska has the highest rate (9.3 per 100,000), which exceeds the rate for motor vehicle-related deaths in Alaska and is more than twice the drowning rate in the next

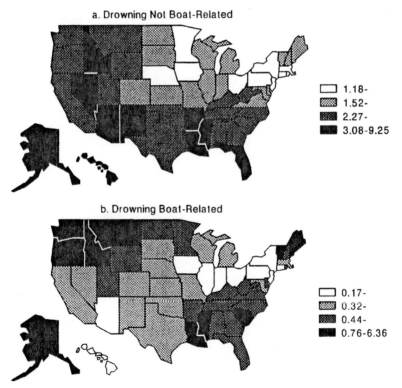

a. Drowning Not Boat-Related

☐ 1.18-
▨ 1.52-
▩ 2.27-
■ 3.08-9.25

b. Drowning Boat-Related

☐ 0.17-
▨ 0.32-
▩ 0.44-
■ 0.76-6.36

Figure 13-5. Death Rates from Drowning by State, per 100,000 Population, 1980–1986

Table 13-2.   Recreational Boat Fatalities by Body
of Water, 1987

Body of Water	Number	Percentage
Lake/pond/reservoir	499	48
River/stream/creek	269	26
Bay/harbor/intercoastal waterway	166	16
Great Lakes	33	3
Ocean/gulf	56	6
Other	2	0
Unknown	11	1
Total	1,036	100

highest state, Louisiana (3.9). A major factor in the extremely high rate in
Alaska is the very low water temperature, which reduces the chance of survival. In warm climates, regional differences may reflect the amount of
swimming in hazardous places and the prevalence of swimming pools. The
latter would especially influence rates among young children, who account
for the majority of drownings in home pools (Metropolitan Life Insurance
Company 1977b).

Drownings involving boats occur most often in lakes and ponds (Table
13-2). The highest rates are in the South and Northwest. Overall, the pattern
is similar to other drownings, except for California and several southwestern
states, which have low rates for drownings involving boats and high rates for
other drownings. The rate in Alaska is 6.4, more than four times the rate in
Louisiana, which has the second highest rate. In addition to the low water
temperature in Alaska, travel by boat as well as fishing and other occupational exposures are common.

The geographic distribution of drowning related to boats is of particular
interest because most states with high rates also have high drowning rates
among motor vehicle occupants. (See Chapter 17.)

TEMPORAL VARIATION

More than any other type of injury death, drowning occurs disproportionately on Saturdays and Sundays, when 40 percent of all drownings occur
(Figure 4-14). Although this pattern reflects the increase in recreational
boating and swimming on weekends, it also is influenced by alcohol use,
which is a prominent factor in adult and adolescent drownings (Dietz and
Baker 1974; Wintemute, et al. 1990). Drowning is also among the most
seasonal of injuries. Two-thirds of all nonboat drownings and one-half of

those involving boats occur during May through August, when both recreational and occupational use of boats are highest (Figure 4-15).

HISTORICAL TRENDS

During the past 60 years, the rate for deaths usually categorized as drowning (i.e., excluding those involving boats) has decreased by 68 percent (Figure 13-6). Most of this decrease occurred between 1930 and 1950. In contrast, the rate for water transport deaths (boat-related deaths, which are primarily drownings) has changed very little. Increases in recreational boat usage may have counteracted any improvements in boats, flotation devices, boating practices, and rescue capability that occurred during these decades.

Since the late 1970s, rates for both boat-related and nonboat-related drowning have decreased significantly for both sexes and all racial groups. Comparing 1980–1986 with 1977–1979, one sees there was an overall reduction of 20 percent. The largest decreases in age-specific drowning rates were for ages 5–19 (Figure 13-7).

Deaths associated with scuba diving decreased from a high of 147 in 1976 to a low of 66 in 1988, then jumped to 114 in 1989 and a similarly high

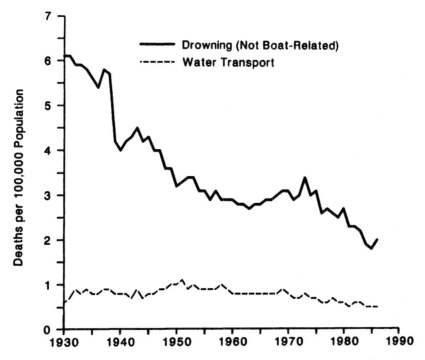

Figure 13-6.   Death Rates from Drowning by Year and Circumstances, 1930–1986

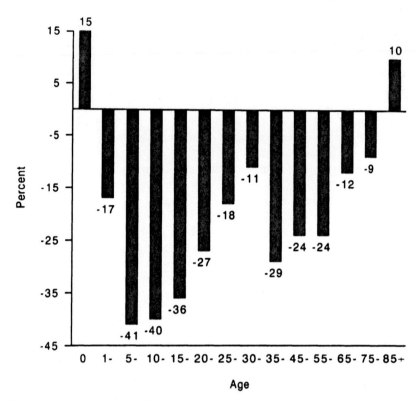

Figure 13-7.   Percentage Change in Death Rates from Drowning by Age, 1984–1986 Compared with 1977–1979

number in 1990 (McAniff 1991). The recent increase was partly associated with an increase in deaths among participants aged 50 or older.

PREVENTIVE MEASURES

It is estimated that a residential swimming pool is 14 times as likely as a car to be involved in the death of a child less than 5 years of age (Baxter et al. 1984). The rapid increase in home pools underscores the need for "child-proof" swimming pools. The effectiveness of designs that separate young children from home swimming pools is indicated by data from two Australian cities where swimming pools are equally common. In Canberra, where childproof fences were required around home swimming pools, the drowning rate for children was found to be one-ninth the rate in Brisbane, where such fences were not required (Pearn and Nixon 1977). Childproof fencing 4.5 to 5 feet high is recommended around swimming pools (Wintemute 1990). In-ground pools without four-sided fencing have been shown to be 1.6 times as likely to be involved in drownings and near-drownings as pools that are less well protected (Present 1987). There is no comparable evidence to support a recommendation for the use of pool covers, and in some cases the devices are believed to have contributed to drownings (Shinaberger et al. 1990).

In addition to "childproofing" swimming pools, hot tubs, and other manmade structures, drowning prevention involves a variety of other strategies (Dietz and Baker 1974). Training in water survival should include not only swimming, floating, and boating skills but also the use of essential equipment such as helmets for kayaking and white water rafting, personal flotation devices for all boaters, and parkas with flotation capability for cold water boating. Because the ability to swim a little could lead to overconfidence or to swimming in places with hazardous currents or undertow, research is needed on the relationships among swimming training, perception of swimming ability, and the likelihood of drowning (Schuman et al. 1977). Training in cardiopulmonary resuscitation (CPR) is strongly recommended for all owners of swimming pools, since a large proportion of drowning deaths could be prevented if resuscitation were initiated immediately, rather than waiting for a rescue squad (Present 1987; Quan et al. 1990; Wintemute et al. 1987). In Sacramento County, California, 40 percent of pool owners support required CPR certification for all pool owners (Wintemute and Wright 1990).

Other preventive measures include changing the speed capabilities and design of small boats and improving ability to locate and rescue people at risk of drowning. The important role of alcohol in drownings, including those related to boats, must be taken into consideration in planning and choosing preventive strategies. High BACs have been reported in 40 to 50 percent of adult drownings (Dietz and Baker 1974; Smith and Kraus 1988; Wintemute 1990). Alcohol use in connection with aquatic activities such as boating and swimming was reported by 36 percent of men and 11 percent of women surveyed (Howland et al. 1990). The association between alcohol and drowning is higher with increasing age, with motor vehicle involvement, and for males (Wintemute et al. 1988). Although alcohol is no longer advertised in connection with automobiles, advertisements for alcohol that depict aquatic settings are still common and may contribute to misconceptions regarding the safety of combining alcohol use with swimming and boating.

REFERENCES

Baxter, L., V. Brown, P. Present, R. Rauchschwalbe, and C. Young (1984). *Infant drownings in swimming pools/spas*. Washington, DC: Consumer Product Safety Commission.

Budnick, L.D., and D.A. Ross (1985). Bathtub-related drownings in the United States, 1979–81. *American Journal of Public Health* 75:630–633.

Dietz, P.E., and S.P. Baker (1974). Drowning—epidemiology and prevention. *American Journal of Public Health* 64:303–312.

Howland, J., T. Mangione, R. Hingson, S. Levenson, and M. Winter (1990). A pilot survey of aquatic activities and related consumption of alcohol, with implications for drowning. *Public Health Reports* 105:415–419.

McAniff, J.J. (1991). *U. S. underwater diving fatality statistics, 1988.* Kingston, RI: The University of Rhode Island National Underwater Accident Data Center.

Metropolitan Life Insurance Company (1977a). Accidental drownings by age and activity. *Statistical Bulletin* 58(May):3–5.

Metropolitan Life Insurance Company (1977b). Swimming pool drownings. *Statistical Bulletin* 58(July–August):4–6.

O'Carroll, P.W., E. Alkon, and B. Weiss (1988). Drowning mortality in Los Angeles County, 1976 to 1984. *Journal of the American Medical Association* 260:380–383.

Pearn, J., and J. Nixon (1977). Are swimming pools becoming more dangerous? *Medical Journal of Australia* 2:702–704.

Present, P. (1987). *Child drowning study: A report on the epidemiology of drownings in residential pools to children under age five.* Washington, DC: Consumer Product Safety Commission.

Quan, L., K.R. Wentz, E.J. Gore, and M.K. Copass (1990). Outcome and predictors of outcome in pediatric submersion victims receiving prehospital care in King County, Washington. *Pediatrics* 86:586–593.

Quan, L., E.J. Gore, K. Wentz, J. Allen, and A.H. Novack (1989). Ten-year study of pediatric drownings and near-drownings in King County, Washington: Lessons in injury prevention. *Pediatrics* 83:1035–1040.

Schuman, S.H., J.R. Rowe, H.M. Glazer, and J.S. Redding (1977). Risk of drowning: An iceberg phenomenon. *Journal of the American College of Emergency Physicians* 6:139–143.

Shinaberger, C.S., C.L. Anderson, and J.F. Kraus (1990). Young children who drown in hot tubs, spas, and whirlpools in California: A 26-year study. *American Journal of Public Health* 80:613–614.

Smith, G.S., and J.F. Kraus (1988). Alcohol and residential, recreational, and occupational injuries: A review of the epidemiologic evidence. *Annual Review of Public Health* 9:99–121.

United States Coast Guard (1988). *Boating statistics 1987.* Technical Report COMDTPUB P16754.1. Washington, DC: U.S. Department of Transportation.

Waller, A.E., S.P. Baker, and A. Szocka (1989). Childhood injury deaths: National analysis and geographic variations. *American Journal of Public Health* 79: 310–315.

Wintemute, G.J. (1990). Childhood drowning and near-drowning in the United States. *American Journal of Diseases of Children* 144:663–669.

Wintemute, G.J., J.F. Kraus, S.P. Teret, and M. Wright (1987). Drowning in childhood and adolescence: A population-based study. *American Journal of Public Health* 77:830–832.

Wintemute, G.J., J.F. Kraus, S.P. Teret, and M. Wright (1988). The epidemiology of drowning in adulthood: Implications for prevention. *American Journal of Preventive Medicine* 4:343–348.

Wintemute, G.J., S.P. Teret, J.F. Kraus, and M. Wright (1990). Alcohol and drowning: An analysis of contributing factors and a discussion of criteria for case selection. *Accident Analysis and Prevention* 22:291–296.

Wintemute, G.J., and M.A. Wright (1990). Swimming pool owners' opinions of strategies for prevention of drowning. *Pediatrics* 85:63–69.

14

Asphyxiation by Choking and Suffocation

Deaths attributed to mechanical suffocation and asphyxiation by foreign materials in the respiratory tract number 4,700 annually. Among children younger than 1 year they account for almost 40 percent of all unintentional injury deaths.

The category "aspiration of food" includes not only asphyxiation by solid food but also the presence in the respiratory tract of regurgitated food. The latter phenomenon, which may occur in the last phases of dying from a variety of causes, accounts for three-fourths of all deaths coded as asphyxiation by food in the first year of life and half of such deaths among older children (Harris et al. 1984). In Georgia, death certificates for two-thirds of all food asphyxiation cases cited regurgitated food as the cause (Dabis et al. 1985).

The ICD (and hence NCHS mortality data) does not differentiate between asphyxiation by regurgitated food and by food entering the airway while eating. Therefore, the analyses presented here include all deaths coded in this general category, referring to them as aspiration of food. Some cases of sudden infant death syndrome (SIDS, or "crib death"), which annually causes 3,500 deaths among children 1–3 months old, may erroneously be categorized as asphyxiation, but this practice is changing as SIDS becomes better recognized.

Deaths categorized as "mechanical suffocation" include asphyxiation resulting from the mouth and nose being covered (for example, by a plastic bag), entrapment in an airtight enclosed space such as a refrigerator or storage tank, unintentional hanging, and being covered by fallen earth or other materials.

AGE AND SEX

Death rates from airway obstruction by food or other foreign materials are highest among children and the elderly (Figure 14-1). Among children younger than 1 year, the great majority of deaths attributed to these causes occur in the first 6 months (Figure 14-2).

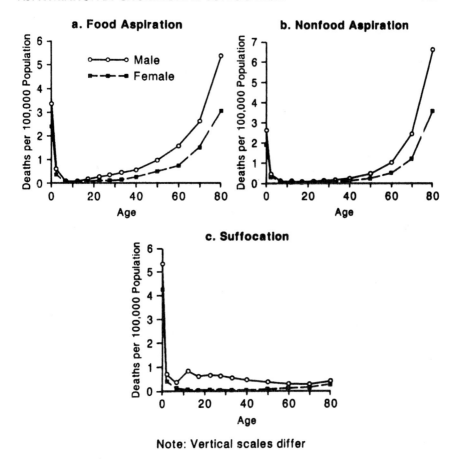

Note: Vertical scales differ

Figure 14-1. Death Rates from Food and Nonfood Aspiration and Suffocation by Age and Sex, 1980–1986

The number of childhood deaths from choking on solid food has been estimated at about 75 per year. Most occur before age 4, with the highest incidence in children less than 2 years old (Harris et al. 1984). The probability that any product will cause fatal choking depends on whether it is likely to be put into the mouth and also on its size, shape, and consistency. Fatal choking in children typically involves round products; pieces of hot dog predominate among obstructing foods, and candies, nuts, and grapes are the others most commonly recorded (Baker and Fisher 1980; Harris et al. 1984). Especially prominent among the nonfood items reported are round or pliable objects such as undersized infant pacifiers, small balls, and uninflated or underinflated balloons.

The largest numbers and highest death rates from choking on food or nonfood material occur among older people, with 2,500 deaths annually of people aged 65 or older. About 270 deaths occur each year in residential institutions such as nursing homes and extended care facilities. Poor denti-

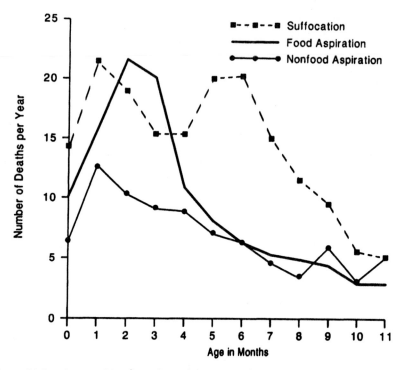

Figure 14-2.   Average Number of Deaths per Year from Food and Nonfood Aspiration and Suffocation by Month of Age, 1980–1986

tion, use of sedative or hypnotic drugs, and diseases affecting motor coordination or mental function may be predisposing factors. Among noninstitutionalized adults, airway obstruction is often caused by a large piece of meat (Mittleman and Wetli 1982). The term "cafe coronary," used to describe adult death from food in the airway, reflects both the suddenness of onset and the fact that some deaths occur in restaurants, where both alcohol use and social inhibitions (such as reluctance to remove unchewable food from the mouth in public) probably play a role. Of the cases where the place of death is stated on the death certificate, more than one-half occur at home and only one-tenth in public places such as restaurants. These figures indicate the need for widespread ability to deal with this emergency in the home and elsewhere.

Suffocation is the fifth most common cause of unintentional injury death among boys aged 10–14, whose death rate from suffocation exceeds that for any group except infants. The male to female ratio of suffocation rates is about 14 to 1 at this age, whereas for all ages combined it is about 3 to 1.

In children less than 5 years old, a CPSC review of almost 300 strangulation incidents revealed that usually clothing or a string around the child's neck became caught on an object. One-tenth of the cases involved pacifiers that had cords attached to them (Rutherford and Kelly 1981). Other products that have resulted in child strangulations include window blind cords, accordion-style gates, crib hammocks, and the lids of toy chests.

A 20-year review of suffocation and strangulation deaths among California children examined the specific events in relation to age. Crib strangulation and suffocation from becoming wedged between crib mattress and frame were most common at 6–8 months of age. Entrapment in refrigerators occurred primarily among children aged 2–7 years. Suffocation by fallen earth at construction sites occurred most often at ages 8–12 years (Kraus 1985). Fallen earth caused 106 deaths in 1988 for all ages combined, and it is especially important among boys aged 10–14. Traumatic asphyxia, the result of chest compression, often involves young children crushed by household furniture and men working beneath automobiles when a jack slips (Sklar et al. 1988).

RACE AND PER CAPITA INCOME

Death rates for blacks and whites are similar for asphyxiation by food and suffocation, but the rates are 50 percent higher among blacks for airway obstruction by nonfood objects. Native Americans have high rates for all three causes of death. Death rates are highest in low-income areas for each of these three causes of death (Figure 14-3), with approximately a twofold difference in rates between the lowest- and highest-income areas.

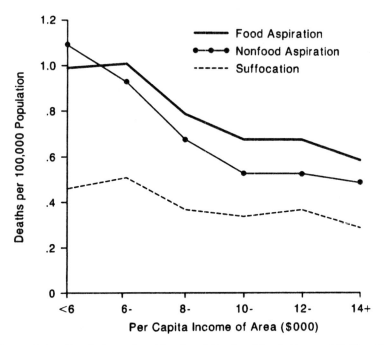

Figure 14-3. Death Rates from Food and Nonfood Aspiration and Suffocation by Per Capita Income of Area of Residence, 1980–1986

URBAN/RURAL AND GEOGRAPHIC DIFFERENCES

Rates of suffocation and of asphyxiation by food or other materials in the respiratory tract do not show a consistent urban/rural pattern. The rates are highest in the most rural areas.

Airway obstruction by nonfood material is most common in southern states, and suffocation rates are highest in western states (Figure 14-4). Re-

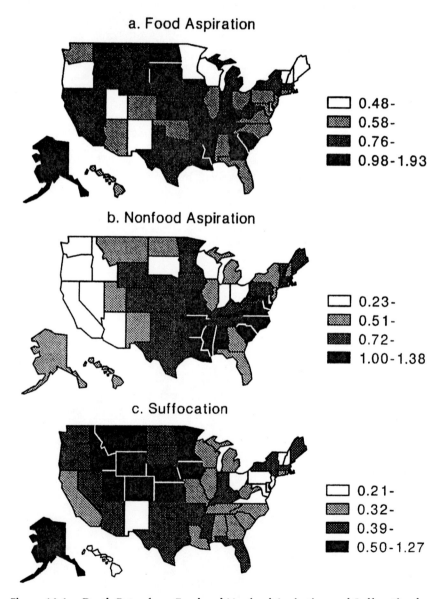

Figure 14-4.   Death Rates from Food and Nonfood Aspiration and Suffocation by state, per 100,000 Population, 1980–1986

gional patterns in rates of food-related deaths may be partly due to variations in the certification of death when post-mortem examination reveals regurgitated food in the respiratory tract (Harris et al. 1984).

SEASON AND DAY OF WEEK

Death rates from suffocation are higher in the summer, and rates from choking are higher in winter. Choking on food or nonfood objects is slightly more common on weekends, possibly because of the frequent association with alcohol use.

HISTORICAL TRENDS

Between 1977–1979 and 1984–1986, the death rate from choking on nonfood materials increased by 68 percent. This was the largest increase seen for any group of injury deaths with the exception of poisoning by cocaine or opiates (see Table 3-3). Death rates for children decreased, but an overall increase occurred because of substantial increases in death rates for the population aged 65 or older (Figure 14-5). For both men and women, the rate more than doubled for ages 75 and older.

During the same period, the overall death rates from suffocation and food asphyxiation declined by 5 percent and 20 percent, respectively. Rates increased, however, for some adult age groups, especially those 75 or older (Figure 14-5).

Changing practices in coding SIDS deaths contributed to the reductions of about 85 percent between 1968 and 1978 in deaths during the first year of life that were coded as either aspiration of food or suffocation. Since 1977–1979, there have been decreases of about 20–50 percent among children aged 0–9 in deaths coded as aspiration or suffocation.

Childhood deaths have decreased from entrapment in refrigerators or freezers, suffocation by plastic bags, and burial by falling earth at construction sites. Some reduction in refrigeration entrapment and suffocation may have resulted from redesign of refrigerators or state laws regarding their disposal (Kraus 1985). Further research is needed to determine the extent to which changes in death rates reflect CPSC regulations designed to reduce choking and strangulation by children's products such as pacifiers, small toys, and cribs.

PREVENTIVE MEASURES

The problem of fatal choking in the elderly has received little attention despite the large numbers of deaths. The type of meat served to the elderly in hospitals and nursing homes and the correct fit of their dentures may be amenable to intervention.

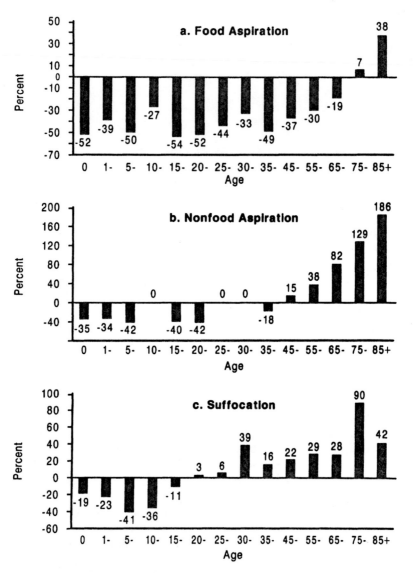

Figure 14-5.   Percentage Change in Death Rates from Food and Nonfood Aspiration and Suffocation by Age, 1984–1986 Compared with 1977–1979

Measures to prevent asphyxiation in children include the thoughtful design and packaging of all products likely to be used by or near young children, with attention to their size, shape, consistency, and likelihood of separating into hazardous pieces. Labels of toys posing a choking hazard for young children should specify the hazard rather than merely stating that a toy is "designed for children age 3 or older" (Langlois et al. 1991). Manufactured foods such as hot dogs and hard candies should be designed to avoid or minimize the characteristics associated with fatal choking (Baker and Fisher 1980; Feldman and Simms 1980). In addition, information about the foods that are hazardous to young children should be widely disseminated.

REFERENCES

Baker, S.P., and R.S. Fisher (1980). Childhood asphyxiation by choking or suffocation. *Journal of the American Medical Association* 244:1343–1346.

Dabis, F., T. McKinley, G. Smith, and R.K. Sikes (1985). Choking and aspiration of food in Georgia, 1977–1983. Atlanta, GA: Centers for Disease Control, unpublished manuscript.

Feldman, K.W., and R.J. Simms (1980). Strangulation in childhood: Epidemiology and clinical course. *Pediatrics* 65:1979–1985.

Harris, C.S., S.P. Baker, G.A. Smith, and R.M. Harris (1984). Childhood asphyxiation by food: A national analysis and overview. *Journal of the American Medical Association* 251:2231–2235.

Kraus, J.F. (1985). Effectiveness of measures to prevent unintentional deaths of infants and children from suffocation and strangulation. *Public Health Reports* 100:231–240.

Langlois, J.A., B.R.A. Wallen, S.P. Teret, L.A. Bailey, J.H. Hershey, and M.O. Peeler (1991). *Toys with small parts: The impact of specific warning labels.* Baltimore, MD: The Johns Hopkins Injury Prevention Center.

Mittleman, R.E., and C.V. Wetli (1982). The fatal cafe coronary: Foreign-body airway obstruction. *Journal of the American Medical Association* 247:1285–1288.

Rutherford, G.W., Jr., and S. Kelly (1981). Accidental strangulations (ligature) of children less than 5 years of age. Washington, DC: U.S. Consumer Product Safety Commission.

Sklar, D.P., B. Baack, P. McFeeley, T. Osler, E. Marder, and G. Demarest (1988). Traumatic asphyxia in New Mexico: A five-year experience. *American Journal of Emergency Medicine* 6:219–223.

15

Poisoning

Poisoning results from either brief or long-term exposure to a chemical agent. In general, this book addresses only acute poisonings. The mechanism of injury depends on the chemical agent itself and on whether it is injected, ingested, inhaled, or absorbed through the skin. Basic preventive approaches, comparable to those for preventing other injuries, include eliminating or reducing the manufacture or sale of an agent, reducing the length of exposure or the concentration of the poison to noninjurious doses, preventing access to the substance, changing its chemical formulation, and providing appropriate emergency and therapeutic measures.

Poisoning causes about 13,000 deaths each year in the United States, more than 99 percent of them among adults. Almost half of all poisoning deaths are ruled suicidal (Table 15-1).

Included with unintentional poisonings are an unknown number of deaths in which the intent of the person was not obvious. Both intentional and unintentional poisoning will be discussed in this chapter because the agents are often the same, the intent may not be known, and preventive

Table 15-1. Poisoning Deaths, 1987

Agent	Unintentional	Suicide	Undetermined	Total[a]
Barbiturates	30	187	20	237
Antidepressants and tranquilizers	185	938	154	1,277
Heroin	595	b	b	595
Cocaine	777	b	b	777
Other or unspecified drugs and medications	2,183	1,766	926	4,875
Alcohol	347	b	b	347
Other or unspecified solids or liquids	298	215	46	559
Motor vehicle exhaust	402	2,684	102	3,188
Other or unspecified gases or vapors	498	531	67	1,096
Total	5,315	6,321	1,315	12,951

Source: National Center for Health Statistics, 1987.
[a]Table excludes 39 homicides by poisoning, 4,938 deaths coded as alcohol dependence or abuse, and 2,026 deaths coded as other or unspecified drug abuse or dependence (1987).
[b]Not separately identifiable.

measures are sometimes similar (Hassall and Trethowan 1972). In general, data from hospitals and poison control centers are not categorized by the presumed intent of the person.

Almost a quarter of a million people are admitted to hospitals each year for treatment of poisoning (Rice, MacKenzie, and associates 1989). Almost 1.4 million poisoning exposures were reported in 1988 to the 64 reporting centers, which serve two-thirds of the U.S. population (Litovitz et al. 1989). Sixty percent of all calls to poison centers involve children younger than 5 years, although this age group constitutes only 0.4 percent of all fatal poisonings. Only 545 fatal poisonings (less than 5 percent of all deaths) were reported to poison control centers, because death often occurs without help having been sought.

CARBON MONOXIDE

Carbon monoxide in motor vehicle exhaust is the most prominent single agent in poisoning deaths (Table 15-1). Because its affinity for hemoglobin is far greater than that of oxygen, carbon monoxide can kill very quickly by precluding the uptake of oxygen by red blood cells. Colorless and odorless, it may produce unconsciousness with little or no warning. These characteristics increase the deadliness of carbon monoxide, whether in motor vehicle exhaust or housefires, or in other circumstances where it is not properly dissipated, diluted, or separated from people.

Unintentional poisoning by motor vehicle exhaust sometimes occurs when people are working in enclosed garages or when fumes seep into working or living quarters connected to garages. Occasionally, exhaust fumes enter a vehicle while it is moving. Most often, fatal poisoning occurs when cars are parked with the engine running to provide heat for the occupants; defects in the exhaust system and car body then allow fumes to enter (Baker et al. 1972). Suicidal poisoning usually takes place in a garage or involves connecting the exhaust system to the occupant compartment of a vehicle.

Among women, the death rate from unintentional poisoning by motor vehicle exhaust rises very sharply to a peak at ages 15–19, then declines rapidly (Figure 15-1). Among men, it peaks at ages 20–24 and increases again after age 75. A similar increase in the rate of suicide by motor vehicle exhaust suggests that some suicides in elderly men may have been certified as "accidental." Suicide by motor vehicle exhaust, which is about five times as common as unintentional poisoning by this means, has a striking age pattern among females, for whom the death rate peaks in the 45–54 age group (Figure 3-3).

Unintentional poisoning by motor vehicle exhaust is rare among Asians. Whites and blacks have similar rates of unintentional deaths but the suicide rate from motor vehicle exhaust is nine times as high for whites as blacks. This white to black ratio, which is higher than for any other injury cause,

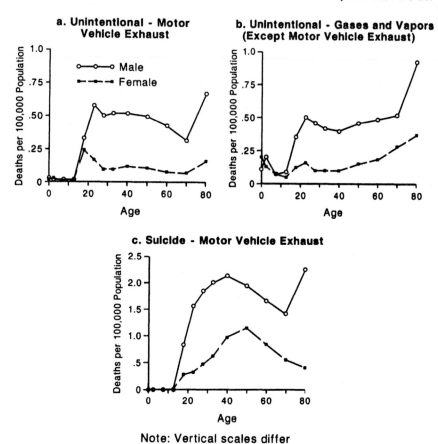

Figure 15-1.   Death Rates from Unintentional and Suicidal Poisoning by Gases and Vapors, by Age and Sex, 1980–1986

remains even when variations in per capita income and place of residence are taken into account.

The high death rate from unintentional poisoning by motor vehicle exhaust in low-income areas may be related to deterioration of old vehicles, which is a major factor in these poisonings. The death rate from suicide by vehicle exhaust, however, is lowest in low-income areas.

Motor vehicle exhaust death rates are slightly higher in more rural areas in the case of unintentional poisoning, whereas suicide rates are low in rural areas (Figure 15-2). For both suicide and unintentional deaths, rates tend to be high in more northern states (Figure 15-3), where garages may offer more opportunity for this means of suicide and where the colder climate increases the use of car heaters. The role of cold weather is further illustrated by the fact that deaths from unintentional poisoning by motor vehicle exhaust are more than three times as common in December–February as in June–

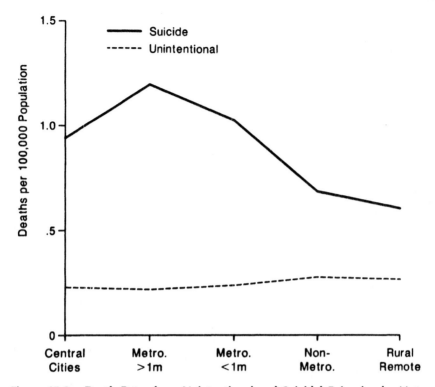

Figure 15-2.   Death Rates from Unintentional and Suicidal Poisoning by Motor Vehicle Exhaust, by Place of Residence, 1980–1986

August (Figure 4-15). Suicide, on the other hand, shows little seasonal variation.

Between 1930 and 1986, the death rate from unintentional poisoning by gases and vapors dropped by 79 percent, due mainly to reductions in poisoning by domestic gas. Since 1947, poisonings by domestic gas and by motor vehicle exhaust have been distinguished from one another in the national mortality data for "poisoning by gases and vapors." Between 1947 and 1986 there was a 99 percent decrease in the rate of unintentional death from gas piped to homes, with the steepest drop during the 1950s (Figure 15-4). In addition to increased use of electric stoves, coal gas (which had a higher carbon monoxide content) was gradually replaced by natural gas as a fuel for cooking. Natural gas does not contain concentrations of carbon monoxide likely to cause fatal poisoning if the gas is emitted from a stove or other appliance without being ignited. By 1988, only 36 unintentional deaths and 16 suicides were attributed to poisoning by domestic piped gas, which in 1947 caused about 1,000 unintentional deaths and 1,200 suicides. In England and Wales, similar dramatic changes occurred in both categories of deaths (and in the total number of suicides) as the carbon monoxide

a. Unintentional - Motor Vehicle Exhaust

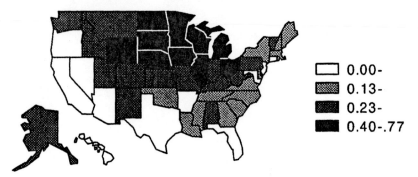

☐	0.00-
▨	0.13-
▦	0.23-
■	0.40-.77

b. Unintentional - Except Motor Vehicle Exhaust

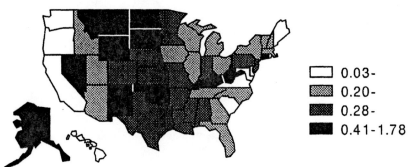

☐	0.03-
▨	0.20-
▦	0.28-
■	0.41-1.78

c. Suicide - Motor Vehicle Exhaust

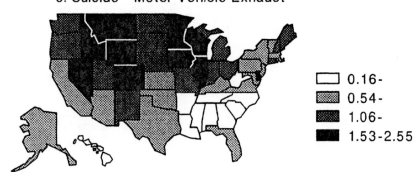

☐	0.16-
▨	0.54-
▦	1.06-
■	1.53-2.55

Figure 15-3. Death Rates from Poisoning by Gases and Vapors by State, per 100,000 Population, 1980–1986

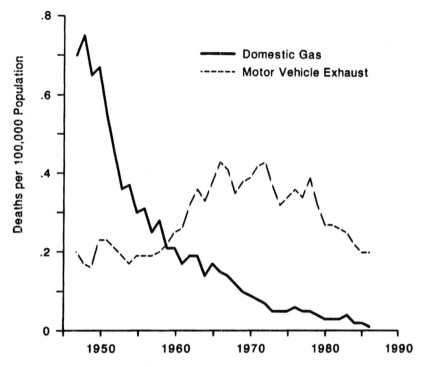

Figure 15-4. Death Rates from Unintentional Poisoning by Domestic Piped Gas and Motor Vehicle Exhaust by Year, 1947–1986

content of piped gas was reduced (Alphey and Leach 1974; Hassall and Trethowan 1972).

From 1955 to 1965 the death rate from unintentional poisoning by motor vehicle exhaust doubled. Then, after remaining fairly constant for about a decade, the number of deaths steadily decreased from 717 deaths in 1979 to 372 in 1988. Measures to prevent entry of carbon monoxide into the passenger compartment (for example, by reducing the rusting through of cars and exhaust systems, locating tailpipes appropriately, and inspecting older vehicles to identify hazardous defects) may have helped to reduce these deaths. The fact that many cars now have fan-driven ventilation systems that function whenever the ignition is on may also have contributed to the decreased mortality. Reduction in the carbon monoxide content of auto exhaust through emission controls, imposed in the United States but not in Great Britain, has coincided with a decrease in unintentional poisoning by exhaust gas in the United States and no decrease in Great Britain (Lester and Clarke 1989).

Carbon monoxide from nonvehicular sources causes about 350 unintentional deaths annually. In West Virginia, such deaths were usually caused by poorly vented heating or cooking appliances using methane, butane, or propane (Baron et al. 1989). West Virginia has the fifth highest rate (0.44) of nonmotor vehicle poisoning by gas or vapor. Alaska's rate (1.78) is seven times the U.S. rate.

OPIATES AND COCAINE

Substances classified as "drugs and medications" cause more than 80 percent of all fatal poisonings by solids and liquids. Of the drugs specifically identified by ICD E-codes for injury and poisoning, the most common by far are opiates (heroin)[1] and cocaine,[2] which caused 798 and 1087 deaths, respectively, in 1988, up from 595 and 777 deaths in 1987.

Fatal opiate poisoning is predominantly the result of heroin overdose. Many heroin deaths are not classified with unintentional deaths because, since 1971, the ICD codes have classified cases involving drug dependence as "natural" death due to drug dependence or abuse rather than as "accidental" deaths. In 1987, 1,062 deaths were classified as due to dependence on heroin, cocaine, or unspecified drugs and 3,232 as drug abuse (Table 15-2). Deaths in these categories are not included in our analyses, but deaths from heroin dependence have been shown to follow the same time trends as unintentional opiate poisoning (Samkoff and Baker 1982). Whether a drug overdose is coded as "accidental" or as a "natural" death depends on the information available to the medical examiner or coroner as well as on the data recorded on the death certificate. Opiate and cocaine poisoning are such large components of fatal poisoning that recognition of these coding problems is important.

Death rates from unintentional poisoning by opiates are especially high for males (the sex ratio is almost 6 to 1) and for ages 25–34 (Figure 15-5). A comparable peak at ages 25–34 is seen for poisonings by other and unspecified substances and may represent the inclusion of some opiate deaths among unspecified poisonings.

Table 15-2.   Deaths from Alcohol or Drug Poisoning, Dependency, and Abuse, 1987

Agent and ICD Code[a]	Alcohol	Heroin and Other Opiates	Cocaine and Local Anesthetics	Unspecified Drug
Poisoning (injuries) (E860, E850.0, E855.2)	347	595	777	—
Alcohol/drug dependence (303, 304.0, 304.2, 304.9)	4,262	25	8	1,029
Nondependent abuse of drug (305.0, 305.5, 305.6, 305.9)	676	11	50	737
Total	5,285	631	835	1,766

[a]International Classification of Diseases, 9th edition.

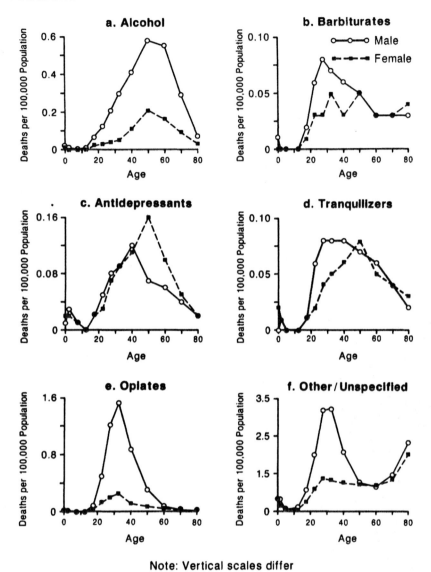

Note: Vertical scales differ

Figure 15-5.   Death Rates from Unintentional Poisoning by Solids and Liquids by Age, Sex, and Type of Drug, 1980–1986

The opiate poisoning death rate among blacks is almost twice that of whites, reflecting the racial composition of large cities, where the death rate from opiate poisoning is especially high. In central cities, the death rate is 15 times the rate in the most rural areas. When place of residence is taken into consideration, little difference between blacks and whites is seen in death rates from opiate poisoning (Baker et al. 1984). Rates of fatal cocaine

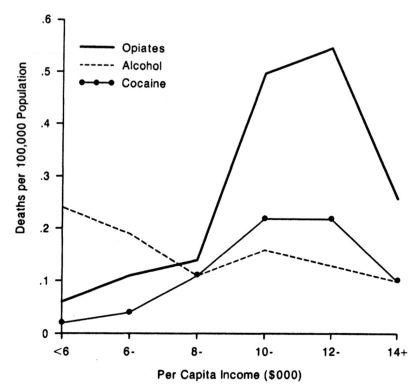

Figure 15-6.   Death Rates from Unintentional Poisoning by Opiates, Cocaine, and Alcohol by Per Capita Income of Area of Residence, 1980–1986

poisoning are as high in other metropolitan areas as in central cities; the death rates in nonmetropolitan areas are only half the rates of MSAs.

Opiate and cocaine poisoning are among the few causes of death for which mortality is lowest in low-income counties (Figure 15-6). For both drugs, death rates are highest in middle-income areas. In central cities as well as in metropolitan and rural areas, counties with high per capita income generally have rates of fatal opiate poisoning several times as high as places with low income.

Since 1970, fluctuations in opiate-poisoning mortality in the United States appear to have coincided with variations in the flow of heroin into the country. When the heroin supply was interrupted in 1972 and again in 1976, there were corresponding decreases in heroin-related mortality (Samkoff and Baker 1982). Opiate deaths than tripled between 1980 and 1986, to a rate that approached the 1975 high (Figure 15-7); deaths numbered 322 in 1980 and 930 in 1986, before dropping to 595 in 1987 and increasing to 798 the following year.

Cocaine poisoning deaths increased dramatically during the 1980s, from 109 in 1980 to 777 in 1987 and 1,087 in 1988.[2] A large increase took place between 1985 and 1986, in association with the crack cocaine epidemic. The

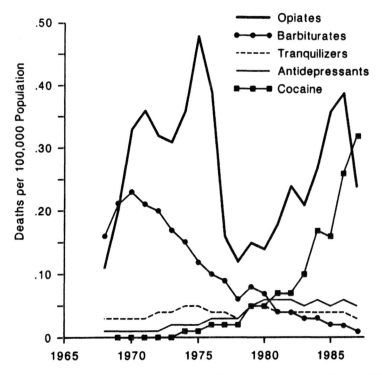

Figure 15-7. Death Rates from Unintentional Poisoning by Type of Drug and Year, 1968–1987

prevalence of recent cocaine use in fatally injured motor vehicle occupants in New York City also increased (Marzuk et al. 1990), but a causal relationship between cocaine use and motor vehicle crash involvement has not been established.

Data from the Drug Abuse Warning Network of the National Institute on Drug Abuse, reflecting emergency room admissions in 431 participating hospitals in 21 metropolitan areas, indicate a fourfold increase between 1985 and 1988 in the number of emergency room cases in which cocaine was mentioned (Adams et al. 1990). The trend was not uniform among cities; the increase was less than twofold in San Francisco and Los Angeles (where cocaine use may have increased rapidly in an earlier period), while a tenfold increase was reported in Baltimore and Philadelphia.

OTHER DRUGS

Psychotherapeutic drugs (primarily antidepressants and tranquilizers) are also important (Table 15-1). Additional poisonings by these agents are undoubtedly included in the large numbers of fatal poisonings by unspecified agents. Among all teenagers admitted to Maryland hospitals in

1979–1982 for poisoning, the most common agents were aspirin and its substitutes, benzodiazepines, alcohol, and antidepressants. Most cases of teenage poisoning were categorized as suicide attempts. Female teenagers had higher rates than males; the sex difference was especially great for aspirin poisoning (Trinkoff and Baker 1986).

Unintentional barbiturate poisoning deaths show a peak at ages 25–29 for men (Figure 15-5); beginning at about age 45, women have almost the same rates as men. Similarly, tranquilizers have higher unintentional death rates among men prior to age 45. Female death rates from antidepressants are much higher than male rates for ages 45–64, a pattern rarely seen for other causes of unintentional injury death. For both tranquilizers and antidepressants, the high death rates in women at about age 50 suggest the possibility that the deaths coded as unintentional include many that are actually of suicidal intent, since that is the age at which the suicide rate in women is highest.

There is little difference between whites and blacks in death rates from unintentional poisoning by barbiturates and psychotherapeutic drugs. In general, drug poisoning deaths do not show strong or consistent relationships with per capita income.

Central cities have the highest death rates from all types of drug poisoning. For poisoning by barbiturates, the urban to rural ratio is 3 to 1. For all drugs combined, the urban to rural ratio is approximately 2 to 1.

Geographic patterns differ for the various types of poisoning (Figure 15-8). California and Nevada rank in the highest group in all categories of drug poisoning except alcohol, for which they rank thirteenth and eleventh, respectively. The rates for many other states are based on small numbers of deaths, so that many of the differences are not statistically significant.

Several markedly different trends in death rates from drugs occurred during recent decades (Figure 15-7). The most dramatic increases were in deaths from opiate and cocaine poisoning, which increased threefold and fivefold, respectively, between 1980 and 1986. In contrast, deaths from barbiturates rose slightly in the late 1960s and then dropped steadily to nearly zero by 1987.

ALCOHOL

Alcohol use often accompanies or contributes to poisoning by drugs or carbon monoxide, decreasing protective inhibitions and awareness of hazards and acting additively or synergistically with other poisons. Alcohol may also prove fatal by itself when consumed in sufficient quantities. About 350 deaths annually are attributed to poisoning by alcohol. In addition, about 5,000 deaths each year are attributed to acute or chronic alcoholism or alcohol abuse but are not coded with injuries (Table 15-2). If the many effects of chronic, heavy use were included, the total number of deaths due to alcohol poisoning would be even greater.

a. Opiates

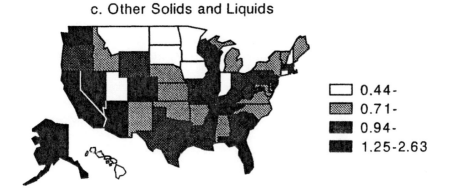

☐	0.00-
▨	0.04-
▨	0.08-
■	0.19-1.32

b. Alcohol

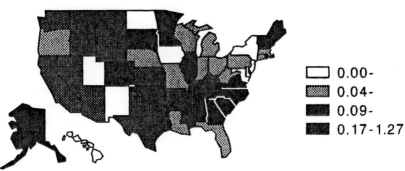

☐	0.00-
▨	0.04-
▨	0.09-
■	0.17-1.27

c. Other Solids and Liquids

☐	0.44-
▨	0.71-
▨	0.94-
■	1.25-2.63

Figure 15-8. Death Rates from Unintentional Poisoning by Solids and Liquids by State, per 100,000 Population, 1980–1986

The death rate from acute alcohol poisoning among males is more than three times the female rate, with a peak at about age 50 for both sexes (Figure 15-5). Death rates are highest for Native Americans and blacks (0.59 and 0.38 per 100,000 population, respectively); the rate for whites is less than one-third as high (0.12), and that for Asians is much lower (0.02).

Hospitalizations related to alcohol showed contrasting racial patterns among Maryland teenagers: Admission rates for alcohol poisoning were twice as high among whites as blacks (Trinkoff and Baker 1986). Death rates from alcohol poisoning are especially high in some southern states (Figure 15-8), with the rate in North Carolina more than eight times the national rate. Virginia's rate is second highest and more than double the rate for Georgia, which ranks third. Research is needed to examine the effect of alcohol control policies and laws in various states on the amounts and types of alcohol consumption and on poisoning by alcohol or by contaminants of illicitly produced alcohol.

CHILDHOOD POISONING

For every poisoning death among children younger than 6 years, about 20,000 ingestions are reported to poison control centers (Table 15-3; Litovitz et al. 1989). Although reports from these centers underestimate the total number of poisonings, they provide information on the relative frequency of ingestions that are of sufficient concern to result in calls to poison control centers. Forty-one percent of reports and 70 percent of deaths in 1988 involved drugs and medicines. The next largest number of reports was for ingestion of cleaning and polishing agents. Ingestion of plants is also a common cause of reports but rarely causes death. Based on the ratio of reports to deaths, the most lethal agents were antidepressants, anticonvulsants, and cardiovascular drugs. Together, these three groups of drugs comprised less than 2 percent of reported poisonings in this age group but 25 percent of the deaths.

Since 1960, poisoning deaths among children younger than 5 years have decreased dramatically. The rate for poisoning by solids and liquids was 2.2 per 100,000 in 1960 and 0.2 in 1988 (Table 15-4). During this period, the number of deaths from lead poisoning dropped from 78 to 0. Deaths from kerosene and other petroleum products dropped from 48 to 4, while deaths from aspirin dropped from 144 to 3.

An especially steep decline in childhood poisoning death rates occurred after childproof packaging was required on all drugs and medications beginning in 1973. The 50 percent decrease in poisoning by all drugs and medications in the first three years (1973–1976) was substantially greater than the decrease in poisonings by other solids and liquids (Figure 15-9), most of which were not required to be packaged in childproof containers (Walton 1982). The declines have continued; between 1977–1979 and 1984–

Table 15-3. Reported and Fatal Poisoning among Children Aged 0–5, 1988

Agent	Reports to Poison Control Centers	Deaths	Ratio of Reports to Deaths
Narcotics	1,007	0	a
Aspirin (salicylates)	5,565	3	1,855
Other analgesics	70,669	0	a
Antidepressants	2,887	3	962
Anticonvulsants	2,201	2	1,101
Cardiovascular drugs	9,076	6	1,513
Hormones	14,037	1	14,037
Other drugs	238,204	15	15,781
Cleaning/polishing agents	87,393	1	87,393
Petroleum products	26,317	4	6,579
Pesticides/fertilizers	27,233	1	27,233
Other solids/liquids	273,303	7	39,043
Plants	85,754	0	a
Total	843,646	43	19,620

Sources: T. L. Litovitz, B. F. Schmitz, and K. C. Holm. 1988 annual report of the American Association of Poison Control Centers National Data Collection System. *American Journal of Emergency Medicine* 7 (1989): 495–545, and National Center for Health Statistics.
aRatio is infinitely large because no deaths.

1986, the 42 percent decline in poisoning death rates for children aged 1–4 exceeded that for any other major cause of childhood injury death.

Although childhood poisoning is no longer a major problem in terms of the total number of deaths, it is worthy of attention. Some groups of children, notably black and Native American, have death rates that are several times the national average. When nonfatal cases are considered, the

Table 15-4. Causes of Fatal Poisoning among Children Aged 0–4, 1960 and 1988

Agent	1960	1988
Aspirin	144	3
Lead	78	0
Petroleum products	48	4
Caustics and cleaning agents	23	2
All other solids and liquids	152	30
Total	445	59
Death rates per 100,000 population	2.2	0.2

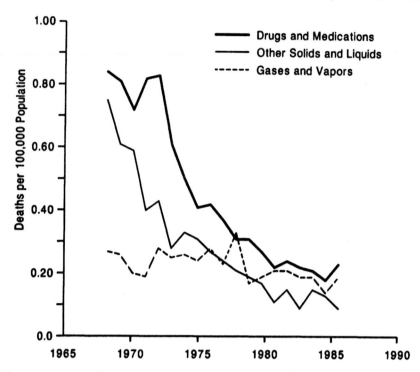

Figure 15-9. Death Rates from Poisoning of Children Aged 0–4 by Year and Category of Poisoning, 1968–1986

number of children and families affected each year by poisoning is very large. Chronic lead poisoning remains a problem of substantial proportions because of its long-term health effects (Needleman 1989).

Deaths and illnesses from poisoning can be further reduced by attention to the formulation, packaging, and use of poisonous agents (Barry 1975). Dramatic reductions in childhood poisoning deaths have resulted from changes in products (for example, reductions in the lead content of paint), packaging (such as childproof or single-dose packages), and energy sources (for example, increased availability of electricity, which reduced the use of kerosene). In addition, development of poison control centers has no doubt contributed to the remarkable decline in poisoning mortality in recent decades. The success of this broad approach, which did not depend on changing the behavior of children or parents, illustrates what can be achieved with intensive efforts and the use of appropriate preventive measures.

NOTES

1. The numbers cited for opiates include deaths from methadone, a synthetic analogue of morphine, as well as heroin, a natural derivative of opium. Deaths from

these substances cannot be distinguished in vital statistics data, but a survey of nonsuicide narcotic deaths in four major U.S. cities revealed that 96 percent were due to heroin.

2. Cocaine poisoning deaths are coded under ICD-E 855.2 "poisoning by local anesthetics." Other drugs so coded, such as lidocaine and procaine, rarely cause death. Therefore, all deaths coded E 855.2 are termed "cocaine poisoning" in this book.

The effect on mortality of the crack cocaine epidemic that began in the mid-1980s was not recognized when data analyses for the second edition of this book were planned. As a result, cocaine was not included in the detailed analyses presented in the Appendix.

REFERENCES

Adams, E.H., A.J. Blanken, L.D. Ferguson, and A. Kopstein (1990). Overview of selected drug trends. Rockville, MD: National Institute on Drug Abuse.

Alphey, R.S., and S.J. Leach (1974). Accidental death in the home. *Royal Society of Health Journal* 3:97–102, 144.

Baker, S.P., B. O'Neill, and R. Karpf (1984). *The injury fact book*. Lexington, MA: Lexington Books.

Baker, S.P., R.S. Fisher, W.C. Masemore, and I.M. Sopher (1972). Fatal unintentional carbon monoxide poisoning in motor vehicles. *American Journal of Public Health* 62:1463–1467.

Baron, R.C., R.C. Backer, and I.M. Sopher (1989). Fatal unintended carbon monoxide poisoning in West Virginia from nonvehicular sources. *American Journal of Public Health* 79:1656–1658.

Barry, P.Z. (1975). Individual versus community orientation in the prevention of injuries. *Preventive Medicine* 4:47–56.

Hassall, C., and W.H. Trethowan (1972). Suicide in Birmingham. *British Medical Journal* 1:717–718.

Lester, D., and R.V. Clarke (1989). Effects of the reduced toxicity of car exhaust on accidental deaths: A comparison of the United States and Great Britain. *Accident Analysis and Prevention* 21:191–196.

Litovitz, T.L., B.F. Schmitz, and K.C. Holm (1989). 1988 annual report of the American Association of Poison Control Centers National Data Collection System. *American Journal of Emergency Medicine* 7:495–545.

Marzuk, P.M., K. Tardiff, A.C. Leon, M. Stajic, E.B. Morgan, and J. Mann (1990). Prevalence of recent cocaine use among motor vehicle fatalities in New York City. *Journal of the American Medical Association* 263:250–256.

McGuire, F.L., H. Birch, L.A. Gottschalk, J.F. Heiser, and E.C. Dinovo (1976). A comparison of suicide and nonsuicide deaths involving psychotropic drugs in four major U.S. cities. *American Journal of Public Health* 66:1058–1061.

Needleman, H.L. (1989). The persistent threat of lead: A singular opportunity. *American Journal of Public Health* 79:643–645.

Rice, D.P., E.J. MacKenzie, and associates. (1989). *Cost of injury in the United State: A report to Congress*. San Francisco: Institute for Health and Aging, University of California and Injury Prevention Center, The Johns Hopkins University.

Samkoff, J.S., and S.P. Baker (1982). Recent trends in fatal poisoning by opiates in the United States. *American Journal of Public Health* 72:1251–1256.

Trinkoff, A.M., and S.P. Baker (1986). Poisoning hospitalizations and deaths among children and teenagers. *American Journal of Public Health* 76:657–660.

Walton, W.W. (1982). An evaluation of the Poison Prevention Packaging Act. *Pediatrics* 69:363–370.

16

Introduction to Motor Vehicle Crashes

Chapters 8 through 15 highlighted information on many of the major causes of injury death. As important as these are, they are overshadowed by the large numbers of deaths resulting from motor vehicle use. Crashes[1] of motor vehicles are the leading cause of death in the United States for people aged 1–34 (Karpf and Williams 1983). From age 5 to 29, *more than one-fifth of deaths from all causes* are caused by motor vehicles. Motor vehicle crashes account for more than 40 percent of *all* mortality among people in their late teens. They cause more deaths of people aged 1–75 than any other injury-producing event. Figure 16-1 illustrates the similarity between males and

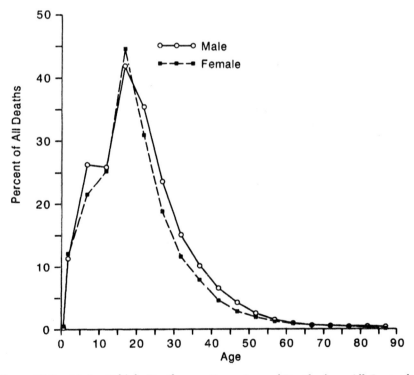

Figure 16-1. Motor Vehicle Deaths as a Percentage of Deaths from All Causes by Age and Sex, 1986 (*Source:* R.S. Karpf and A.F. Williams (1983). Teenage drivers and motor vehicle deaths. *Accident Analysis and Prevention* 15:55–63.)

211

females in the *proportions* of their deaths that are associated with motor vehicles; this similarity is remarkable in view of the fact that motor-vehicle-related death *rates* are much higher for males than for females.

For the entire U.S. population, motor vehicles are associated with more than 500,000 hospital admissions annually (Rice, MacKenzie, and associates 1989) and with 57 percent of all head-injury–associated deaths (Sosin et al. 1989). Motor vehicles have also been found to cause 44 percent of all brain injuries diagnosed by a physician (Kraus et al. 1975), 20 percent of facial injuries treated in emergency rooms (Karlson 1982), and 56 percent of acute spinal cord injuries (Kraus et al. 1975). The annual cost of motor vehicle-related injuries in 1985 dollars is estimated at $48.7 billion, including indirect costs (lost productivity) (Rice, MacKenzie, and associates 1989).

Motor vehicle crashes are also the leading cause of work-related injury deaths; between one-fifth and one-third of all occupational injury fatalities involve road vehicles (see Chapter 9). Nonfatal occupational injuries related to motor vehicles are not well documented, but among 30,000 municipal workers they accounted for one-eighth of all injuries and one-sixth of the costs of all injuries (Runyan and Baker 1988).

In the 1980s, motor vehicle crashes on public roads (sometimes referred to as "in traffic" crashes) have caused between 44,000 and 52,000 deaths and between 4 million and 5 million injuries each year (NCHS 1982; NSC 1982). Approximately half a million of these injuries require hospital admission (Rice, MacKenzie, and associates 1989), involving an average of six days of hospitalization (NHTSA 1988). For most of the population, motor vehicle crashes constitute the single most important component of the overall injury problem.

Yet, motor vehicles are an integral part of our lives. They transport people and goods, provide recreational opportunities, and are used by millions of Americans on their jobs. Although motor vehicles thus provide mobility for much of our society, their widespread use and the speeds at which they travel create the potential (although not the necessity) for injury and death to their occupants and other road users.

Most injuries from motor vehicles result when mechanical energy is conveyed to people in amounts or at rates that exceed their injury thresholds. Contrary to the popular belief that the human body is very fragile, with adequate protection it can withstand high forces without injury. In addition to DeHaven's work (see Chapter 10), early evidence also was provided by Colonel John Stapp, who withstood deceleration in a rocket sled from 632 to 0 mph in 1.4 seconds without serious injury. This was possible because of the relatively long stopping distance involved, the high resistance of the body to transient forces, and the use of a belt harness system that spread the forces over a large body area (Stapp 1955).

Understanding motor vehicle crash injuries and possible countermeasures can be aided by a model developed by Haddon (Haddon 1968, 1980a, 1980b). In what has become known as the "Haddon matrix," the time sequence of a crash is divided into three phases—precrash, crash, and postcrash—and these interact with three sets of crash factors—human,

Table 16-1. Examples of Factors Related to the Likelihood of Injury

Phases	Factors		
	Human	Vehicle	Physical and Social Environment
Precrash	Alcohol intoxication Fatigue Experience and judgment Driver vision Amount of travel	Brakes, tires Center of gravity Jackknife tendency Ease of control Load weight Speed capability	Laws related to alcohol and driving Visibility of hazards Road curvature and gradient Surface coefficient of friction Divided highways, one-way streets Intersections, access control Signalization Speed limits

Crash	Seat belt use
	Age
	Sex
	Osteoporosis
		Speed at impact
		Vehicle size
		Automatic
		  restraints
		Hardness and
		  sharpness of
		  contact surfaces
		Load containment
			Speed limits
			Recovery areas
			Guard rails
			Characteristics of fixed objects
			Median barriers
			Roadside embankments

Postcrash	Age
	Physical condition
		Fuel system
		  integrity
			Emergency communication and
			  transport systems
			Distance to and quality of medical
			  services
			Rehabilitation programs

vehicle, and environment—in a nine-cell matrix (Table 16-1). Each cell of the matrix offers opportunities for intervention to reduce motor vehicle crash injuries. For a thorough discussion of the matrix see Haddon (1968, 1980b). The *precrash phase* includes all of the events that determine whether a crash actually takes place—for example, whether the driver was impaired by alcohol, the vehicle had deficient brakes, or the road lighting was inadequate. The *crash phase* includes factors that determine whether injury occurred in the crash and, if so, its type and severity—for example, whether the occupant was wearing a seat belt, how large the car was, and whether the signpost it struck was designed to yield on impact. The *postcrash phase* includes everything that determines the consequences of the injury—for example, how quickly bleeding can be stopped, whether or not a fire occurs after the crash, how fast the emergency medical system responds, and the availability of good medical care and rehabilitation services.

For decades, most intervention efforts focused on the precrash phase, especially efforts to change driving behavior in order to prevent crashes from occurring. Although there is an important role for this approach, concentration exclusively on any one matrix cell is inappropriate. Moreover, many efforts to reduce injuries by changing human behavior have had little success. In the last 20–25 years, a more balanced approach has been adopted, one that incorporates many countermeasures aimed at changing events in the crash and postcrash phases, as well as preventing crashes through measures aimed at driver and pedestrian behavior and vehicle and environmental design.

The basic Haddon matrix approach to identifying countermeasure opportunities can be adapted to other types of injuries and has been applied to such diverse problems as drowning, burns, rape, asphyxiation by food, and injuries from machines (Dietz 1977; Dietz and Baker 1974; Feck et al. 1978; Haddon 1980a; Harris et al. 1984).

The 10 basic strategies described in Chapter 7 provide an alternative framework for considering motor vehicle injuries and relevant countermeasures. For detailed discussions of the subject of crash injury prevention see Haddon (1980a, 1980b, 1975), Haddon and Baker (1981), Haddon et al. (1964), IIHS (1981), and Robertson (1983).

Two data sources provide detailed national information on virtually all traffic deaths: the NCHS mortality file and the Fatal Accident Reporting System (FARS) of the National Highway Traffic Safety Administration (NHTSA). These sources agree closely as to the total number of deaths. NCHS data are used for all analyses by race, place of residence, or income level in *The Injury Fact Book* because FARS data do not indicate race and generally specify place of residence only for drivers. In other respects, FARS records provide greater detail and therefore are used in most analyses of motor vehicle traffic deaths in Chapters 16–21.

Except where otherwise noted, the information presented in Chapters 16–21 pertains to deaths or injuries that result from crashes on public roads (these are often referred to as "in traffic" crashes). In addition to the 45,000–50,000 such deaths each year, NCHS mortality data include 1,200 people killed by road vehicles in nontraffic situations—for example, off road, in driveways, on private roads, and at worksites.

Compared to deaths, nonfatal injuries are not as clearly defined or as easily enumerated. The best national estimates of the incidence of nonfatal injuries are based on samples, such as NCHS's National Health Interview Survey (NHIS) or NHTSA's National Accident Sampling System (NASS). NHIS provides only limited information on motor vehicle crash injuries, which are a subset of an annual national sample of health conditions. NASS, a relatively recent data collection system, is more detailed; it is designed to provide a representative national sample of police-reported crashes. In addition, estimates of the incidence of specific categories of motor vehicle-related injuries have been obtained from several population-based regional studies (Table 16-2).

Hospital-based research reveals significant underreporting of nonfatal injuries by most official statistics. A major study of injuries in northeastern Ohio, for example, found that the number of people injured in traffic

Table 16-2. Estimates of the Incidence of Motor Vehicle Injuries from Population-Based Regional Studies

Types of Injury Studied	Population and Year of Injury	Motor Vehicle Injuries Per 100,000 Study Population Per Year	Total Number Projected to 1980 U.S. Population	Percentage of Injuries Studied Caused by Motor Vehicles
Injury requiring emergency room treatment[a] (Barancik et al. 1983	5 counties in northeastern Ohio, 1977	2,071 injuries	4,690,000	10
Facial injury treated in emergency room[a] (Karlson 1982)	Dane County, Wisconsin, June 1978-May 1979	278 facial injuries including 169 lacerations, 28 fractures	630,000 (383,000) (63,000)	20 20 26
Brain injury diagnosed by a physician[b] (Kraus et al. 1984)	San Diego County California, 1981	79 brain injuries	179,000	44
Acute spinal cord injury[b] (SCI) (Kraus et al. 1975)	18 counties in California, 1970-1971	3 spinal cord injuries	6,800	56
Burns, including scalds, resulting in hospitalization (Feck and Baptiste 1979)	New York State, excluding New York City, 1974-1975	1.6 burns	3,700	6

[a]Also includes hospital admissions and deaths.
[b]All cases were admitted to hospitals and/or died.

collisions and treated in emergency rooms was 43 percent greater than the total number of injured people known from police accident reports (Barancik et al. 1983). Because police reports include many injured people who did not receive emergency room treatment, the actual discrepancy is probably even greater.

Injuries related to motor vehicles but not involving crashes are generally identifiable only from surveys, medical records, or death certificates rather than from police reports. Examples include carbon monoxide poisoning (see Chapter 15), scalds and chemical burns from radiators and batteries, flame burns from ignited upholstery or other fires in cars, broken fingers caught in doors, and injuries in sudden stops (Agran et al. 1985; Feck et al. 1978).

This chapter describes motor vehicle death rates and compares fatalities in major types of crashes. It also provides summaries by income and place of residence. Tabulations by age, sex, and state are introduced here and are presented in greater detail in Chapters 17 through 21. The latter chapters add detailed analyses on the circumstances of crashes, based primarily on data from FARS and NASS.

AGE AND SEX

Motor vehicle death rates vary tremendously by age and sex, with the highest peak in the late teenage years and early twenties (Figure 16-2). After

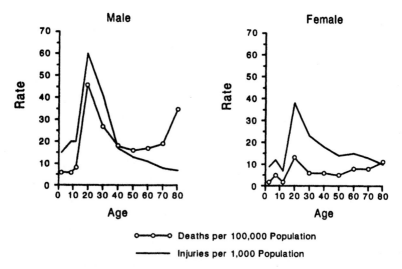

Figure 16-2.   Motor Vehicle Crash Injury and Death Rates by Age and Sex, Northeastern Ohio, Emergency Room Visits in 1977 and Deaths in 1976–1978 (*Source:* J.I. Barancik, and B.F. Chatterjee (1984). Northeastern Ohio Trauma Study: II. Injury rates by age, sex, and cause. *American Journal of Public Health* 74:473–478. Reprinted with the permission of the publisher.)

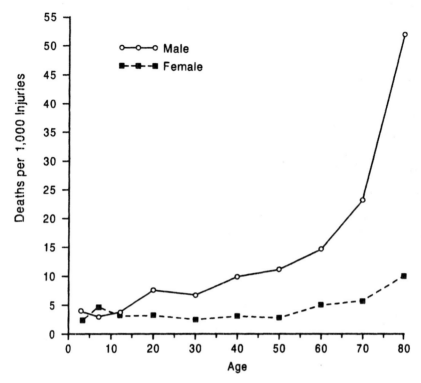

Figure 16-3. Deaths per 1,000 Motor Vehicle Crash Injuries by Age and Sex, Northeastern Ohio, Emergency Room Visits in 1977 and Deaths in 1976–1978 (*Source:* J.I. Barancik, and B.F. Chatterjee (1984). Northeastern Ohio Trauma Study: II. Injury rates by age, sex, and cause. *American Journal of Public Health* 74:473–478. Reprinted with the permission of the publisher.)

that, death rates decline, then increase again beginning at about age 65. Males sustain fatal injuries much more frequently than females, especially in their twenties. The ratio of male to female death rates is 2.8 to 1 for all ages combined and almost 4 to 1 for ages 20–29. The only age at which there is little sex difference is during the first year of life, when almost all the deaths are to vehicle occupants. The drop in occupant death rates after the first year of life (Figure 4-6) is not evident in Figure 16-2 because the latter includes pedestrian deaths, which are a significant cause of death for toddlers.

As in the case of fatality rates, the rates for motor vehicle crash injuries treated in emergency rooms are highest for ages 15–24 (Figure 16-2). Injury rates are higher for males than for females between the ages of 1 and 35, but the male–female differences are not as pronounced for injuries as for deaths. After about age 15, injuries to males tend to be more severe than injuries to females. Then the ratio of deaths to injuries for males jumps sharply, reflecting the greater injury severity, and among adults it is from two to three times as high as the female death to injury ratio (Figure 16-3).

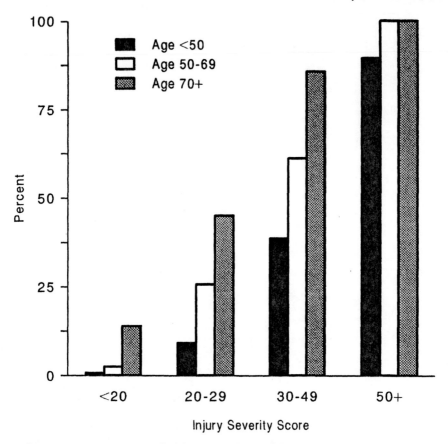

Figure 16-4.   Percentage of Patients Hospitalized for Motor Vehicle Crash Injuries Who Died by Injury Severity Score and Age, Eight Hospitals in Baltimore, 1968–1969

Older people have the highest ratio of deaths to injuries because of their greater susceptibility to complications when injured and their substantially poorer prognosis. This effect is greatest for the least severe injuries. Minor injuries that are rarely fatal in younger people result in significant mortality at ages 70 and older, whereas for the most severe injuries age plays a less important role in survival. Figure 16-4 illustrates this effect, using a measure of injury severity, the Injury Severity Score (ISS), which assesses the overall severity of multiple injuries (AAAM 1990; Baker et al. 1974).

It is common for motor vehicle crash deaths to be discussed as though they all result from similar events—usually two-car crashes with occupant deaths. In fact, many types of motor vehicle crashes occur, and it is misleading to describe them as if they were alike. Crashes can involve occupants of a single vehicle or multiple vehicles of different types, as well as pedes-

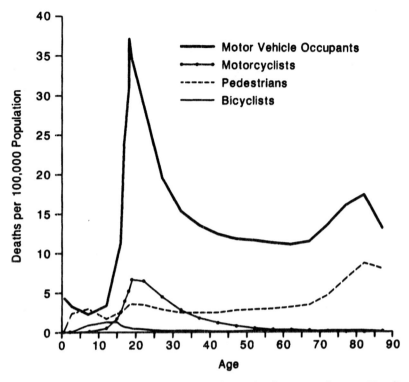

Figure 16-5. Death Rates from Motor Vehicle Crashes by Age and Type of Fatality, 1980–1986

trians, motorcyclists, and bicyclists. Generally, the characteristics of the people involved in different kinds of crashes vary considerably.

Death rates for the various types of crashes show distinctive age patterns (Figure 16-5). The rates by single year of age were shown in Figures 4-3 through 4-6. Bicyclist death rates peak at age 14, occupant rates at age 18, and motorcyclist rates at age 21. Pedestrian death rates are highest after age 70, with lower peaks at ages 6 and 18–21. The relative importance of each category of motor vehicle fatality varies with age (Figure 16-6). For each of the seven broad age groups in Figure 16-6, motor vehicle occupants are the largest category. Pedestrian deaths are prominent among the elderly and among children less than 15 years old, and they account for almost half of all motor vehicle-related deaths of 5–9-year-old children (not separately shown). Among the major types of fatal crashes, bicyclists account for the fewest deaths, but they represent about one-sixth of all motor vehicle-related deaths between the ages of 5 and 14. Among ages 15–34, motorcyclists account for more than one-tenth of such deaths.

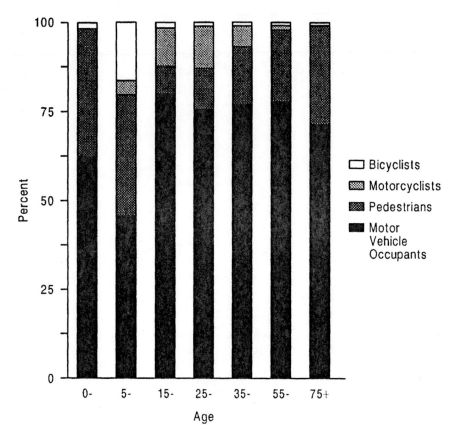

Figure 16-6. Percentage of Motor Vehicle Deaths by Age and Type of Fatality,
1980–1988

RACE AND PER CAPITA INCOME

Death rates from motor vehicle crashes vary tremendously by race and per
capita income. Native Americans have the highest death rates from all types
of motor vehicle crashes combined—42 per 100,000, compared with 20 for
whites, 17 for blacks, and 11 for Asians. In addition, age patterns vary
among racial groups (Figure 16-7). Death rates peak for whites at ages 15–24
and for Native Americans and blacks at ages 20–24. Between ages 30 and 65
the death rates for blacks and Asians are relatively constant, while the rates
for whites and Native Americans decrease. The rates among the elderly
increase for all four racial groups.

Whites have the highest death rates from motorcycle crashes; Native
Americans have only slightly lower rates, and they have the highest rates as
occupants and pedestrians. Asians have the lowest rates in all categories

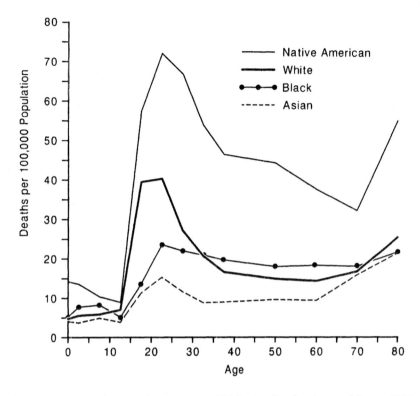

Figure 16-7.   Death Rates from Motor Vehicle Crashes by Age and Race, 1980–1986

(Figure 16-8), although their death rates as occupants and bicyclists have increased in the past decade.

The factors underlying these differences need further exploration. Although racial differences in injury rates have sometimes been attributed to different patterns of alcohol use, additional factors play a role. For example, for Native Americans living on reservations, there is very limited public transportation, most roads are rural and without pedestrian areas, and riding in the open cargo compartment of a pickup truck is a common practice (Simpson et al. 1983).

When analyses for whites and blacks are further separated by age and sex as well as by type of fatality, it is clear that the teenage peaks in occupant and motorcyclist death rates are the highest for white males (Figure 16-9). In contrast, the teenage peaks in bicyclist death rates are virtually the same for black and white males.

The occupant death rate for black males exceeds that for white males from about age 35 to age 74, while at other ages it is higher for white males. For females the occupant death rate for whites is higher at all ages. Pedes-

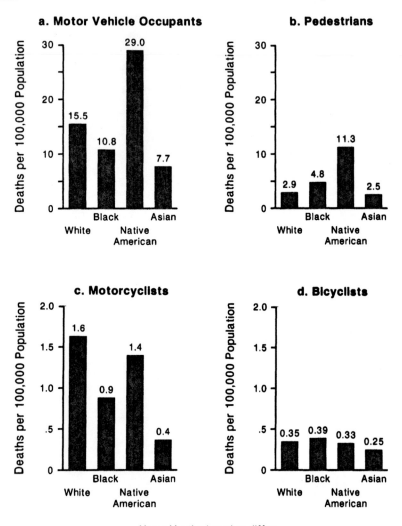

Note: Vertical scales differ

Figure 16-8. Death Rates from Motor Vehicle Crashes by Race and Type of Fatality, 1980–1986

trian death rates are substantially higher for blacks except at ages 15–19 (both sexes) and for 10–14-year-old females.

Motor vehicle death rates generally decrease as income in the area of residence increases (Figure 16-10). For occupants, the death rate in counties where the annual per capita income is less than $6,000 is almost three times the rate in counties where the average income is $14,000 or more. The inverse relationship is true for all major racial groups (Baker et al. 1984).

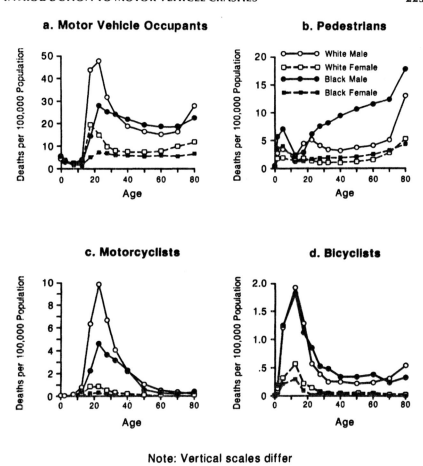

Figure 16-9.   Death Rates from Motor Vehicle Crashes by Age, Race, Sex, and Type of Fatality, 1980–1986

The higher occupant death rates in lower-income areas are not explained by differences in the amount of motor vehicle travel, since the Nationwide Personal Transportation Study (NPTS) found that the amount of travel per person more than doubles as per capita income increases from $4,000 to $20,000 (Carsten and Weber 1981). It is likely that poorly designed and maintained roads in many low-income areas, older vehicles, different driving practices, differences in alcohol use, and inadequate emergency and medical care all contribute to the higher death rates. One observational study found that adult drivers in high-income areas used seat belts at three times the rate of adult drivers in low-income areas. The difference was even greater among teenage drivers (Wells et al. 1990).

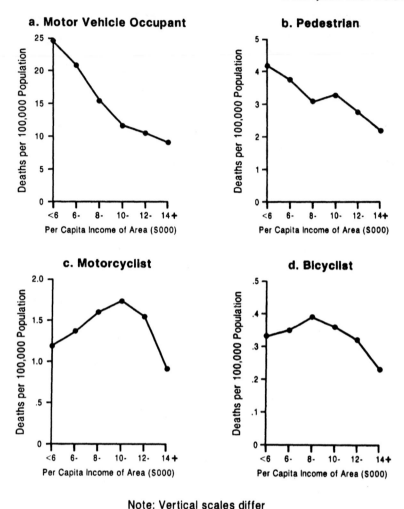

Note: Vertical scales differ

Figure 16-10. Death Rates from Motor Vehicle Crashes by per Capita Income of Area of Residence and Type of Fatality, 1980–1986

URBAN/RURAL AND GEOGRAPHIC DIFFERENCES

Motor vehicle death rates are almost twice as high among residents of the most rural areas as in central cities and metropolitan areas of a million or more, increasing from 17 per 100,000 population to 31 in the most rural areas. These differences reflect the major contribution of occupant deaths; death rates of pedestrians and motorcyclists are highest for residents of central cities (Figure 16-11). In the late 1970s, the most recent period for which rates have been calculated by race and census tract, occupant death

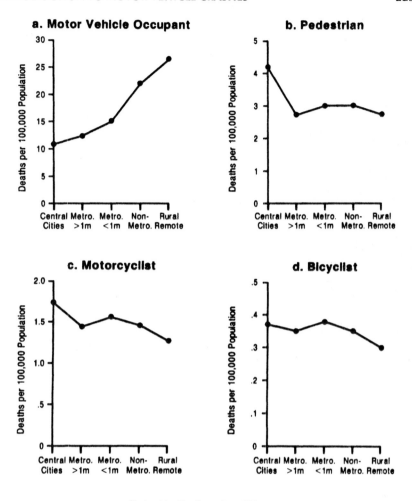

Note: Vertical scales differ

Figure 16-11.   Death Rates from Motor Vehicle Crashes by Place of Residence and Type of Fatality, 1980–1986

rates among whites in the most rural areas were three times the rates in the largest cities, and for blacks there was a fivefold difference. Pedestrian death rates were highest in large cities for whites, but the reverse was true for blacks. For motorcyclists, death rates were highest among whites in metropolitan areas, whereas for bicyclists rates were highest among black residents of very rural areas (Baker et al. 1984).

In addition to differences by population density, there are large differences in motor vehicle death rates among states. The geographic patterns in these rates differ among the four major categories of motor vehicle-

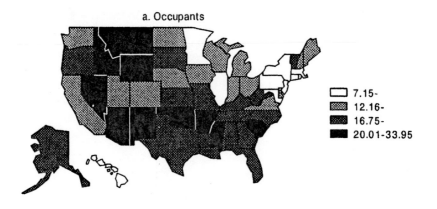

a. Occupants

7.15-
12.16-
16.75-
20.01-33.95

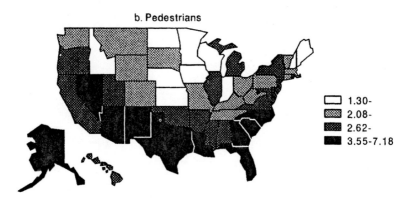

b. Pedestrians

1.30-
2.08-
2.62-
3.55-7.18

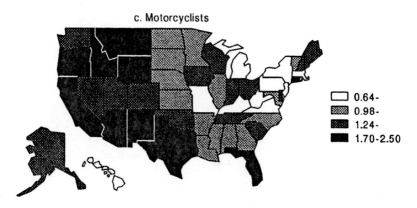

c. Motorcyclists

0.64-
0.98-
1.24-
1.70-2.50

Figure 16-12. Death Rates from Motor Vehicle Crashes by State, per 100,000 Population, 1980–1986

d. Bicyclists

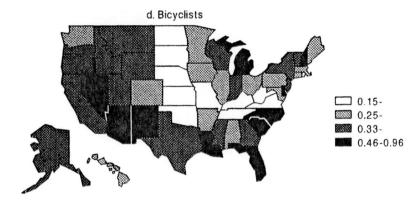

	0.15-
	0.25-
	0.33-
	0.46-0.96

Figure 16-12.   Continued

related deaths (Figure 16-12). Occupant death rates are generally lowest in the Northeast and highest in western and southern states. Pedestrian death rates are especially high in the Southeast and Southwest and in states such as New York with large urban populations; motorcyclist death rates are generally highest in western states. Bicyclist deaths, however, show less clear regional patterns.[2]

In general, geographic patterns for rates calculated for resident deaths per 100,000 population are similar to those for deaths per 100 million vehicle miles traveled in each state, indicating that variations in the amount of travel do not substantially account for the geographic variations shown in Figure 16–12.

HISTORICAL TRENDS

During the past half century, the overall motor vehicle death rate per 100,000 population has not shown the major changes that are apparent for many other causes of death (Figure 4-16). Rates for some separate categories of motor vehicle deaths, however, have changed dramatically (Figure 16-13). The pedestrian death rate, for example, decreased by more than half between 1930 and 1960. The motorcyclist death rate increased fivefold from 1960 to 1980, then decreased by 18 percent. The occupant death rate has varied over time, but in 1986 it was only 5 percent lower than in 1930 (Table 4-2).

Although motor vehicle deaths are increasingly viewed as a public health problem, they are also viewed as a transportation problem. The latter viewpoint usually focuses on deaths per vehicle mile traveled rather than on the population-based death rates. As travel has increased (Figure 16-14), the mileage-based death rate has declined steadily from about 16 deaths per

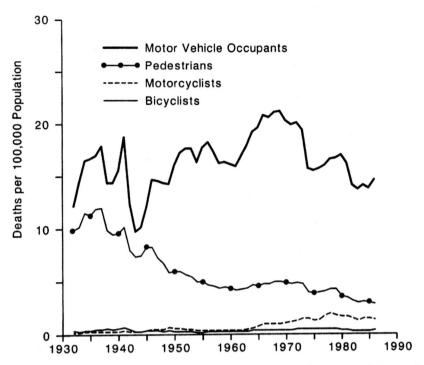

Figure 16-13. Death Rates from Motor Vehicle Crashes by Year and Type of Fatality, 1932–1986

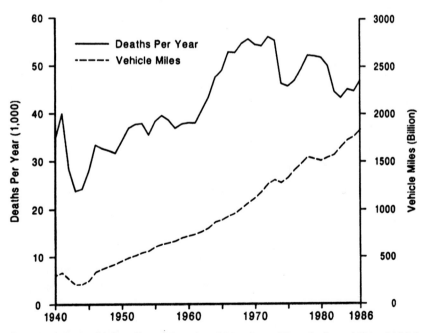

Figure 16-14. Vehicle Miles of Travel and Number of Deaths from Motor Vehicle Injuries, 1940–1986

100,000 vehicle miles of travel in the early 1930s to a rate of less than 3 by 1982.

Vehicle mileage is a useful indicator of exposure to risk for some purposes, but has significant limitations; for example, vehicle mileage is a poor indicator of pedestrian exposure. Even for motor vehicle occupants the exposure to risk varies with both the amount and type of travel; death rates associated with rural mileage, for example, are higher than rates associated with relatively low-speed urban mileage. Some of these effects were illustrated in 1974 when total vehicle travel decreased by about 1.5 percent compared with 1973 as a result of gasoline shortages, but deaths declined by more than 16 percent (Figure 16-14). In this case, substantial decreases in average travel speeds also occurred as a result of the adoption of 55 mile per hour speed limits. Studies have shown that the lower speed limits were responsible for about half of the reduction in deaths occurring after 1973 (Mela 1977).

NOTES

1. The terms *crash* and *collision* are used interchangeably in this book. Unless otherwise specified, both terms include multiple-vehicle, single-vehicle, motorcycle, bicycle, and pedestrian collisions, as well as other motor vehicle crashes.

2. Figure 16-12, based on FARS data for the state in which the crash occurred, differs from death rates in the Appendix, based on NCHS data for the place of residence of the deceased.

REFERENCES

Agran, P.F., D.E. Dunkle, and D. Winn (1985). Noncrash motor vehicle accidents: Injuries to children in the vehicle interior. *American Journal of Diseases of Children* 139:304–306.

Association for the Advancement of Automotive Medicine (1990). *The Abbreviated Injury Scale, 1990 revision*. Des Plaines, IL: AAAM.

Baker, S.P., B. O'Neill, W. Haddon, Jr., and W.B. Long (1974). The Injury Severity Score: A method for describing patients with multiple injuries and evaluating emergency care. *Journal of Trauma* 14:187–196.

Baker, S.P., B. O'Neill, and R. Karpf (1984). *The injury fact book*. Lexington, MA: Lexington Press.

Barancik, J.I., B.F. Chatterjee, Y.C. Greene, E.M. Michenzi, and D. Fife (1983). Northeastern Ohio Trauma Study: I. Magnitude of the problem. *American Journal of Public Health* 73:746–751.

Carsten, O., and K. Weber (1981). Child and adult travel exposure and fatality risk. In *Proceedings of the Twenty-Fifth Conference of the American Association for Automotive Medicine*. Arlington Heights, IL: American Association for Automotive Medicine.

Dietz, P.E. (1977). Social factors in rapist behavior. In R. Rada (Ed.), *Clinical aspects of the rapist*. New York: Grune and Stratton.

Dietz, P.E., and S.P. Baker (1974). Drowning: Epidemiology and prevention. *American Journal of Public Health* 64:303–312.

Feck, G.A., M.S. Baptiste, and C.L. Tate, Jr. (1978). *An epidemiologic study of burn injuries and strategies for prevention.* Atlanta, GA: U.S. Department of Health and Human Services, Public Health Service, Centers for Disease Control.

Fife, D., J. I. Barancik, and B. F. Chatterjee (1984). Northeastern Ohio Trauma Study: II. Injury rates by age, sex, and cause. *American Journal of Public Health* 74:473–478.

Haddon, W., Jr. (1968). The changing approach to the epidemiology, prevention, and amelioration of trauma: The transition to approaches etiologically rather than descriptively based. *American Journal of Public Health* 58: 1431–1438.

Haddon, W., Jr. (1975). Reducing the damage of motor-vehicle use. *Technology Review* 77:1–9.

Haddon, W., Jr. (1980a). Advances in the epidemiology of injuries as a basis for public policy. *Public Health Reports* 95:411–421.

Haddon, W., Jr. (1980b). Options for the prevention of motor vehicle crash injury *Israel Journal of Medical Sciences* 16:45–68.

Haddon, W., Jr., and S.P. Baker (1981). Injury control. In D. Clark and B. Mac-Mahon (Eds.), *Preventive and community medicine.* Boston: Little, Brown, pp. 109–140.

Haddon, W., Jr., E.A. Suchman, and D. Klein (1964). *Accident research: Methods and approaches.* New York: Harper & Row.

Harris, C.S., S.P. Baker, G.A. Smith, and R.M. Harris (1984). Childhood asphyxiation by food: A national analysis and overview. *Journal of the American Medical Association* 251:2231–2235.

Insurance Institute for Highway Safety (1981). *Policy options for reducing the motor vehicle crash injury cost burden.* Washington, DC: Insurance Institute for Highway Safety.

Karlson, T.A. (1982). The incidence of hospital-treated facial injuries from vehicles. *Journal of Trauma* 22:303–310.

Karpf, R.S., and A.F. Williams (1983). Teenage drivers and motor vehicle deaths. *Accident Analysis and Prevention* 15:55–63.

Kraus, J.F., M.A. Black, N. Hessol, P. Ley, W. Rokaw, C. Sullivan, S. Bowers, S. Knowlton, and L. Marshall (1984). The incidence of acute brain injury and serious impairment in a defined population. *American Journal of Epidemiology* 119:186–201.

Kraus, J.F., C.E. Franti, R.S. Riggins, D. Richards, and N.O. Borhani (1975). Incidence of traumatic spinal cord lesions. *Journal of Chronic Diseases* 28:471–492.

Mela, D.F. (1977). *Review of information on the safety effects of the 55 mph speed limit in the U.S.* Technical Report DOT HS-802-383. Washington, DC: National Highway Traffic Safety Administration.

National Center for Health Statistics (1982). Persons injured by class of accident and whether activity restricting, 1981. Unpublished data from the National Health Interview Survey.

National Highway Traffic Safety Administration (1988). *National accident sampling system 1986: A report on traffic crashes and injuries in the United States.* Washington, DC: U.S. Department of Transportation.

National Safety Council (1982). *Accident facts, 1982 edition*. Chicago: National Safety Council.

Rice, D.P., E.J. MacKenzie, and associates (1989). *Cost of injury in the United States: A report to Congress*. San Francisco: Institute for Health and Aging, University of California and Injury Prevention Center, The Johns Hopkins University.

Robertson, L.S. (1983). *Injuries: Causes, control strategies, and public policy*. Lexington, MA: Lexington Books.

Runyan, C.W., and S.P. Baker (1988). Occupational motor vehicle injury morbidity among municipal employees. *Journal of Occupational Medicine* 30:883–886.

Simpson, S.G., R. Reid, S.P. Baker, and S.P. Teret (1983). Injuries among the Hopi Indians, a population-based survey. *Journal of the American Medical Association* 249:1873–1876.

Sosin, D.M., J.J. Sacks, and S.M. Smith (1989). Head injury-associated deaths in the United States from 1979 to 1986. *Journal of the American Medical Association* 262:2251–2255.

Stapp, J.P. (1955). Effects of mechanical force on living tissues. I. Abrupt deceleration and windblast. *Journal of Aviation Medicine* 26:268–287.

Wells, J.K., A.F. Williams, and N.J. Teed (1990). Belt use among high school students. Excerpted in *National Association of Secondary School Principals News Leader* 38:8.

17

Motor Vehicle Occupants

Injuries to passenger vehicle occupants are the predominant cause of motor vehicle crash deaths. In recent years more than 70 percent of all traffic-related deaths were to people injured as occupants of passenger vehicles.[1] Among 15- to 24-year-old males, one out of every three deaths from *all* causes (disease as well as injury) results from injuries as a motor vehicle occupant.

Preventing or reducing the severity of occupant injury in crashes is analogous to protecting breakable items that are going to be mailed. The box for mailing should be sturdy—a flimsy box that collapses if dropped will not prevent damage—and it should be sealed so that it does not pop open and spill the contents if it is dropped. The inside of the box should be free of sharp protrusions (e.g., exposed nails), and the contents should be surrounded by energy-absorbing packing so that they cannot rattle around loose inside. This way, if the box is dropped or even partially crushed, the forces reaching the breakable goods will be reduced and spread over a wide area, reducing the likelihood of damage.

Similarly, to protect vehicle occupants, it is important that the passenger compartment be strong and resist intrusion in crashes. To help keep the occupants inside the vehicle, the doors should stay closed and the windshield should *not* pop out in a crash. The inside of the compartment should be free of hard rigid features that could injure an occupant, and, to the extent possible, it should be padded with energy-absorbing materials. Finally, because occupants cannot be completely surrounded by energy-absorbing materials, they should be restrained to prevent them from striking parts of the compartment that could cause injuries. As in the case of packaging breakable items, the objective is to reduce the crash forces reaching the occupants and also to spread the forces that do reach them over as wide an area of the body as possible.

The dimensions and characteristics of the vehicle exterior influence the crash forces that reach the occupant compartment. In frontal crashes, when the front end of the vehicle hits something solid it will begin crushing and absorbing some of the energy, but the occupant compartment does not stop moving forward until the front end is no longer being crushed. In general, this means that the greater the length of the front end that crushes, the lower the deceleration of the occupant compartment.

By using some of the space between the hard structure of the compartment and the occupants, the forces experienced by the occupants can be lowered even further. Energy-absorbing padding on the dashboard and energy-absorbing steering columns, for example, are used to absorb some of the crash forces. To further reduce decelerative forces on the occupants, lap/shoulder belts effectively couple occupants to the compartment, and, because they stretch somewhat during a crash, they actually decelerate the occupants at a lower rate than the compartment itself.

Lap/shoulder belts, when worn correctly, reduce the chances of occupant death in a crash by about 45 percent (Evans 1986; NHTSA 1984). The actual lifesaving benefits of seat belts, however, are severely limited by the fact that many occupants do not wear them. In fact, seat belt use is least common among people who are at greatest risk of being in crashes, such as teenagers and residents of low income areas (O'Neill et al. 1983; Wells et al. 1990; Williams and O'Neill 1979; Williams et al. 1983). Belt use tends to be lower among groups of drivers exhibiting behaviors that increase crash involvement, such as consuming alcohol and driving fast (Preusser et al. 1986, 1988, in press).

Despite extensive efforts to educate and persuade motorists to buckle up, voluntary seat belt use rates have remained low around the world. Only in some jurisdictions with laws requiring use have high levels of belt wearing been achieved. During the 1980s, many states passed laws requiring seat belt use, and by 1990, 37 states had such laws. Where surveys have been conducted in these states, there is an overall usage rate of about 47 percent among occupants covered by the law (Campbell et al. 1988). Most states exempt people in rear seating positions and in large trucks, and some even exempt occupants of pickup trucks and multipurpose vehicles. In general, states with primary belt use law enforcement (i.e., where drivers can be charged with violating a seat belt law even if there is no other traffic violation) have higher usage rates than those with secondary enforcement (i.e., where drivers must first be stopped for a traffic violation). Among the first eight states to pass seat belt laws, fatality rates of front seat occupants declined by almost 10 percent in states with primary enforcement compared with 7 percent in states with secondary enforcement (Wagenaar et al. 1988). In North Carolina, belt use jumped to 78 percent soon after the belt use law was passed but gradually declined to 64 percent. The increased use resulted in a 12 percent reduction in deaths and a 15 percent reduction in serious injuries (Reinfurt and Campbell 1990). In jurisdictions where seat belt laws are not publicized and enforced, belt use levels tend to be only slightly higher than they were before the laws. It has been demonstrated in the United States and Canada that programs of well-publicized enforcement of belt laws can produce use rates in excess of 80 percent (Jonah and Grant 1985; Williams and Lund 1986, 1988; Williams et al. 1987). In addition to laws, strategies to increase seat belt use include incentives, rewards, and reminders, but their long-term effectiveness after termination of such programs has not been demonstrated (Geller 1988).

Seat belts can protect occupants only when they are used. Counter-measures such as seat belts that require some action and cooperation on the part of occupants are termed "active." Many other types of occupant protection features that require no action on the part of occupants are built into modern cars. Examples of such "passive" or automatic protection include energy-absorbing steering columns, padded dashboards and pillars, high-penetration resistant windshields, and nonadjustable head restraints. These features are effective in preventing many injuries, especially in the less serious crashes, but additional protection is needed.

Public health officials and researchers have long advocated other types of automatic protection to prevent injuries, especially in frontal crashes, which are the most common fatal crashes (Figure 17-1). Two basic design approaches have been developed to provide such automatic crash protection in frontal crashes—air bags and automatic seat belts. This kind of auto-matic crash protection for the driver and right front seat passenger has been required for new passenger cars beginning with a phased-in program for 1987 models and for all cars beginning with the 1990 model year. (Manufac-turers choosing to use air bags for the driver side have an additional four years before automatic protection is required for the right front passenger position.) Automatic belts, which are automatically positioned around the occupant when the doors are closed or when the ignition is turned on, are intended to produce higher levels of use than has been achieved with manual belts.

There are three basic automatic belt designs. One has a motorized shoulder belt that moves around a track above the door, and the second has a shoulder belt connected to the door. For both of these designs, lower body restraint in frontal crashes is provided automatically by special energy-absorbing padding in the knee area, but for protection comparable to that provided by a lap/shoulder belt a manual lap belt still needs to be fastened. The third design has both the lap and shoulder portions attached to the door.

In general, cars with automatic belts have higher levels of use than corresponding cars with manual belts. However, in cars with motorized shoulder belts, use of the manual lap belts is low. Cars with the automatic lap/shoulder belts have the lowest levels of use among cars with automatic belts (Reinfurt et al. 1990; Streff and Molnar 1990).

The other approach to automatic crash protection—the air bag—is superior to automatic seat belts. Air bags offer protection to front seat occupants in frontal crashes of moderate and higher severity (IIHS 1979a, 1979b). Cars with air bags are also equipped with lap/shoulder belts. The combination of an air bag plus a lap/shoulder belt is the best occupant protection yet developed, offering additional protection beyond that provided by the belt alone, especially to occupants' faces, heads, and chests in more serious frontal crashes. The percentage of drivers using manual seat belts is as high in cars with air bags as in comparable cars without air bags (Williams et al. 1990).

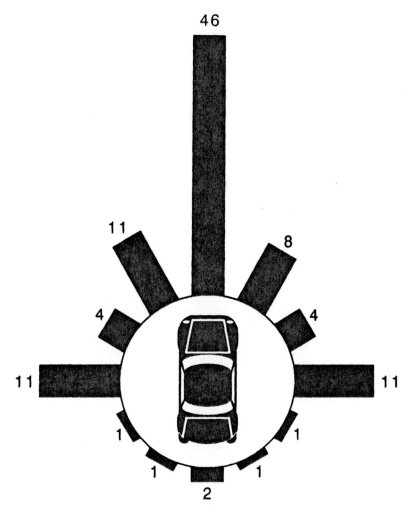

Figure 17-1. Percentage Distribution of Fatally Injured Passenger Vehicle Occupants by Direction of Impact, 1980–1986

The basic components of an air bag system are one or more crash sensors, inflators, and fabric bags. The sensors determine whether a frontal or front-corner crash is of sufficient violence that the air bag should be activated. The inflators, when triggered by the crash sensors, produce harmless nitrogen gas that inflates bags stored out of sight in the center of the steering wheel and in the instrument panel on the passenger side. In a crash, the bags are inflated in a fraction of a second to provide a relatively soft, energy-absorbing cushion between the occupants and the hard structures in front of them.

Because of their small size, infants and small children need special infant or child restraints that are designed to work with adult seat belts.

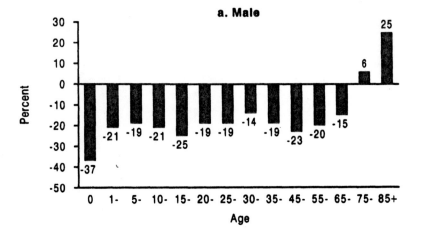

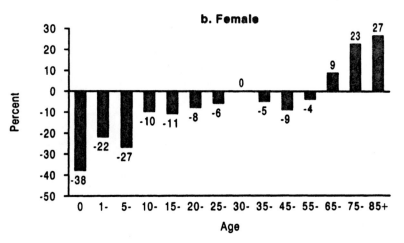

Figure 17-2. Percentage Change in Death Rates for Motor Vehicle Occupants by Age and Sex, 1984–1986 Compared with 1977–1979

For infants, these restraints face rearward and are held in place by the adult seat belt, with the infant belted in a semireclining position. The restraints for older children are typically forward facing with the child sitting upright in a seat with a belt harness and the seat anchored with an adult seat belt. When worn correctly, these restraints are very effective (Partyka 1988). As with seat belts for adults, lack of use of infant and child restraints is a problem. In addition, incorrect use, especially failure to correctly attach the child restraint to the car or to secure the child properly within the seat, greatly reduces their effectiveness.

    Laws requiring restraint use by children have been enacted in all states and have increased observed child restraint use in infants and toddlers from

23 percent in 1981 to 81 percent in 1988; however, child restraints often are not used correctly, and consequently the protection afforded is reduced (Datta and Guzek 1990; Ziegler 1989). In California and Michigan, the law was associated with a decrease in injuries in children less than age 4, including 17–25 percent reductions in head injuries (Agran et al. 1987; Margolis et al. 1988). Nationally, the occupant death rate of children less than 1 year of age decreased by 38 percent between 1980 and 1986 (Figure 17-2). Although it is difficult to prove that the reduction resulted from the adoption of child restraint laws (Wagenaar et al. 1987), the fact that the greatest reduction in death rates occurred in the youngest children is consistent with the greater use of child restraints by this age group.

AGE AND SEX

Very large age and sex differences exist in the death and injury rates for passenger vehicle occupants, with young males having especially high rates. Some of these differences are due to variations in the amount and type of travel and the consequent exposure to risk. Data from the Nationwide Personal Transportation Survey show that the greater amount of travel by males contributes to their high death and injury rates. However, even when variations in the amount of travel are taken into consideration by calculating rates per person mile, the death and injury rates for males are still substantially higher than those for females after about age 10. For both sexes, the peaks for ages 16–19 remain prominent even when amount of travel is controlled for.

The higher death rates for males probably reflect differences in speed, alcohol use, and other variables related to serious crashes and high fatality rates. Compared to fatal crashes of female drivers, those involving male drivers are more likely to be single-vehicle crashes or nighttime crashes, which typically are very severe (Figure 17-3). As drivers, males account for 70 percent of miles driven and 70 percent of drivers in crashes, but 77 percent of the drivers in fatal crashes. Thus, the amount of travel appears to explain more of the sex difference in crash rates than in death rates.

Exposure not only explains some of the variations in death rates but also is a factor that can be manipulated to reduce injuries and deaths. Some states have curfew laws that prohibit driving by beginning young drivers during certain nighttime hours. Such laws have substantially reduced crashes of 16-year-olds (Preusser et al. 1984). Similarly, the very availability of high school driver education courses influences many teenagers to drive sooner than they would otherwise, thereby increasing the amount of driving by this very high-risk group. In some communities, large reductions in teenage crashes followed decreases in licensure and driving by 16-year-olds when high school driver education courses were discontinued (Robertson 1980).

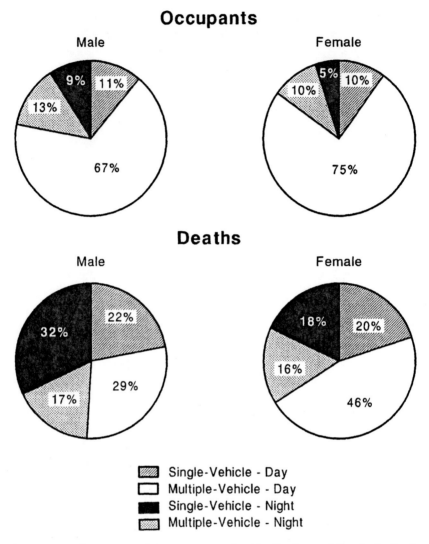

Figure 17-3.   Percentage of Occupants Involved in Crashes and Deaths in Crashes
by Sex, Time of Day, and Number of Vehicles, 1980–1988 (Deaths), 1982–1986
(Crashes)

Fatal crash involvement rates per 10,000 licensed drivers for both multi-
ple- and single-vehicle crashes are highest for 18-year-old drivers and lowest
for drivers aged 45–64 (Figure 17-4). The involvement rate for drivers 70
years and older increases in multiple-vehicle crashes at junctions or intersections. This finding suggests age-related changes in the ability to perceive,
gauge the speed of, and respond to the movements of other vehicles. Despite
such changes, the fatal crash involvement rate of drivers 70 years and older
(2.8 per 10,000 licensed drivers) is lower than the average involvement rate

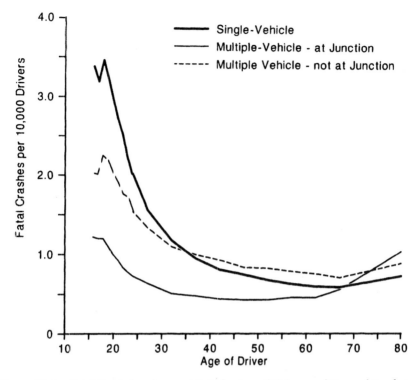

Figure 17-4. Fatal Crash Involvement Rate by Age of Driver and Type of Crash per 10,000 Licensed Drivers, 1980–1987

(3.0) for drivers of all ages combined. The higher mortality rates among elderly drivers compared to middle-aged drivers probably reflect their lower injury thresholds and greater likelihood of complications following injury, as well as increases in certain types of crashes.

URBAN/RURAL AND GEOGRAPHIC DIFFERENCES

Occupant death rates in all types of crashes combined are highest in the southern and western parts of the United States (Figure 16-12a). Mapping by county shows that the counties with the fewest people per square mile have the highest death rates (Baker et al. 1987). The high rates in rural areas in part reflect poorer roads and trauma services but are also strongly influenced by the higher speeds involved in many rural crashes. High blood alcohol concentrations, however, are not more common among occupants killed in rural areas (Mathematical Analyses Division 1989).

The geographic patterns vary for different types of crashes. For example, death rates from collisions with trains, which kill about 600 motor vehicle occupants annually, are highest in the central part of the United States (Figure 17-5a). Most of these states have especially large numbers of

a. Collision With Train

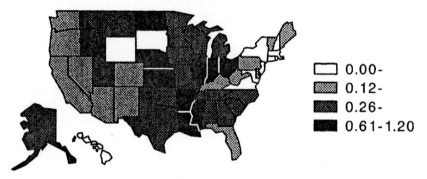

0.00-
0.12-
0.26-
0.61-1.20

b. Multiple-Vehicle Crash

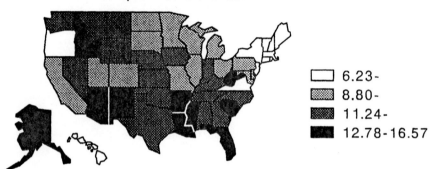

6.23-
8.80-
11.24-
12.78-16.57

c. Collision with Tree

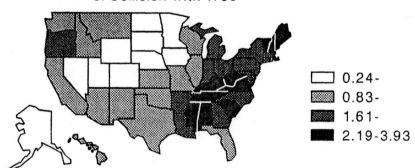

0.24-
0.83-
1.61-
2.19-3.93

Figure 17-5.   Death Rates from Motor Vehicle Crashes by State and Type of Crash, per Billion Vehicle Miles, 1980–1988

d. Collision With Utility Pole

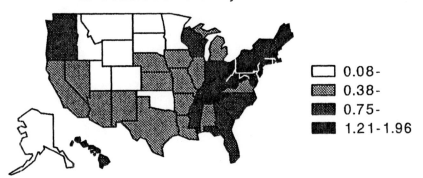

- ☐ 0.08-
- ▨ 0.38-
- ▦ 0.75-
- ■ 1.21-1.96

e. Overturn

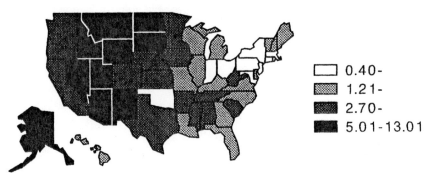

- ☐ 0.40-
- ▨ 1.21-
- ▦ 2.70-
- ■ 5.01-13.01

f. Immersion

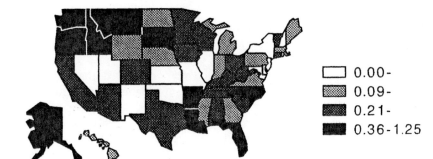

- ☐ 0.00-
- ▨ 0.09-
- ▦ 0.21-
- ■ 0.36-1.25

Figure 17-5. Continued

rail–highway crossings on the same level (referred to as "at grade") with no protection other than warning or stop signs. In New York, where death rates from collisions with trains are very low, the trains pass over or under highways at 42 percent of all public crossings; in addition, 60 percent of the at-grade crossings are protected by gates, flashing lights, or other active warning devices (Federal Railroad Administration 1989). Because of the tremendous forces involved and the high death rates, collisions between trains and motor vehicles must be prevented wherever possible with measures that alter the driving environment, such as elimination of rail–highway intersections at grade or installation of gates that cannot be driven around, rather than relying on motor vehicle drivers' perceptions of risk and their ability to respond adequately.

Death rates for occupants in multiple-vehicle crashes, excluding collisions with trains, are lowest in the northeastern, north central, and Pacific Coast states. They are generally highest in the mountain states (Figure 17-5b). The rates range from 6.2 per billion vehicle miles in Rhode Island to 16.6 in Mississippi.

Collisions with trees, which claim about 3,000 lives each year, are associated with high death rates in the eastern third of the country (Figure 17-5c). Collisions with utility poles, which result in 1,400 deaths annually, also have high rates in eastern states, especially the Northeast (Figure 17-5d). These differences reflect the fact that many roads in the East are bordered with trees and that utility poles often are very close to the road, especially in areas where they were installed early in this century when roads were narrow. It is possible to identify trees, poles, and other structures that are in especially hazardous locations (e.g., sites that combine a downhill gradient with a road curvature of more than six degrees) and to remove, reposition, or shield such fixed objects in ways that protect vehicle occupants (Wright and Robertson 1976). Placing utility poles farther from lanes of travel and burying electrical and telephone lines also reduce or eliminate the risk of collision with poles. Where signs and light supports cannot be moved or shielded with energy-absorbing structures, breakaway structures that yield on impact reduce injuries when crashes occur.

About 8,000 occupants are killed each year in vehicles that overturn. Death rates for such rollover crashes, which are highest in the mountain states (Figure 17-5e), are related not only to the gradient and curvature of roads but also to the absence of recovery areas and guardrails, which would prevent vehicles that leave the roadway from rolling down an embankment or overturning after striking a curb, ditch, or culvert (Wright et al. 1984). Embankments were cited in 1,300 fatalities in 1983, and curbs, ditches, or culverts were cited in 2,000.

Drowning rates associated with vehicle immersion are highest in Alaska, the Northwest, and several southeastern states (Figure 17-5). In Florida, where about 45 motor vehicle occupants drown each year, the number of occupant drownings per 100 million vehicle miles is about twice the national average. In Sacramento County, California, sites where drownings in motor vehicles occur involve roads with a greater mean curvature than control sites

(Wintemute et al. 1990). In many states with high rates of motor vehicle-related drowning, the lack of physical barriers or spatial separation between roads and canals or other bodies of water no doubt contributes to the likelihood of vehicle occupant drownings.

SEASON, DAY, AND TIME

Passenger vehicle occupant fatalities are most common in the summer months and least common in the winter. This seasonal pattern holds true for all regions of the country, including the southern states, but it is most extreme in Alaska where winter days are very short.

Time of day is also an important factor in the incidence of injuries and deaths (Figure 17-6). Forty-four percent of passenger vehicle occupant fatalities occur in crashes between 10:00 P.M. and 3:59 A.M., even though only 22 percent of crashes occur during these nighttime hours. Thirty-two percent of deaths occur in daytime crashes (6:00 A.M. to 5:59 P.M.), even though three-fourths of all passenger miles traveled (Carsten and Weber 1981) and more than 63 percent of crashes reported to the police take place during the day.

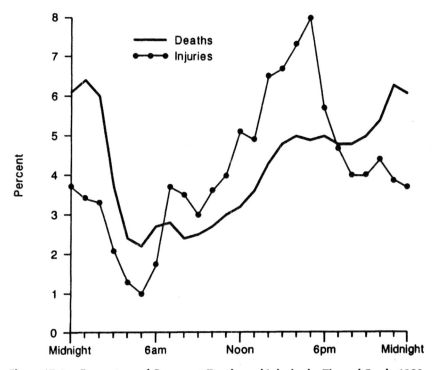

Figure 17-6.   Percentage of Occupant Deaths and Injuries by Time of Crash, 1980–1988

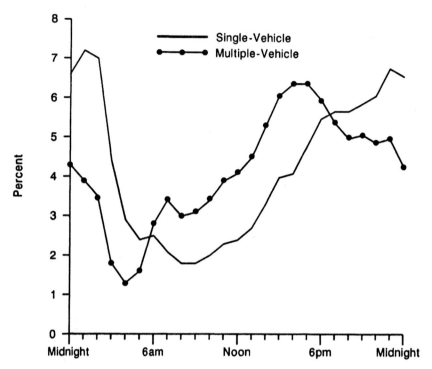

Figure 17-7.   Percentage of Single- and Multiple-Vehicle Fatal Crashes by Time of Crash, 1980–1988

A larger proportion of multiple-vehicle than of single-vehicle crashes occurs during the daytime (Figure 17-7). There is a pronounced peak in deaths from multiple-vehicle crashes from 4:00 to 5:59 P.M. Single-vehicle fatal crashes exhibit a dramatic peak from 11:00 P.M. to 2:59 A.M. and are least common from 8:00 to 9:59 A.M. The temporal pattern for single- versus multiple-vehicle crashes resembles the pattern for deaths versus injuries (Figure 17-6).

Although there is substantial variation in the number of occupant deaths by day of week, with most deaths occurring on weekends, the day-to-day variation is confined mainly to nighttime crashes (Figure 17-8). One-third of all fatal crashes occur between 6:00 P.M. and 5:59 A.M. on Friday and Saturday nights. The occupant death rate per person mile of travel is highest on Fridays and Saturdays and lowest on Tuesdays and Wednesdays.

Seasonal and temporal variations in the incidence of crashes are influenced not only by hours of daylight and corresponding visibility but also by amounts of travel, which are greater in the daytime and during the summer. Alcohol-impaired driving, which is more common at night and is a more important factor in single-vehicle crashes than in multiple-vehicle crashes, contributes significantly to the greater severity of nighttime crashes. The number of deaths per 1,000 occupants in crashes is about four times as great between midnight and 5:59 A.M. as it is during the daytime (Figure 17-9).

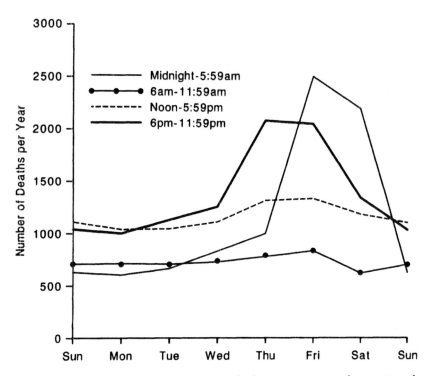

Figure 17-8. Average Number of Motor Vehicle Occupant Deaths per Year by Time and Day of Crash, 1980–1988

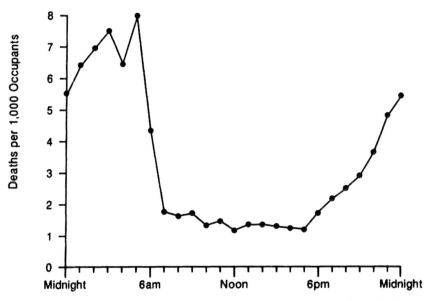

Figure 17-9. Deaths per 1,000 Occupants in Crashes by Time of Crash, 1980–1986

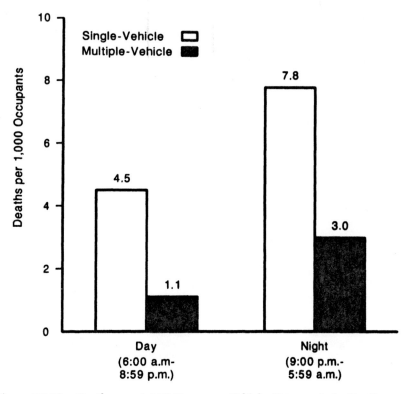

Figure 17-10. Deaths per 1,000 Passenger Vehicle Occupants in Daytime and Nighttime Single- and Multiple-Vehicle Crashes, 1980–1986

TYPES OF CRASHES

Single-vehicle crashes are associated with higher death rates than are multiple-vehicle crashes (Figure 17-10). This is true of daytime as well as nighttime crashes.

More than half of all occupants of passenger cars in fatal crashes as well as half of those in towaway crashes[2] (i.e., those where one or more vehicles is towed from the scene) are in direct-frontal and front-corner impacts (Figure 17-1). The largest proportion are direct-frontal impacts, which account for 46 percent of the fatalities. Rear impacts, which are common in minor, nontowaway crashes, cause only 2 percent of the deaths. The prominence of frontal impacts in serious crashes makes it especially important to provide automatic crash protection that is effective in frontal impacts.

About one-tenth of all occupants in towaway crashes are in vehicles that overturn. These rollover crashes have high death rates—almost three times the rate for nonrollovers (Figure 17-11)—partly because a much larger proportion of occupants (5.4 percent) are ejected from their vehicles in rollovers, compared with only 0.4 percent ejected from vehicles that do not

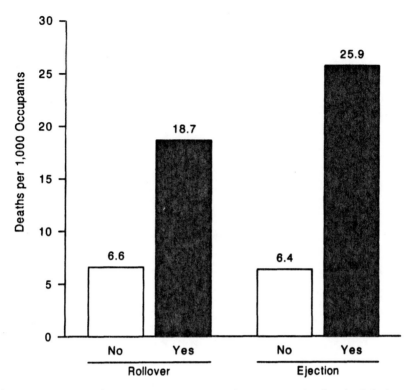

Figure 17-11. Deaths per 1,000 Occupants in Towaway Crashes in Relation to Rollover and Ejection, 1980–1986

roll over. Ejection is associated with a fourfold increase in the risk of death: 25.9 deaths per 1,000 people ejected compared with 6.4 among those not ejected (Figure 17-11). When ejection status is analyzed for different types of crashes, the relative risk of death resulting from ejection ranges from 1.5 to 8.0, with the greatest increase in risk in single-vehicle rollover crashes (Esterlitz 1989). In 1988, 8,300 crash fatalities involved total ejection from the vehicle and 1,900 involved partial ejection (NHTSA 1989a). The ability of a vehicle to keep occupants inside in a crash (whether or not the vehicle overturns) is a major determinant of the likelihood of severe injury or death.

Ejection in noncrash situations is also an important cause of serious injury, especially in children. Hospital data on child passengers injured in noncrash events such as sudden stops revealed that children who fell or were ejected from vehicles were 10 times as likely to have serious injuries as children who remained in the vehicles (Agran, Dunkle, and Winn 1985).

Concern about postcrash fire is often cited as a reason for nonuse of seat belts. Fire occurs in about 3 percent of vehicles involved in fatal crashes, but it is the most harmful event in less than 1 percent (NHTSA 1989a). Because injury greatly increases the difficulty of getting out of a car following a

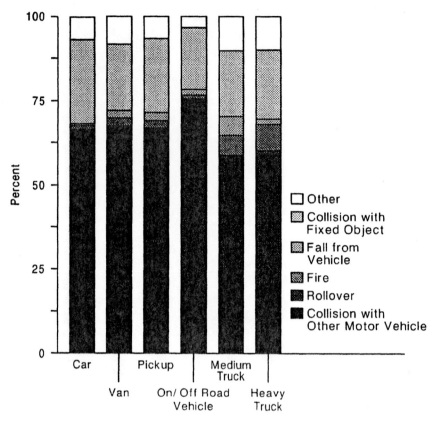

Figure 17-12. Percentage Distribution of Occupant Deaths by Most Harmful Event and Type of Vehicle, 1982–1986

crash, seat belts are likely to help, rather than hinder, one's escape from a burning vehicle.

VEHICLE TYPE AND SIZE

Almost equal proportions of motor vehicle occupant deaths occur in single- and multiple-vehicle crashes. Single-vehicle crashes can be further sub-divided into impacts with fixed objects, rollovers, and other types of events. The mix of crash types varies with the type and size of the vehicle (Figure 17-12); collisions with other vehicles predominate among deaths of pas-senger car occupants, and single-vehicle rollover crashes predominate among deaths of utility vehicle occupants. Rollovers are involved in 16 percent of occupant deaths in passenger cars, 39 percent in heavy trucks, and 59 percent in utility vehicles. Other research has shown that certain small utility vehicles have especially high rates of overturn in crashes (Rein-furt et al. 1981; Smith 1982). Fatal falls from vehicles not involved in crashes are relatively rare for most vehicle types, but account for about 175 occupant deaths annually in pickup trucks and utility vehicles. The relative frequency of each type of crash has important implications for prevention. Carrying passengers in the open beds of pickup trucks can be made illegal. (In Albuquerque, New Mexico, it is illegal to carry unrestrained dogs in an open pickup truck, although there is no such law applying to children.) To reduce the high incidence of rollovers, small vehicles designed for on/off road use could be designed with lower centers of gravity and wider track widths (the width between the wheels) (Robertson 1989).

Vehicle size is a major determinant of the severity of occupant injuries in a crash (IIHS 1987). For both single- and multiple-vehicle crashes, occupant death rates are lowest in large cars. There is no basis for claims that if all cars were small the risk would be substantially reduced, since single-vehicle crashes and collisions with large trucks account for a large proportion of small-car occupant deaths; these would remain even if all cars were small. Furthermore, occupant death and injury rates are higher in collisions between two small cars than in collisions between two large cars (Campbell and Reinfurt 1973).

The high death rates in small cars are not strongly influenced by driver age. The hypothesis that high death rates in small cars reflect age differences among drivers (i.e., that young drivers are more likely to drive small cars as well as to be involved in crashes) is contradicted by the fact that regardless of driver age, death rates per 1,000 occupants in crashes show similar relationships to car size (Baker et al. 1984).

The proportions of crashes involving rollover or ejection vary considerably by size and type of vehicle. For single-vehicle crashes, more than three-fourths of the deaths in utility vehicles involve rollovers, compared with about one-third of the deaths in large passenger cars (Figure 17-13). Among small cars, vans, and pickup trucks, the corresponding proportion is about 55 percent. Similar variations and patterns may be noted for the proportion of fatally injured occupants who were ejected from their vehicles during a crash, with utility vehicles having the highest percentage of occupants ejected and large cars the lowest (Figure 17-14).

TYPE OF ROAD AND SPEED LIMIT

Death rates on various types of roads depend on the amount of travel as well as type of road, which influence both the incidence and severity of crashes. When adjustments are made for the amount of travel by calculating mileage-based rates, rural roads have higher death rates per 100 million miles than do urban roads. This is true for interstates and other limited-access highways and, to an even greater extent, for roads where access is not controlled (Figure 17-15).

Interstate highways have relatively low crash rates because they separate vehicles traveling in opposite directions, greatly reducing head-on and

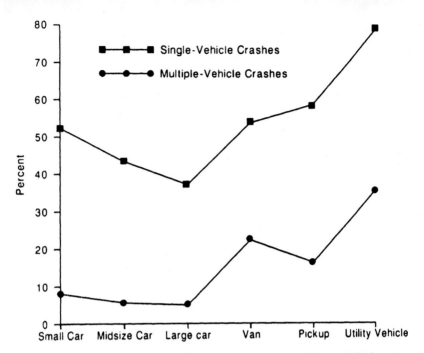

Figure 17-13. Percentage of Fatally Injured Occupants Whose Vehicles Overturned, by Size of Car or Type of Vehicle and Type of Crash, 1982–1986

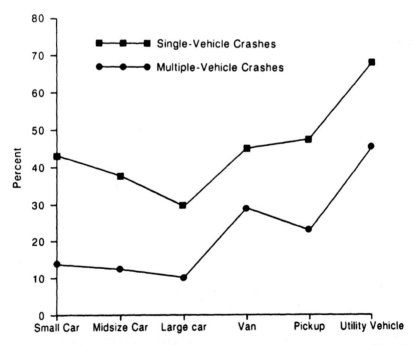

Figure 17-14. Percentage of Fatally Injured Occupants Who Were Ejected, by Size of Car or Type of Vehicle and Type of Crash, 1982–1986

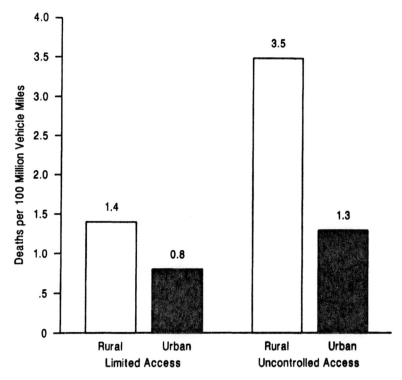

Figure 17-15. Occupant Deaths per 100 Million Vehicle Miles by Type of Road and Urban/Rural Classification, 1988

intersection-type side impact crashes; in addition, they are usually designed with gentler grades and curves and with wider recovery areas. When crashes do occur, the consequences are often severe because the average speed of travel (and therefore the typical impact speed) is greater than on many other roads.

The ratio of occupant deaths to injuries increases dramatically with the speed limit, from about 5 deaths per 1,000 injuries where the limit is 30 mph or less to 31 per 1,000 where the limit is 55 mph (Figure 17-16). The increases in speed limits from 55 to 65 mph on rural interstates that were initiated by 40 states during the late 1980s resulted in an estimated 20–30 percent increase in deaths on those roads and a 40 percent increase in serious injuries (Baum et al. 1989, 1990; NHTSA 1989b; Wagenaar et al. 1990).

ALCOHOL

Alcohol-impaired driving is one of the leading factors in passenger-vehicle crashes resulting in serious and fatal injuries. About 40 percent of all crashes with occupant fatalities involve drivers who have BACs of 0.10 percent or higher (IIHS 1990). In 1989, 53 percent of the drivers killed in

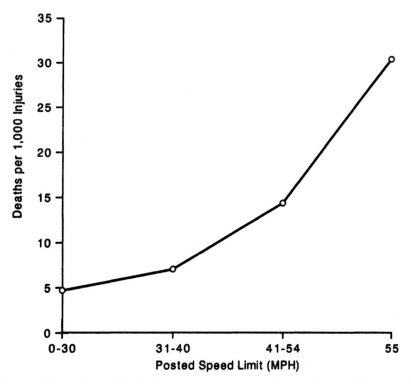

Figure 17-16. Motor Vehicle Occupant Deaths per 1,000 Injuries by Posted Speed Limit, 1980–1984

single-vehicle crashes had illegal BACs. Alcohol-related crashes kill many people in addition to the alcohol-impaired drivers; for example, more than one-fourth of children aged 0–14 killed as motor vehicle occupants were shown to have died in alcohol-related crashes (Margolis et al. 1986).

Alcohol impairs driving skills measurably even at very low BACs (Borkenstein et al. 1974; Moskowitz et al. 1985). The impairment effect increases rapidly with higher BACs. There is also evidence that high BACs can have a negative effect on injury outcome (Anderson 1987).

Research has shown that half or more of the fatally injured drivers in single-vehicle crashes or at-fault drivers in multiple-vehicle crashes had illegal BACs. In contrast, fatally injured drivers who were not at fault and drivers not involved in crashes are much less likely to be intoxicated (Baker and Spitz 1970; Jones and Joscelyn 1978; McCarroll and Haddon 1962; U.S. Congress 1968). A classic study by McCarroll and Haddon found that 50 percent of the drivers killed in single-vehicle crashes had BACs of 0.10 percent or higher, compared with 3 percent of a comparison group of drivers who did not crash but who were matched on the basis of day, time, site, and direction of travel (McCarroll and Haddon 1962). Recent research indicates that for each increase of 0.02 percent in the BAC the likelihood of a fatal crash doubles. At BACs of 0.15 percent or higher, the risk of a crash was 300 to 600 times the risk at BACs of zero or near zero (Zador 1991).

Generally, the more violent the crash the greater the likelihood that alcohol is a factor. Drivers with illegal BACs are involved in only a small percentage of minor "fender-benders" but in about 40 percent of all fatal crashes and 53 percent of single-vehicle fatal crashes. A two-city study found that the proportion of drivers in crashes who had BACs of 0.10 or higher increased from 8 percent of uninjured drivers to 13 percent of drivers with minor injuries and 23 percent of those with serious injuries (Farris et al. 1977).

The likelihood of fatally injured drivers[4] having illegal BACs varies by driver age and time of day of the crash (Figure 17-17). Alcohol involvement is most common in nighttime crashes and among drivers aged 20–49. Alcohol involvement also varies by type of crash (Figure 17-18). Drivers killed in single-vehicle crashes are much more likely to have illegal BACs than drivers killed in multiple-vehicle crashes. (This does not mean that multiple-vehicle crashes are less likely to involve alcohol; usually only fatally injured drivers are tested, so in multiple-vehicle fatal crashes only

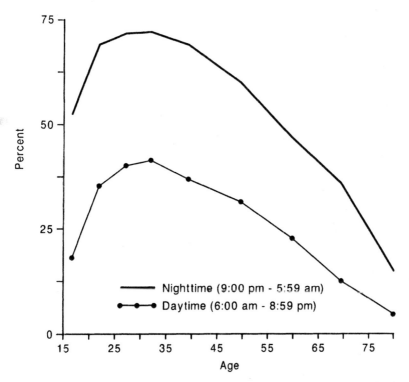

Figure 17-17.   Percentage of Fatally Injured Passenger Vehicle Drivers with Blood Alcohol Concentrations at or above 0.10 Percent by Age and Time of Crash, 1980–1988

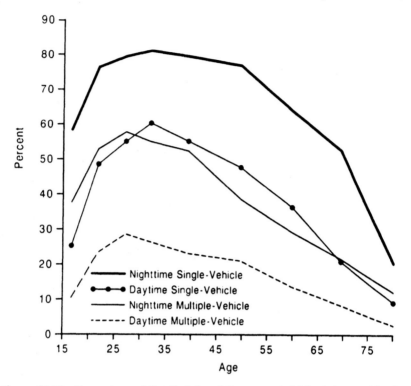

Figure 17-18   Percentage of Fatally Injured Passenger Vehicle Drivers with Blood Alcohol Concentrations at or above 0.10 Percent by Age, Time of Crash, and Type of Crash, 1980–1988

about one-half of the drivers are tested; therefore, surviving drivers with high BACs are often missed. In the 20–64 age group, more than 75 percent of the drivers killed in nighttime single-vehicle crashes have BACs of 0.10 percent or higher.)

Further subdivision of the data by sex reveals that about 80 percent of males aged 20 to 55 killed in nighttime crashes have BACs of at least 0.10 percent. Fatal crashes of male drivers more often involve alcohol than those of females (Figure 17-19). In single-vehicle crashes in which the driver is killed, female drivers in daytime crashes have the lowest alcohol involvement and male drivers in nighttime crashes have the highest.

The very frequent and longstanding involvement of alcohol in serious and fatal motor vehicle crashes illustrates the difficulty of reducing deaths and injuries by changing human behavior. The major contribution of alcohol to motor vehicle deaths and injuries, both in the United States and in virtually all other industrial societies, has led to programs, laws, and enforcement activities intended to deter people from driving while intoxicated and thereby to reduce the incidence of such deaths and injuries (Ross 1982).

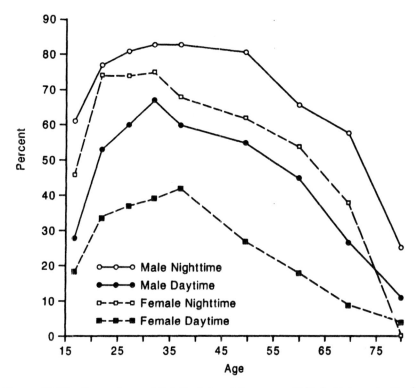

Figure 17-19.   Percentage of Fatally Injured Passenger Vehicle Drivers in Single-Vehicle Crashes with Blood Alcohol Concentrations at or above 0.10 Percent by Age, Sex, and Time of Crash, 1980–1988

The basis of most efforts to curb alcohol-impaired driving is a wide range of laws proscribing the behavior. In the 1980s, several hundred state laws aimed at this problem were passed; as a result of these laws, as well as changes in public attitudes about "drunk" driving and decreases in per capita alcohol consumption, important reductions in alcohol-related fatal crashes occurred. In 1980, 53 percent of the fatally injured drivers of passenger vehicles had BACs of 0.10 percent or greater; by 1989, this percentage had declined to 40 percent (IIHS 1990). Laws that established a legal minimum age of 21 for purchasing alcohol (DuMouchel et al. 1987; Williams 1986) and laws permitting the administrative suspension of driving licenses of persons who fail or refuse a chemical test for alcohol were important factors in this progress (Zador et al. 1989).

The greatest long-term reduction in the alcohol problem has occurred in the state of New South Wales, Australia, which in 1982 adopted legislation permitting the police to stop motorists at random and test them for alcohol (Homel 1988). The enforcement of this legislation is unusually intense for a traffic law: About one-third to one-half of all licensed drivers are tested for alcohol at random each year. The payoff has been a 20 percent reduction in motor vehicle deaths, with the proportion of fatally injured motorists with BACs of 0.05 percent or greater dropping from 42 percent to a little over 30 percent. Similar legislation will be adopted throughout Australia by the end of 1991. It is important to note that despite the very intensive enforcement, 30 percent of the fatalities continue to involve drivers with BACS that are illegal in Australia, illustrating the difficulty of changing behaviors related to drinking and driving. A comparable program in the United States would cost about $150 million per year; although the cost per life saved would be small if the program were as effective as in Australia, enforcement efforts of this magnitude are unknown in this country.

HISTORICAL TRENDS

During recent decades, motor vehicle occupant death rates have reflected improvements in roads and vehicles and changes in patterns of use, speed limits, and the economy. Since the mid-1960s, occupant death rates per 100 million vehicle miles have declined (Figure 17-20), in part because of state and local highway safety legislation and programs, as well as federal motor vehicle safety standards, which began in 1967–1968. Federal standards for

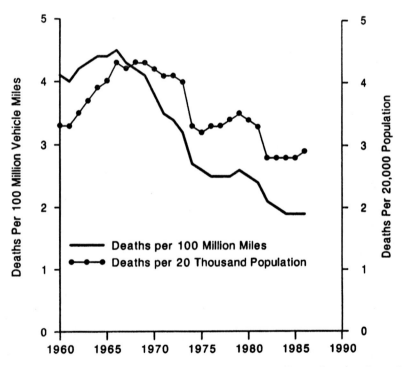

Figure 17-20.   Motor Vehicle Occupant Death Rates Based on Mileage and Population, 1980–1986

vehicles require virtually all new passenger cars sold in the United States to meet performance requirements to reduce the likelihood of crashes (e.g., standards for brakes), of injuries when crashes occur (e.g., standards for windshields and restraint systems), and of postcrash injuries (e.g., standards to make fuel systems less likely to leak and start postcrash fires). Research studies have documented the substantial reductions in deaths and injuries in cars designed to meet the requirements of these standards (Crandall et al. 1986; GAO 1986; NHTSA 1976; Robertson 1981).

Gasoline shortages and the subsequent nationwide institution of 55 mph speed limits in 1974 caused a dramatic decline in highway deaths. This was partly due to a decrease in the amount of travel, but the reduced travel speeds directly accounted for about half of the reduction (NRC 1984). In ways that are still not fully understood, general economic trends also influence motor vehicle deaths (Figure 3-17).

The char. 's in occupant death rates between the two three-year periods—197 1979 and 1984–1986—are shown in Figure 17-2. Generally, the death rates have improved but with female rates decreasing less than male rates. The greatest reductions occurred among children younger than 1 year (a 37 percent reduction in both sexes). The increases in rates among the elderly differ markedly from the trend from 1968 to 1979 when there were large decreases in the rates for ages 65 and older (Baker et al. 1984).

NOTES

1. Passenger vehicles are defined here as cars, light trucks, vans, and utility vehicles such as Jeep CJs. Occupants include drivers and passengers.

2. In general, much better information is available for towaway crashes, and they are more likely to be reported to the police. Some analyses in this book are restricted to towaway crashes, which represent a subset of all crashes and overlap with the subset of fatal crashes.

3. In almost all jurisdictions, a BAC of 0.10 percent by weight or higher in a driver is considered an offense in its own right (i.e., it is illegal *per se* to drive with a BAC of 0.10).

4. Information on the BACs of nonfatally injured drivers involved in crashes resulting in death and/or serious injury to others are not routinely obtained in any jurisdiction. Consequently, statistics on alcohol involvement tend to be confined to fatally injured drivers whose BACs are measured as part of an autopsy. FARS data from 13 states where more than 80 percent of the fatally injured drivers are tested for alcohol were used for the alcohol analyses in this book.

REFERENCES

Agran, P.F., D.E. Dunkle, and D.G. Winn (1985). Motor vehicle childhood injuries caused by noncrash falls and ejections. *Journal of the American Medical Association* 253:2530–2533.

Agran, P.F., D.E. Dunkle, and D.G. Winn (1987). Effects of legislation on motor vehicle injuries in children. *American Journal of Diseases of Children* 141:959-964.

Anderson, T.E. (1987). *Effect of acute alcohol intoxication in injury tolerance and outcome.* Warren, MI: General Motors Research Laboratories.

Baker, S.P., and W.U. Spitz (1970). Age effects and autopsy evidence of disease in fatally injured drivers. *Journal of the American Medical Association* 214:1079-1088.

Baker, S.P., B. O'Neill, and R. Karpf (1984). *The injury fact book.* Lexington, MA: Lexington Books.

Baker, S.P., R.A. Whitfield, and B. O'Neill (1987). Geographic variations in mortality from motor vehicle crashes. *New England Journal of Medicine* 316:1384-1387.

Baum, H.M., A.K. Lund, and J.K. Wells (1989). The mortality consequences of raising the speed limit to 65 mph on rural interstates. *American Journal of Public Health* 79:1392-1395.

Baum, H.M., J.K. Wells, and A.K. Lund (1990). Motor vehicle crash fatalities in the second year of 65 mph speed limits. *Journal of Safety Research* 21:1-8.

Borkenstein, R.F., R.F. Crowther, R.O. Shumute, W.B. Ziel, R. Zylman, and A. Dale (1974). The role of the drinking driver in traffic accidents (Grand Rapids Study). *Blutalkohol* 2, Supp. 4.

Campbell, B.J., and D.W. Reinfurt (1973). *Relationship between driver crash injury and passenger car weight.* Chapel Hill: University of North Carolina, Highway Safety Research Center.

Campbell, B.J., J.R. Stewart, and F.A. Campbell (1988). *Changes in death and injury associated with safety belt laws, 1985-1987.* Chapel Hill, University of North Carolina, Highway Safety Research Center.

Carsten, O., and K. Weber (1981). Child and adult travel exposure and fatality risk. In *Proceedings of the Twenty-Fifth Conference of the American Association for Automotive Medicine.* Arlington Heights, IL: American Association for Automotive Medicine, pp. 323-333.

Crandall, R.W., H.K. Gruenspecht, T.E. Keeler, and L.B. Lave (1986). *Regulating the automobile.* Washington, DC: The Brookings Institution.

Datta, T.K., and P. Guzek (1989). *Restraint system use in 19 U.S. cities. 1989 Annual Report.* Washington, DC: National Highway Traffic Safety Administration.

DuMouchel, W., A.F. Williams, and P. Zador (1987). Raising the alcohol purchase age: Its effects on fatal motor vehicle crashes in twenty-six states. *Journal of Legal Studies* 16:249-266.

Esterlitz, J.R. (1989). Relative risk of death from ejection by crash type and crash mode. *Accident Analysis and Prevention* 21:459-468.

Evans, L. (1986). The effectiveness of safety belts in preventing fatalities. *Accident Analysis and Prevention 18: 229-241.*

Farris, R., T.B. Malone, and M. Kirkpatrick (1977). *A comparison of alcohol involvement in exposed and injured drivers.* Washington, DC: National Highway Traffic Safety Administration.

Federal Railroad Administration, Office of Safety (1989). *Rail-highway crossing accident/incident and inventory bulletin, No. 11, calendar year 1988.* Washington, DC: U.S. Department of Transportation.

Geller, E.S. (1988). A behavioral science approach to transportation safety. *Bulletin of the New York Academy of Medicine* 64(7):632–661.

General Accounting Office (1986). *Motor vehicle safety: Enforcement of federal standards can be enhanced.* Washington, DC: United States General Accounting Office.

Homel, R. (1988). *Policing and punishing the drinking driver. A study of general and specific deterrence.* New York, Springer-Verlag.

Insurance Institute for Highway Safety (1979a). Air bags: A special issue. *Status Report* 14 (August 21):1–19.

Insurance Institute for Highway Safety (1979b). The human costs of air bag delay: 39,000 lives might have been saved. *Status Report* 14 (September 7):1–8.

Insurance Institute for Highway Safety (1987). Special issue: Small passenger vehicles a problem. *Status Report* 22(2):1–7.

Insurance Institute for Highway Safety (1990). Alcohol. In *Fatality facts 1990.* Arlington, VA: Insurance Institute for Highway Safety.

Jonah, B.A., and B.A. Grant (1985). Long-term effectiveness of selective traffic enforcement programs for increasing seat belt use. *Journal of Applied Psychology* 2:257–263.

Jones, R.K., and K.B. Joscelyn (1978). *Alcohol and highway safety 1978: A review of the state of knowledge.* Report No. UM-HSRI-78-5. Ann Arbor: University of Michigan Highway Safety Research Institute.

Margolis, L.H., J. Kotch, and J.H. Lacey (1986). Children in alcohol-related motor vehicle crashes. *Pediatrics* 77:870–872.

Margolis, L.H., A.C. Wagenaar, and W. Liu (1988). The effects of a mandatory child restraint law on injuries requiring hospitalization. *American Journal of Diseases of Children* 142:1099–1103.

Mathematical Analyses Division (1989). *Alcohol involvement in fatal traffic crashes, 1988.* Washington DC: National Highway Traffic Safety Administration.

McCarroll, J.R., and W. Haddon, Jr. (1962). A controlled study of fatal automobile accidents in New York City. *Journal of Chronic Diseases* 15:811–826.

Moskowitz, H., M.M. Burns, and A.F. Williams (1985). Skills performance at low blood alcohol levels. *Journal of Studies on Alcohol* 46:482–485.

National Highway Traffic Safety Administration (1976). *Effectiveness, benefits, and costs of federal safety standards for protection of passenger car occupants.* Washington, DC: U.S. Department of Transportation.

National Highway Traffic Safety Administration (1984). Federal motor vehicle safety standard: Occupant crash protection. 49 *CFR* Part 571. Washington, DC: U.S. Government Printing Office.

National Highway Traffic Safety Administration (1989a). *Fatal Accident Reporting System 1988.* Technical Report DOT HS-807-507. Washington, DC: U.S. Department of Transportation.

National Highway Traffic Safety Administration (1989b). *Report to Congress on the effects of the 65 mph speed limit through 1988.* Washington, DC: National Highway Traffic Safety Administration.

National Research Council, Transportation Research Board (1984). *55: A decade of experience.* Washington, DC: National Academy of Sciences.

O'Neill, B., A.F. Williams, and R.S. Karpf (1983). Passenger car size and driver seat belt use. *American Journal of Public Health* 73:588–590.

Partyka, S.C. (1988). *Lives saved by child restraints from 1982 through 1987.* Washington, DC: National Highway Traffic Safety Administration.

Preusser, D.F., A.F. Williams, and A.K. Lund (1986). Seat belt use among New York bar patrons. *Journal of Public Health Policy* 7:470-479.

Preusser, D.F., A.F. Williams, and A.K. Lund (In press). Characteristics of belted and unbelted drivers. *Accident Analysis and Prevention.*

Preusser, D.F., A.K. Lund, A.F. Williams, and R.D. Blomberg (1988). Belt use by high-risk drivers before and after New York's seat belt use law. *Accident Analysis and Prevention* 20:245-250.

Preusser, D.F., A.F. Williams, P.L. Zador, and R.D. Blomberg (1984). The effect of curfew laws on motor vehicle crashes. *Law and Policy* 6:115-128.

Reinfurt, D.W., and B.J. Campbell (1990). Evaluating the North Carolina safety belt wearing law. *Accident Analysis and Prevention* 22:197-210.

Reinfurt, D.W., C.L. St. Cyr, and W.W. Hunter (1990). Usage patterns and misuse rates of automatic seat belts by system type. In *Proceedings of the Association for the Advancement of Automotive Medicine.* Des Plaines, IL: Association for the Advancement of Automotive Medicine, pp. 163-180.

Reinfurt, D.W., L.K. Li, C.L. Popkin, B. O'Neill, P.F. Burchman, and J.K. Wells (1981). *A comparison of the crash experience of utility vehicles, pickup trucks and passenger cars.* Chapel Hill: University of North Carolina, Highway Safety Research Center.

Robertson, L.S. (1980). Crash involvement of teenage drivers when driver education is eliminated from high school. *American Journal of Public Health* 70:599-603.

Robertson, L.S. (1981). Automobile safety regulations and death reductions in the United States. *American Journal of Public Health* 71:818-822.

Robertson, L.S. (1989). Motor vehicle injuries: The law and the profits. *Law, Medicine & Health Care* 17:69-72.

Ross, H.L. (1982). *Deterring the drinking driver: Legal policy and social control.* Lexington, MA: Lexington Books.

Smith, S.R. (1982). *Analysis of fatal rollover accidents in utility vehicles.* Washington, DC: National Highway Traffic Safety Administration.

Streff, F.M., and L.J. Molnar (1990). *Direct observation of safety belt use in Michigan: Spring 1990.* Ann Arbor: University of Michigan Transportation Research Institute.

U.S. Congress, House of Representatives, Committee on Public Works (1968). *1968 Alcohol and highway safety report: A study transmitted by the Secretary of the Department of Transportation to the Congress, in accordance with requirements of section 204 of the Highway Safety Act of 1966, Public Law 89-564.* 90th Congress, 2nd session.

Wagenaar, A.C., R.G. Maybee, and K.P. Sullivan (1988). Mandatory seat belt laws in eight states: A time-series evaluation. *Journal of Safety Research* 19:51-70.

Wagenaar, A.C., F.M. Streff, and R.H. Schultz (1990). Effects of the 65 mph speed limit on injury morbidity and mortality. *Accident Analysis and Prevention* 22:571-585.

Wagenaar, A.C., D.W. Webster, and R.G. Maybee (1987). Effects of child restraint laws on traffic fatalities in eleven states. *Journal of Trauma* 27:726-732

Wells, J.K., A.F. Williams, N.J. Teed, and A.K. Lund (1990). Belt use among high school students. Excerpted in *National Association of Secondary School Principals News Leader* 38:8.

Williams, A.F. (1986). Raising the legal purchase age in the United States: Its effects on fatal motor vehicle crashes. *Alcohol, Drugs, and Driving* 2(2);1–12.

Williams, A.F., and A.K. Lund (1986). Seat belt use laws and occupant crash protection in the United States. *American Journal of Public Health* 76:1438–1442.

Williams, A.F., and A.K. Lund (1986). Seat belt use laws and occupant crash protection in the United States. *American Journal of Public Health* 76:1438–1442.

Williams, A.F., and A.K. Lund (1988). Mandatory seat belt use laws and occupant crash protection in the United States: Present status and future prospects. In J.D. Graham, (Ed.), *Preventing automobile injury*. Dover, MA: Auburn House Publishing Company, pp. 51–72.

Williams, A.F., and B. O'Neill (1979). *Seat belt laws: Implications for occupant protection*. SAE Technical Paper No. 790683. Warrendale, PA: Society of Automotive Engineers.

Williams, A.F., D.F. Preusser, R.D. Blomberg, and A.K. Lund (1987). Seat belt use law enforcement and publicity in Elmira, New York: A reminder campaign. *American Journal of Public Health* 77:1450–1451.

Williams, A.F., J.K. Wells, and A.K. Lund (1983). Voluntary seat belt use among high school students. *Accident Analysis and Prevention* 15:161–165.

Williams, A.F., J.K. Wells, and A.K. Lund (1990). Seat belt use in cars with air bags. *American Journal of Public Health* 80:1514–1516.

Wintemute, G.J., J.F. Kraus, S.P. Teret, and M.A. Wright (1990). Death resulting from motor vehicle immersions: The nature of the injuries, personal and environmental contributing factors, and potential interventions. *American Journal of Public Health* 80:1068–1070.

Wright, P.H., J.W. Hall, and P. Zador (1984). Low cost countermeasures for ameliorating run-off-the-road crashes. *Transportation Research Record* 926. Washington, DC: Transportation Research Board, pp. 1–7.

Wright, P.H., and L.S. Robertson (1976). Priorities for roadside hazard modification: A study of 300 fatal roadside object crashes. In *Proceedings of the Twentieth Conference of the American Association for Automotive Medicine*. Arlington Heights, IL: American Association for Automotive Medicine, pp. 114–127.

Zador, P. (1991). Alcohol-related relative risk of fatal driver injury in relation to driver age and sex. *Journal of Studies on Alcohol* 52:302–310.

Zador, P.L., A.K. Lund, M. Fields, and K. Weinberg (1989). Fatal crash involvement and laws against alcohol impaired driving. *Journal of Public Health Policy* 10:467–485.

Ziegler, P.N. (1989). Use of child safety seats. *Research Notes*. Washington, DC: National Highway Traffic Safety Administration.

18

Large Trucks

Crashes and crash injuries involving large trucks (those weighing more than 10,000 pounds when empty) are of special interest for three reasons. First, crash involvement rates for large trucks exceed those for passenger vehicles when mileage and type of road are controlled for (Figure 18-1; Preusser and Stein 1987). Second, more than 5,000 deaths occur each year in crashes involving large trucks (Table 18-1). In such crashes, other road users have especially high fatality rates; 84 percent of the deaths involve persons who were sharing the road with the large truck. Third, truck drivers have the

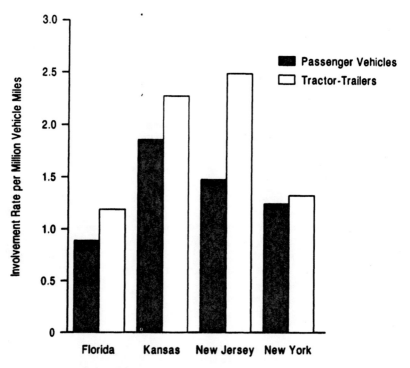

Figure 18-1. Crash Involvement Rates of Passenger Vehicles and Tractor-Trailers on Toll Roads

Table 18-1. Persons Killed in Crashes Involving Large Trucks, by Truck Type, 1988

Truck Type	Occupant of Large Truck	Occupant of Other Vehicle	Pedestrian	Motorcyclist or Bicyclist	Total	Percentage of Total
10,000–19,499 lb.[a]	33	155	26	5	219	4.1
19,500–25,999 lb.[a]	16	104	10	2	132	2.5
26,000 + lb. (single unit)	50	295	44	7	396	7.4
Combination	707	3363	316	40	4426	83.0
Unknown	30	118	9	0	157	3.0
Total	836	4035	405	54	5330	100.0
Percentage of Total	15.7	75.7	7.6	1.0		100.0

[a]Gross vehicle weight rating, single-unit trucks

eighth highest occupational death rate among 347 occupations studied (Leigh 1987).

The risk of crashes of large trucks has often been underestimated because about one-half of their mileage is on relatively safe interstate highways, compared with less than one-fourth of passenger vehicle mileage (FHWA 1989). As a result, their overall crash involvement rate is low when no adjustment is made for category of road. On comparable roads, however, tractor-trailers have higher rates of crashes than passenger vehicles. The high crash involvement of large trucks involves many factors, including driver fatigue and impairment, poor truck brakes, excessive speed, and some road designs that are inadequate for large trucks.

In addition to high crash rates, fatality rates are high when crashes involve large trucks—largely reflecting the tremendous energy exchanges during the crash phase because of the mass of the truck. Head-on crashes between trucks and passenger vehicles are especially unforgiving for the occupants of the passenger vehicles. However, the forces on the passenger car occupants could be greatly reduced if an energy-absorbing structure were added to truck front-ends (Jones 1987). Similarly, passenger vehicle occupants would be at less risk in truck crashes if truck sides and rear ends were designed to prevent passenger vehicles from underriding them (Gloyns and Rattenbury 1989). Although NHTSA proposed a federal standard in 1981 to equip trucks with lower, sturdier rear end guards, similar to those used in Europe, no final action has been taken.

The high death rates per 100,000 truck drivers reflect not only the many miles that they drive and the high rates of crashes but also the lack of occupant crash protection afforded by most trucks. Federal occupant protection standards have typically been delayed or not applied in the case of trucks; passive protection is needed, including attention to the steering assembly (a factor in many truck driver deaths) and impact protection that would reduce penetration or extreme deformation of the cab (Baker et al. 1976).

This chapter emphasizes combination vehicles (tractors pulling one or more trailers), because they are involved in 83 percent of fatalities resulting from crashes of large trucks (Table 18-1).

FREIGHT SHIPMENT

The mode of transport selected for shipment of freight is an important determinant of injury and death rates, since the death rate per billion ton miles varies greatly among the various modes (Table 18-2). Analysis of data from the late 1960s showed that highway transport of freight was associated with the highest rate, about 11 deaths per billion ton miles for federally regulated carriers; this was more than four times the rate for rail transport (NTSB 1971). In some geographic areas or for certain types of freight, there may be little choice as to mode of transport. However, the large differences

Table 18-2.   Surface Freight Transportation Fatality Rates,
1963–1968

Transport Mode	Deaths per Billion Ton Miles
Highway (federally regulated carriers)	10.9
Rail	2.5
Marine	0.31
Petroleum pipeline	0.01

Source: National Transportation Safety Board, 1971.

among modes in the human costs of freight transport—that is, the cost in lost lives—should be considered in policy related to development and use of transportation systems. Shipment of hazardous materials by any mode creates the potential for extensive loss of life. Prevention of such disasters is discussed by Waller (1985).

TRUCK DRIVER CHARACTERISTICS

When other factors are controlled for, young drivers are at greatest risk of being involved in crashes. Involvement rates are especially high for drivers less than 30 years of age when driving a double (a tractor pulling two trailers) (Stein and Jones 1988). For both single-unit trucks and combination vehicles, fatal crash involvement rates decrease with driver age until about age 30, then stay relatively constant (Figure 18-2). Drivers younger than 21 have an involvement rate that is six times the rate for all drivers (Campbell and Wolfe 1988); their rates are more than twice those for drivers aged 21–24 in both urban and rural areas, during both night and day and on freeways as well as other roads.

Fatigue plays an important role in truck crashes. The problem is exacerbated by employment pressures and economic incentives for truck drivers to drive for long hours without adequate rest. Crash involvement rates increase after about six hours of driving, and after eight hours the risk is almost twice the risk in the first two hours (Jones and Stein in press). Drivers using sleeper berths to acquire their off-duty rest time in two shifts are three times as likely to be involved in crashes as drivers who accumulate their required eight hours of rest in one period (Hertz 1988).

The role of alcohol in fatal crashes of large trucks has decreased in recent years. FARS data show that in 1988, BACs of 0.10 percent or higher were found in only 8 percent of drivers of tractor-trailers who were fatally injured in single-vehicle crashes compared with 16 percent in 1980 (IIHS 1990b). Among 359 on-duty tractor-trailer drivers who were tested for alcohol and other drugs at a truck weighing station, only 2 had alcohol in their blood, and these were at levels below 0.04 percent. The drugs most

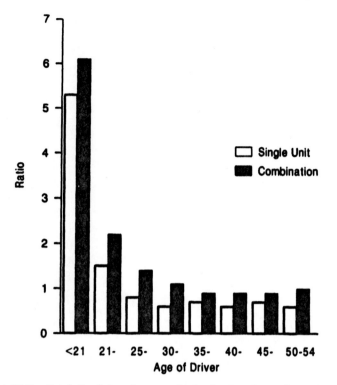

Figure 18-2. Fatal Crash Involvement Ratios by Truck Configuration and Age of Driver (*Source:* After K.L. Campbell and A.C. Wolfe (1988) *Fatal accident involvement rates by driver age for large trucks*. Ann Arbor: University of Michigan Transportation Research Institute, p. 18.)

commonly detected were stimulants and marijuana, which were found in 17 and 15 percent, respectively, of the truck drivers (Lund et al. 1988). In a study of fatally injured truck drivers, 33 percent were found to have one or more drugs of abuse in their system; 20 percent had stimulants, 13 percent had marijuana, and 11 percent had alcohol (NTSB 1990).

VEHICLE TYPE AND SIZE

Truck configuration has been shown by case-control research to be a major factor affecting crash involvement on interstate highways. A truck tractor pulling one trailer is about twice as likely to be involved in a crash as a single-unit truck, and a double is three times as likely as a tractor pulling a single trailer (Stein and Jones 1988). Since doubles travel primarily on safer, limited-access roads, their unadjusted rate of crash involvement for all types of roads is lower than the average for heavy trucks. When differences in road type are adjusted for, doubles have a higher rate of crashes than average (Campbell et al. 1988).

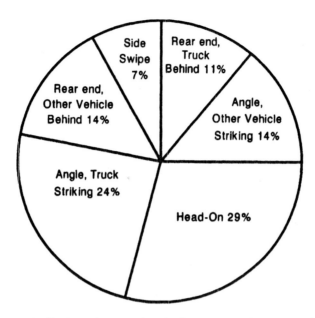

Figure 18-3. Distribution of Types of Multiple-Vehicle Collisions Involving Heavy Trucks, 1988

CIRCUMSTANCES OF CRASHES

The largest proportion of fatal collisions between heavy trucks and other vehicles involves side impact crashes, including angle and side swipe impacts (45 percent); the second largest category is head-on crashes (29 percent); and rear-end crashes comprise the remainder (25 percent) (Figure 18-3).

Of the fatally injured occupants of heavy trucks, 62 percent are killed in single-vehicle crashes. For both single- and multiple-vehicle crashes, frontal impacts (11 o'clock to 1 o'clock) cause 56 percent of all truck occupant fatalities.

Rollovers or overturns are involved in one-fourth of the crashes that are fatal to truck occupants (NHTSA 1989). The likelihood that a tractor-trailer will overturn increases with the loaded weight of the vehicle (Fancher et al. 1989). Overturns are especially likely on ramps and other curved roadways; on New York City limited-access highways, 75 percent of tractor-trailer overturns occurred on curved roadways compared with 34 percent of control sites (Schwartz and Retting 1986). Collisions involving jackknifed tractor-trailers occurred at increased frequency on wet roadways and among trucks that were empty or lightly loaded (Figure 18-4).

Truck brakes have been implicated in as many as one-third of all serious crashes of heavy trucks (NHTSA 1987). Heavy trucks require a greater stopping distance than cars. At 55 mph, a loaded tractor-trailer required 196 feet to stop versus 133 feet for a car (Jones 1985). Antilock brakes—which enable trucks to stop in shorter distances and provide improved steering

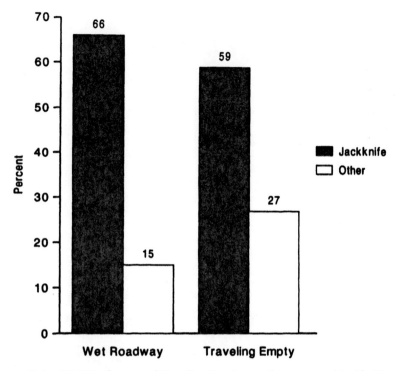

Figure 18-4.   Wet Roadways and Traveling Empty as a Percentage of Jackknife and Other Collisions in Tractor-Trailers on New York City Freeways (*Source:* S.I. Schwartz and R.A. Retting (1986). New York City heavy truck crashes: 1983–1985 findings. *Institute of Transportation Engineers 56th annual meeting compendium of technical papers.* Washington, DC: Institute of Transportation Engineers, p. 249.)

control on wet and slippery surfaces—could eliminate many jackknife crashes, but they are only being tested on a limited number of tractor-trailers in the United States (IIHS 1990a). Such brakes are required in new trucks in Europe. The problems related to the poor designs of most truck brakes are exacerbated by bad maintenance practices of many truck owners and operators (NHTSA 1987). Defective brakes are found commonly in truck inspection programs and were reported in 26 percent of trucks hauling hazardous waste (IIHS 1986). In a case-control study, 49 percent of tractor-trailers that struck the rear of other vehicles had brakes with defects severe enough to have required a truck to be taken out of service compared with 12 percent of comparison tractor-trailers (Jones and Stein in press).

RADAR DETECTORS

Use of radar detectors has been shown to be greater in tractor-trailers than in other vehicles and to be correlated with higher speeds of travel (Ciccone et al. 1987; Freedman et al. 1990; Teed and Williams 1990). Research in seven eastern states, where the speed limit was 55 mph, revealed that twice as many trucks with radar detectors were exceeding 70 mph as were those without. Forty percent of tractor-trailers were using radar detectors; among trucks carrying hazardous materials, an even greater proportion (46 percent) used detectors (Williams et al. 1990). Subsequent measurement of radar detector use on interstate highways throughout the United States found that half of all trucks (including those carrying hazardous materials) were using radar detectors (Teed and Williams 1990). Two states (Connecticut and Virginia) and the District of Columbia ban the use of radar detectors in all vehicles, and New York State bans them in commercial vehicles; a federal regulation to ban their use in interstate commercial vehicles is under consideration.

TIME OF DAY AND TYPE OF ROAD

Comparison of the times and locations of fatal truck crashes with the National Truck Trip Information Survey indicates that rates of fatal crashes are more than three times as high at night (9:00 P.M. to 6:00 A.M.) as during other hours. Fatal crash involvement rates are substantially lower on limited-access highways than on other roads. On limited-access highways the rates are higher in urban areas, but on other roads the rates are generally higher in rural areas (Campbell et al. 1988).

GEOGRAPHIC DISTRIBUTION

Death rates from crashes involving tractor-trailers range from less than 1 death per billion vehicle miles in Rhode Island, Hawaii, and Massachusetts to more than 5 per billion miles in Mississippi, Arkansas, and Montana. Rates are generally highest in southern, central, and mountain states (Figure 18-5). (The denominator for these rates is billions of miles traveled by all types of vehicles combined, since the majority of deaths in these crashes occur in vehicles other than the tractor-trailers.)

TIME TRENDS

The number of tractor-trailer occupants killed in crashes decreased from 887 in 1980 to 648 in 1989, a 27 percent decrease. Deaths of others in collisions involving tractor-trailers increased from 3,525 to 3,761 in the same period, an increase of 2 percent, with an intermediate low of 3,372 in 1982 (IIHS 1990b).

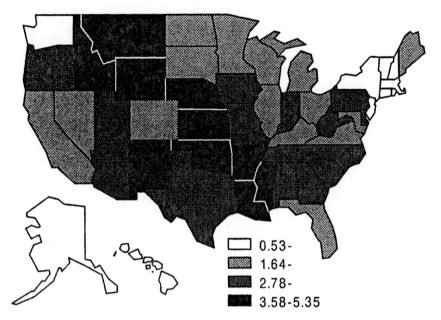

Figure 18-5.   Death Rates from Crashes Involving Large Trucks by State and Type of Crash, per Billion Vehicle Miles, 1982–1988.

REFERENCES

Baker, S.P., J. Wong, and R.D. Baron (1976). Professional drivers: Protection needed for a high-risk occupation. *American Journal of Public Health* 66:649–653.

Campbell, K.L., and A.C. Wolfe (1988). *Fatal accident involvement rates by driver age for large trucks.* Ann Arbor: University of Michigan Transportation Research Institute.

Campbell, K.L., D.F. Blower, R.G. Gattis, and A.C. Wolfe (1988). *Analysis of accident rates of heavy-duty vehicles.* Ann Arbor: University of Michigan Transportation Research Institute.

Ciccone M.A., M. Goodson, and J. Pollner (1987). Radar detectors and speed in Maryland and Virginia. *Journal of Political Science and Administration* 15:277–284.

Fancher, P.S., K.L. Campbell, and D.F. Blower (1989). *Vehicle design implications of the Turner proposal.* SAE Paper No. 892461. Warrendale, PA: Society of Automotive Engineers.

Federal Highway Administration (1989). *Highway statistics 1988.* FHWA-PL-89-003. Washington, DC: Federal Highway Administration.

Freedman, M., A.F. Williams, N. Teed, and A.K. Lund (1990). Radar detector use and speeds in Maryland and Virginia. Arlington, VA: Insurance Institute for Highway Safety.

Gloyns, P.F., and S.J. Rattenbury (1989). Cars in conflict with larger vehicles—the problem of under-run. *SAE Technical Paper Series* No. 890746. International Congress and Exposition, Detroit MI.

Hertz, R.P. (1988). Tractor-trailer driver fatality: The role of nonconsecutive rest in a sleeper berth. *Accident Analysis and Prevention* 20:431–439.

Insurance Institute for Highway Safety (1986). Hazardous materials regulations: "Inadequate and needlessly confusing." *Status Report* 21(10):1.

Insurance Institute for Highway Safety (1990a). Antilock brakes for trucks. *Status Report* 25:5:1–11.

Insurance Institute for Highway Safety (1990b). In *Fatality facts 1990*. Arlington, VA: Insurance Institute for Highway Safety.

Jones, I.S. (1985). Truck air brakes: Current standards and performance. *Proceedings of the 29th Conference of the American Association for Automotive Medicine*. Morton Grove IL: American Association for Automotive Medicine.

Jones, I.S. (1987). The benefits of energy absorbing structures to reduce the aggressivity of heavy trucks in collision. Eleventh International Conference on Experimental Safety Vehicles. Washington DC: U.S. Department of Transportation, National Highway Traffic Safety Administration.

Jones, I.S., and H.S. Stein (In press). Effect of driver hours in service on tractor-trailer crash involvement. *Accident Analysis and Prevention*.

Jones, I.S., and H.S. Stein (1989). Defective equipment and tractor-trailer crash involvement. *Accident Analysis and Prevention* 21:469–481.

Leigh, J.P. (1987). Estimates of the probability of job-related death in 347 occupations. *Journal of Occupational Medicine* 29:510–519.

Lund, A.K., D.F. Preusser, R.D. Blomberg, and A.F. Williams (1988). Drug use by tractor-trailer drivers. *Journal of Forensic Sciences* 33:648–661.

National Highway Traffic Safety Administration (1989). *Fatal Accident Reporting System 1988*. Technical Report DOT HS-807-507. Washington, DC: U.S. Department of Transportation.

National Highway Traffic Safety Administration (1987). *Heavy Truck Safety Study*. Washington, DC: U.S. Department of Transportation.

National Transportation Safety Board (1971). *Special study: Fatality rates for surface freight transportation, 1963 to 1968*. Report No. NTSB-STS-71-4. Washington, DC: National Transportation Safety Board.

National Transportation Safety Board (1990). *Safety study: Fatigue, alcohol, other drugs, and medical factors in fatal-to-the-driver heavy truck crashes*. Washington, DC: National Transportation Safety Board.

Preusser, D.F., and H.S. Stein (1987). Comparison of passenger vehicle and truck crash rates on toll roads. *ITE Journal* 39–44.

Schwartz, S.I., and R.A. Retting (1986). New York City heavy truck crashes: 1983–1985 findings. *Institute of Transportation Engineers 56th annual meeting compendium of technical papers*. Washington, DC: Institute of Transportation Engineers. pp. 245–253.

Stein, H.S., and I.S. Jones (1988). Crash involvement of large trucks by configuration: A case control study. *American Journal of Public Health* 78:491–98.

Teed, N., and A.F. Williams (1990). *Radar detector use in trucks in 17 states*. Arlington, VA: Insurance Institute for Highway Safety.

Waller, J.A. (1985). *Injury control: A guide to the causes and prevention of trauma*. Lexington, MA: Lexington Books.

Williams, A.F., N. Teed, M. Freedman, and A.K. Lund (1990). *Radar detector use in large trucks*. Arlington VA: Insurance Institute for Highway Safety.

19

Pedestrians

Pedestrian deaths, the second largest category of motor vehicle deaths, include almost half of the traffic deaths for ages 3–9 and more than one-fourth for ages 75 or older. In 1988, almost 7,000 people were killed as pedestrians, representing about one-seventh of all traffic-related deaths.

Analyses in this chapter, except where otherwise specified, are for pedestrians injured on public roads, often referred to as "in traffic." Nontraffic locations such as private driveways, however, are the site of more than 125 deaths of young children each year, with the highest rate in 1-year-olds. Typically such deaths occur when a car or van is backing up (Brison et al. 1988).

AGE AND SEX

Unlike motor vehicle occupant deaths, the highest pedestrian death rates are for the elderly, with lower peaks seen for children and teenagers (Figure 16-5). Nonfatal injury rates are highest for children aged 5–14. As with other causes of injury, the high pedestrian death rates for the elderly in part reflect the high fatality rates among those injured. In addition, when adjustment is made for exposure, elderly pedestrians are more likely to be injured than younger adults (Haddon et al. 1961; Smeed 1976).

Seventy percent of the pedestrians killed are males. After age 18, the male to female ratio of death rates is about 3 to 1. Among children, the sex difference is apparent beginning in the second year of life.

One-fifth of all collisions that are fatal to adult pedestrians occur at intersections, compared with less than one-tenth in the case of children younger than 5 years (NHTSA 1989). Among children, 84 percent who are killed as pedestrians are in the roadway but not at an intersection.

URBAN/RURAL, INCOME, AND GEOGRAPHIC DIFFERENCES

Pedestrian collisions are predominantly an urban phenomenon. Six out of seven injuries to pedestrians and three out of four deaths occur in urban areas. However, the ratio of deaths to injuries is higher in rural areas,

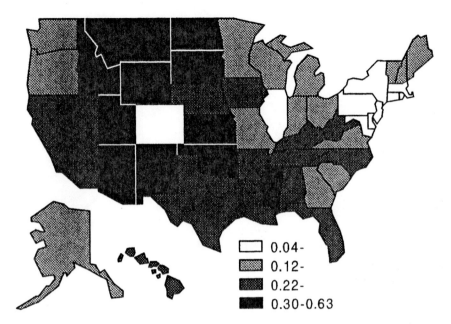

Figure 19-1. Death Rates for Pedestrians (Nontraffic) by State, per 100,000 Population 1980–1986

reflecting the generally higher impact speeds in rural areas and the reduced access to trauma centers (Mueller et al. 1988). The overall death rate in central cities is substantially higher than in other areas. For blacks, however, the reverse is true (Baker et al. 1984).

Pedestrian death rates on public roads are generally highest in southern and southwestern states and range from 1.5 per 100,000 in Iowa to 6.9 per 100,000 in New Mexico (Figure 16-12). Nontraffic pedestrian deaths, however, are highest in the mountain states (Figure 19-1). City children in low income areas have higher rates of pedestrian injuries than those in more affluent areas (Pless et al. 1987; Rivara and Barber 1985).

SEASON AND TIME

The number of pedestrian deaths per month increases throughout the year to a peak in October through December (Figure 19-2). More than 70 percent of all pedestrian deaths occur between 3:00 P.M. and 2:59 A.M. with the highest incidence from 6:00 to 9:59 P.M. (Figure 19-3). Nonfatal injuries more closely reflect the periods of greatest pedestrian activity, predominantly the daytime, with the highest incidence at about 4:00 P.M.

The peak hour for pedestrian fatalities changes with the seasonal variation in the hour of dusk. Each month, the peak hour occurs about an hour after the average time of sunset. Pedestrian conspicuousness, street lighting,

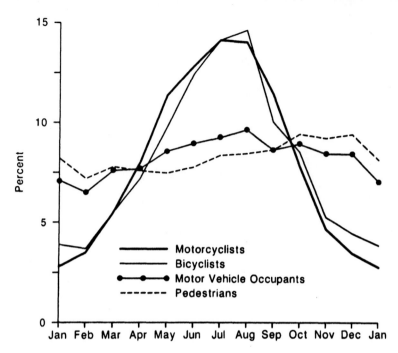

Figure 19-2. Percentage of Deaths of Motor Vehicle Occupants, Pedestrians, Motorcyclists, and Bicyclists by Month, 1980–1988

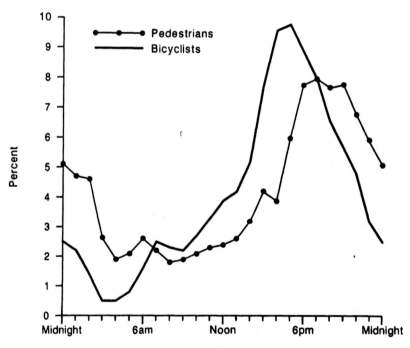

Figure 19-3. Percentage of Pedestrian and Bicyclist Deaths by Time of Day, 1980–1988

other visibility factors, and variations in weather probably play important roles.

ALCOHOL

As with passenger vehicle occupant deaths, alcohol impairment plays a major role in adult pedestrian fatalities (Baker et al. 1974; Haddon et al. 1961; IIHS 1990; U.S. Congress 1968). Blood alcohol concentrations of 0.10 percent or greater are found in 59 percent of pedestrians 16 years and older killed in nighttime crashes. Moreover, because most drivers involved in pedestrian fatalities are not tested for alcohol, the contribution of alcohol to pedestrian deaths is undoubtedly even greater (Baker et al. 1974). Throughout ages 20–64, more than half of pedestrians who are fatally injured at night have high BACs (Figure 19-4). Pedestrians in this age range, who are more likely to be impaired than elderly pedestrians, are greatly overrepresented among nighttime fatalities.

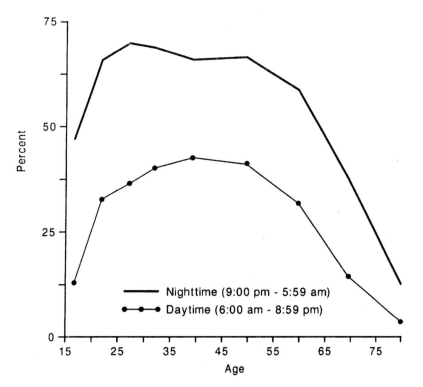

Figure 19-4. Percentage of Fatally Injured Pedestrians with Blood Alcohol Concentrations at or above 0.10 Percent by Age and Time of Day, 1980–1988

VEHICLE FACTORS

Vehicle size and design are major factors in pedestrian injuries. In Great Britain, the death rate among pedestrians struck by various types of vehicles was found to range from 4 per 1,000 for bicycles to 106 per 1,000 for heavy trucks. Of people struck by cars, 31 per 1,000 were killed (Ashton 1982). In Maryland, the number of pedestrians killed per 10,000 vehicles was twice as high for cars with wheelbases greater than 120 inches compared with those with wheelbases less than 111 inches (Robertson and Baker 1976).

Impacts with pedestrians usually involve the front structures of vehicles. Other circumstances include children running into the sides of cars and pedestrians being struck by mirrors or other protruding structures or run over by the rear wheels of trucks or buses. The dynamics of the collision depend on many factors, including the vehicle's shape, speed at impact, braking action, contact point, and the height of the pedestrian relative to the bumper and the front of the hood. A pedestrian may be run over (this is especially common when the vehicle is a truck or the pedestrian is a child), but more often the most serious injuries are sustained as a result of the pedestrian being thrown onto the hood, windshield, or top of the car. Serious injuries to the head, pelvis, and legs are especially common; the severity of these injuries, especially to the head, can be influenced by the design and materials of parts of the vehicle against which pedestrians may be thrown (Ashton 1982; Ashton et al. 1977; MacLaughlin and Kessler 1990).

ROAD DESIGN AND SPEED LIMIT

Each year about 500 pedestrians are struck and killed while on crosswalks; many others are struck and killed while on sidewalks and median strips or traffic islands (NHTSA 1989). These deaths, representing about one-tenth of all pedestrian deaths, point to the inadequate protection provided by pedestrian areas that are on the same level as roadways but not physically separated from vehicle traffic. Even in urban areas, the great majority of pedestrian fatalities occur on major thoroughfares rather than neighborhood streets (Rivara et al. 1989).

Separation of pedestrians from motorized traffic is sometimes achieved with overpasses and underpasses and/or barriers at the sides of roads. More often, separation is absent or merely temporal, as with traffic lights. Permitting right turns at red lights has resulted in significant increases in pedestrian collisions at signalized intersections, especially in urban areas (Preusser et al. 1981; Zador 1982). Engineering changes, including extending the time available for pedestrians to cross with a green light, have been shown to reduce injuries and deaths among elderly pedestrians on a major urban boulevard (Retting 1988).

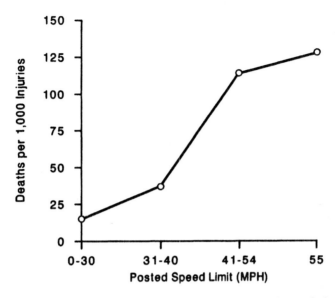

Figure 19-5. Pedestrian Deaths per 1,000 Injuries by Posted Speed Limit, 1980–
1984

The speed of vehicles involved in pedestrian impacts is a major determinant of the severity and outcome of injury. This is reflected in the much higher ratio of deaths to injuries where speed limits are higher (Figure 19-5). The ratio of deaths to injuries is about nine times as high where the speed limit is 55 mph as on roads where it is 30 mph or less. In addition, the speed of vehicle travel influences the likelihood that a pedestrian will be struck because a driver cannot stop quickly enough. Braking and other avoidance maneuvers have been shown to reduce the severity of urban pedestrian injuries in children and teenagers; the same study found that even in residential zones, almost 20 percent of the vehicles were traveling at more than 30 mph when they struck pedestrians (Pitt et al. 1990).

HISTORICAL TRENDS

Pedestrian death rates declined by more than half between 1935 and 1955. The trend roughly paralleled occupant death rates from the early 1930s until after World War II (Figure 16-13). Subsequently, as motor vehicle ownership and use increased, pedestrian death rates continued to decline for another decade, possibly because fewer people walked to their destinations. The reductions in vehicle mileage, changes in travel patterns, and lower speed limits following the 1974 gas shortage substantially reduced pedestrian as well as occupant deaths. Although the overall trend since the late 1970s has been downward, the death rates increased somewhat in males

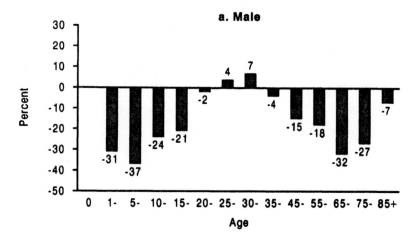

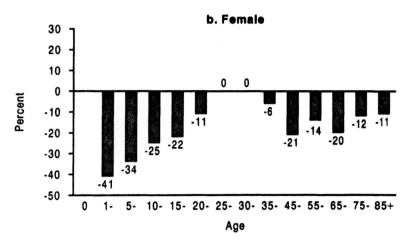

Figure 19-6.   Percentage Change in Death Rates for Pedestrians by Age and Sex, 1984–1986 Compared with 1977–1979

aged 25–34 (Figure 19-6). Otherwise the trends were roughly similar in the two sexes.

REFERENCES

Ashton, S.J. (1982). Vehicle design and pedestrian injuries. In A.J. Chapman, F. M. Wade, and H.C. Foot (Eds.), *Pedestrian accidents*, New York: John Wiley.

Ashton, S.J., J.B. Pedder, and G.M. Mackay (1977). Pedestrian leg injuries, the bumper and other front structures. Presented at the International Research Committee on the Biokinetics of Impacts, 3rd International Conference on Impact Trauma, Berlin.

Baker, S.P., B. O'Neill, and R. Karpf (1984). *The injury fact book*. Lexington, MA: Lexington Books.

Baker, S.P., L.S. Robertson, and B. O'Neill (1974). Fatal pedestrian collisions. *American Journal of Public Health* 64: 319–325.

Brison, R.J., K. Wicklund, and B.A. Mueller (1988). Fatal pedestrian injuries to young children: A different pattern of injury. *American Journal of Public Health* 78:793–795.

Haddon, W., Jr., P. Valien, J.R. McCarroll, and C.J. Umberger (1961). A controlled investigation of the characteristics of adult pedestrians fatally injured by motor vehicles in Manhattan. *Journal of Chronic Diseases* 14:655–678.

Insurance Institute for Highway Safety (1990). Alcohol. In *Fatality facts 1990*. Arlington, VA: Insurance Institute for Highway Safety.

MacLaughlin, T.F., and J.W. Kessler (1990). Pedestrian head impact against central hoods of motor vehicles—test procedures and results. *34th Stapp car crash conference proceedings*. Warrendale PA: Society of Automotive Engineers, Inc., pp. 113–121.

Mueller, B.A., F.P. Rivara, and A.B. Bergman (1988). Urban-rural location and the risk of dying in a pedestrian-vehicle collision. *Journal of Trauma* 28:91–94.

National Highway Traffic Safety Administration (1989). *Fatal Accident Reporting System 1988*. Technical Report DOT HS-807-507. Washington, DC: U.S. Department of Transportation.

Pitt, R., B. Guyer, C. Hsieh, and M. Malek (1990). The severity of pedestrian injuries in children: An analysis of the pedestrian injury causation study. *Accident Analysis and Prevention* 22:549–559.

Pless, I.B., R. Verreault, L. Arsenault, J.Y. Frappier, and J. Stulginkas (1987). The epidemiology of road accidents in childhood. *American Journal of Public Health* 77:358–360.

Preusser, D.F., W.A. Lead, K.B. DeBartolo, and R.D. Blomberg (1981). The effect of right-turn-on-red on pedestrian and bicyclist accidents. Technical Report DOT HS-806-182. Washington, DC: National Highway Traffic Safety Administration.

Retting, R.A. (1988). Urban pedestrian safety. *Bulletin of the New York Academy of Medicine* 64:810–815.

Rivara, F.P., and M. Barber (1985). Demographic analysis of childhood pedestrian injuries. *Pediatrics* 76:375–381.

Rivara, F.P., D.T. Reay, and A.B. Bergman (1989). Analysis of fatal pedestrian injuries in King County, WA, and prospects for prevention. *Public Health Reports* 104:293–297.

Robertson, L.S., and S.P. Baker (1976). Motor vehicle sizes in 1440 fatal crashes. *Accident Analysis and Prevention* 8:167–175.

Smeed, R.J. (1976). Pedestrian accidents. *In Proceedings of the International Conference on Pedestrian Safety, Vol. 2*. Haifa, Israel: Technion.

U.S. Congress, House of Representatives. Committee on Public Works (1968). *1968 Alcohol and highway safety report: A study transmitted by the Secretary of the Department of Transportation to the Congress, in accordance with requirements of section 204 of the Highway Safety Act of 1966, Public Law 89-564*. 90th Cong., 2nd sess.

Zador, P.L. (1982). Right-turn-on-red laws and motor vehicle crashes. *Accident Analysis and Prevention* 14:219–234.

20

Motorcyclists

Motorcyclist deaths, numbering almost 3,500 in 1988, comprise 7 percent of all traffic deaths. For males in their twenties, one out of every seven motor vehicle fatalities is a motorcycle driver or passenger. Analyses of FARS and NASS data indicate that for every death there are 50 injuries reported to the police. In addition, many injuries are not reported to the police (Kraus et al. 1975a). This is especially likely when no other motor vehicle is involved.

Motorcyclists generally travel at speeds similar to or greater than passenger vehicle occupants but lack the stability and protection of a four-wheel enclosed vehicle. It is therefore not surprising that the death rate per 100 million person miles of travel is more than 35 times the rate for cars (Table 8-1). The number of deaths per vehicle mile of travel is 19 times the rate for passenger cars (IIHS 1990).

AGE AND SEX

About one-half of all motorcyclist deaths occur in the 20–29-year-old age group and more than 90 percent among ages 15–39. Death rates are highest for ages 18–24 (Figures 4-5 and 20-1). The death rate is 11 times as high for males as for females. Males killed as motorcycle operators outnumber by about 17 to 1 those killed as passengers. For females, the difference is in the opposite direction; female passengers outnumber operators by about 4 to 1.

The best population-based data on nonfatal injuries are from California. These show a very sharp peak in incidence at age 18 (Kraus et al. 1975a). FARS and NASS data indicate that injuries are more apt to be fatal in older motorcyclists. For ages 35–44, there are approximately 70 deaths per 1,000 reported injuries, compared with 32 per 1,000 for ages 25–34 and 16 per 1,000 for ages 15–24.

GEOGRAPHIC DIFFERENCES AND HELMET LAWS

Differences among states in motorcyclist death rates are determined to a large extent by two factors: amount of motorcycle travel and helmet use.

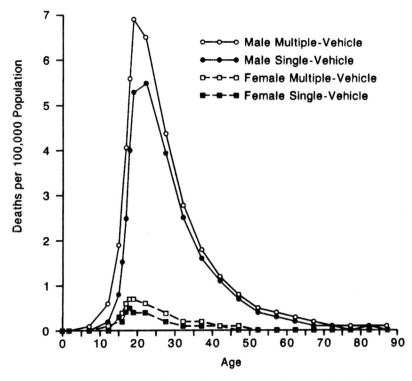

Figure 20-1. Motorcyclist Death Rates by Age, Sex, and Type of Crash, 1980–1986

Laws requiring helmet use by all motorcyclists have been shown by a variety of studies to reduce motorcyclist deaths by about 30 percent. Despite this reduction, many states repealed or weakened their helmet laws in the 1970s and subsequently experienced a substantial drop in helmet use and an increase of about 40 percent in deaths (Watson et al. 1980). This repeal or weakening of helmet use laws occurred in about half of the states, as a result of the revocation of a federal requirement that states without helmet laws would lose some federal highway construction funds.

In states with no helmet law or a law applying only to younger motorcyclists (usually those younger than 18 or 19 years of age), helmet use is typically about 50 percent; in states with helmet use laws for all motorcyclists, use is close to 100 percent. In recent years a number of states have reinstated helmet use laws. When Louisiana and Texas did so, use rose by 95 percent in both states (Lund et al. in press; McSwain et al. 1985). Louisiana's reinstatement was followed by a reduction in the rate of deaths per 1,000 crashes from 38 to 29. California, the state with the most motorcycle fatalities, is one of only three states never to have had a helmet law for all motorcyclists. Such a law was passed by the state legislature in 1988 and 1989, but on both occasions the governor vetoed the bill. In 1991, a helmet law was again passed by the legislature and was signed by the new governor; California's first helmet law for all motorcyclists goes into effect on January 1, 1992.

Improved testing, licensing, and education programs are frequently advocated as alternatives to helmet laws, but there is no evidence that they reduce motorcycle crashes (IIHS 1988).

SEASON, DAY, AND TIME

Because motorcycles expose their riders to the weather, motorcycle use is seasonal, and the pattern of deaths reflects this (Figure 19-2). The number of motorcyclist deaths per month ranges from a low of about 100 in January to a monthly average of 500 in June, July, and August. This seasonal pattern differs from the pattern for car occupants and pedestrians and more closely resembles that for bicyclists, for whom use is also seasonal.

Weekends have the highest incidence of motorcyclist fatalities; 56 percent occur on Friday, Saturday, and Sunday. As in the case of motor vehicle occupant and pedestrian fatalities, most motorcyclist deaths occur during the evening or night. The peak time begins at about 4:00 P.M., which is earlier than the peak for passenger vehicle occupant deaths, and extends to about 2:00 A.M. (Figure 20-2).

TYPES OF CRASHES AND VEHICLES

Collisions with other motor vehicles are involved in 54 percent of all motorcyclist deaths. Characteristics related to the likelihood of motorcycle crashes and injuries include speed at the time of the collision, stability, and conspicuity (Freedman and Davit 1982; Hurt and Thom 1981; Kraus et al. 1975b). The importance of conspicuity is underscored by the fact that more than half of the drivers of vehicles that collide with motorcycles say they did not see the motorcycle in time to avoid the collision (Hurt and Thom 1981). All motorcycles sold in the United States now come with the headlights wired to be on whenever the motorcycle is in use; the daytime use of headlights by motorcyclists has reduced their crash involvement (Zador 1985).

The characteristics of the motorcycle itself, such as the absence of adequate leg protection, and of other structures likely to be impacted by motorcyclists in crashes, such as hardness, degree of curvature or sharpness, and lack of energy attenuation, influence the severity of motorcyclist injuries. About 8 motorcycle occupant deaths per 10,000 registered motorcycles occur each year (IIHS 1990). This ratio is four times as high as for passenger vehicles. Assuming that a motorcycle is used for as many years as a car, this means that the average motorcycle manufactured is four times as likely as a

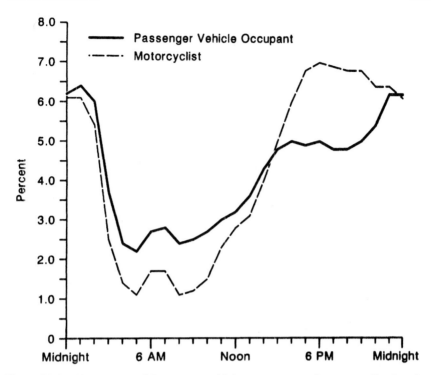

Figure 20-2. Percentage of Passenger Vehicle Occupant and Motorcyclist Deaths by Time of Day, 1980–1988

car to have one of its users killed. The potential benefit to be realized from motorcycle modifications that reduce crashes and injuries is therefore substantial.

Motorcycles patterned after those designed for racing have been shown to have rates of fatal and severe crashes that are twice the rates of other motorcycles (Kraus et al. 1988). The introduction of racing design models in California, with advertising that emphasized high speed and rapid acceleration, was associated with a substantial increase in the motorcycle fatality rates from 1983 to 1986.

ALCOHOL

The likelihood of alcohol involvement in fatal motorcycle crashes varies markedly with operator age, type of crash, and time of crash (Figure 20-3). Fatally injured motorcycle drivers, like passenger car drivers, are most likely to have illegal BACs if they are killed in nighttime single-vehicle crashes. About 80 percent of the drivers aged 25–54 killed in such crashes have BACs

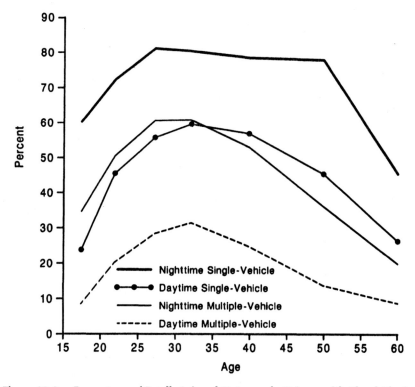

Figure 20-3. Percentage of Fatally Injured Motorcycle Drivers with Blood Alcohol Concentrations at or above 0.10 Percent by Age, Time of Day, and Type of Crash, 1980–1986

of 0.10 percent or higher. Research in Maryland indicated that for the majority of motorcyclists who were found in postmortem examinations to have illegally high BACs, the police reports did not indicate that the motorcyclists had been drinking (Baker and Fisher 1977).

HISTORICAL TRENDS

During the 1970s, no major cause of death from injury or disease experienced an increase as great as that for motorcyclist mortality. During the 1980s, however, there was a decrease in both registered motorcycles and motorcyclist deaths (NSC 1989). The number of deaths declined from 4,961 in 1980 to 3,036 in 1989, a 39 percent decrease (IIHS 1990). The peak in death rates occurred during 1980 and 1981, so that the overall rate for 1984–1986 was very close to the rate for 1977–1979. Between these two periods, death rates declined for people younger than 20 years of age and increased for ages 25 and older (Figure 20-4).

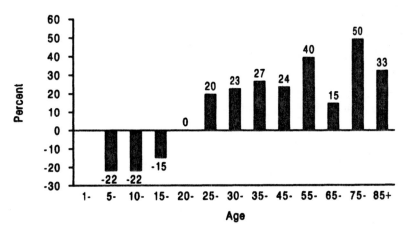

Figure 20-4. Percentage Change in Motorcyclist Death Rates by Age, 1984–1986 Compared with 1977–1979

REFERENCES

Baker, S.P., and R.S. Fisher (1977). Alcohol and motorcycle fatalities. *American Journal of Public Health* 67:246–249.

Freedman, M., and P.S. Davit (1982). *Improved conspicuity to the sides and rear of motorcycles and mopeds. Final Report* (DOT HS-806-377). Washington DC: National Highway Traffic Safety Administration.

Hurt, H.H., and D.R. Thom (1981). *Motorcycle accident cause factors and identification of countermeasures, Final Report* (DOT HS-5-01160). Washington, DC: National Highway Traffic Safety Administration.

Insurance Institute for Highway Safety (1988). Two studies question value of motorcycle licensing program. *Status Report* 23(8):1–2.

Insurance Institute for Highway Safety (1990). Motorcycles. In *Fatality facts 1990.* Arlington, VA: Insurance Institute for Highway Safety.

Kraus, J.F., S. Arzemanian, C.L. Anderson, S. Harrington, and P. Zador (1988). Motorcycle design and crash injuries in California, 1985. *Bulletin of the New York Academy of Medicine.* 64 (7):788–803.

Kraus, J.F., R.S. Riggins, and C.E. Franti (1975a). Some epidemiologic features of motorcycle collision injuries: I. Introduction, methods and factors associated with incidence. *American Journal of Epidemiology* 102:74–98.

Kraus, J.F., R.S. Riggins, and C.E. Franti (1975b). Some epidemiologic features of motorcycle collision injuries: II. Factors associated with severity of injuries. *American Journal of Epidemiology* 102:99–109.

Lund, A.K., A.F. Williams, and K.N. Womack (In press). Motorcycle helmet use in Texas. *Public Health Reports.*

McSwain, N.E., A. Willey, and T.H. Janke (1985). The impact of re-enactment of the motorcycle helmet law in Louisiana. In *Proceedings of the Twenty-Ninth Conference of the American Association for Automotive Medicine.* Arlington Heights, IL: American Association for Automotive Medicine.

National Safety Council (1989). *Accident facts—1989 edition*. Chicago: National
    Safety Council.
Watson, G.S., P.L. Zador, and A. Wilks (1980). The repeal of helmet use laws and
    increased motorcycle mortality in the United States, 1975–1978. *American
    Journal of Public Health* 70:579–585.
Zador, P.L. (1985). Motorcycle headlight use laws and fatal motorcycle crashes in
    the United States, 1975–1983. *American Journal of Public Health* 75:43–46.

21

Bicyclists

About 900 bicyclists were killed in 1988, comprising 2 percent of all traffic deaths. Forty percent of bicyclist deaths occur in the 5–14-year-old age group. For this age group, injuries to bicyclists cause about 15 percent of all traffic deaths and 20 percent of all brain injuries (Kraus et al. 1987). About 90 percent of all bicyclist deaths involve collisions with motor vehicles. Nonfatal injuries, however, generally are caused by falls from bicycles, which are rarely reported to the police (Waller 1971). U.S. emergency rooms treat more than 500,000 bicyclists each year, of whom about 15 percent have been struck by vehicles (CDC 1987).

AGE AND SEX

Two-thirds of bicycle-related injuries are in children less than 15 years old. The death rate rises rapidly beginning at about age 4 and is highest at ages 12–14. Of all bicyclists killed, however, 58 percent are aged 15 or older, and 41 percent are aged 20 or older. Among bicyclists with brain injury, the severity of the injury and the proportion of cases involving motor vehicles increase with age (Kraus et al. 1987). The male to female ratio of death rates for all ages combined is about 5 to 1 (Figures 3-4 and 4-6).

In Seattle, the incidence of bicycle-related head injuries was highest at ages 5–9 (283 per 100,000 population), and the incidence of all bicyclist injuries was highest at ages 10–14 (809 per 100,000 population). Injury rates per 100 miles ridden were also highest in these two age groups, 30.0 and 18.1, respectively (Thompson et al. 1990).

Among children aged 1–18 who were treated for bicycle-related injuries in Philadelphia, 44 percent of the cases involved loss of control of the bicycle and 17 percent involved bicyclists who had been hit by a car. Ten percent were pedestrians who had been struck by a bicycle (Selbst et al. 1987).

The proportion of bicyclists judged to be at fault in collisions with motor vehicles declines with age. In Maryland it decreased from 92 percent in children less than 13 years old to 34 percent in cyclists aged 25 or older (Williams 1976). Among adult bicyclists surveyed in Kansas City, 46 percent had been in bicycle-related crashes, 20 percent of which involved collisions with motor vehicles (Kiburz et al. 1986)

GEOGRAPHIC DIFFERENCES

Regional differences in bicyclist death rates are less pronounced than for other deaths related to motor vehicles (Figure 16-12). Similarly, variation by degree of urbanization shows no pronounced pattern. Death rates are lowest in areas of high per capita income (0.23 per 100,000, compared with 0.36 for the entire population).

SEASON, DAY, AND TIME

The seasonal distribution of bicyclist deaths is similar to that of motorcyclist deaths (Figure 19-2). Almost two-thirds occur during the five-month period from May through September.

Unlike motorcyclist deaths, the peak time of day is from 3:00 P.M. to 7:59 P.M. (Figure 19-3). This period begins after school hours and is substantially earlier than the peak for pedestrians. The importance of visibility is suggested by the fact that among all injury-producing collisions between bicyclists and motor vehicles during twilight or darkness, 28 percent involve the motor vehicle striking the bicycle from the rear or making a left turn in front of an oncoming bicycle (Williams 1976).

About one-third of all bicyclist deaths occur on the weekend between 6:00 P.M. Friday and midnight Sunday. Because half of the fatally injured bicyclists are children, who are less likely than adults to either ride at night or use alcohol, this weekend effect is less pronounced than for other types of motor vehicle deaths. However, alcohol has been identified as an important contributor to deaths of bicyclists aged 15 or older (Kraus et al. 1987).

HISTORICAL TRENDS

Adult bicyclists have made up an increasing proportion of bicyclist fatalities in recent years. In 1989, 43 percent of the fatalities occurred among people aged 21 or older compared with 31 percent in 1980 (IIHS 1990). Death rates for adult bicyclists aged 25 and older increased greatly for 1984–1986 compared with those for 1977–1979 (Figure 21-1). The greatest increase, about 90 percent, occurred in the 35–44-year-old age group. For this age group, the increase in the death rate from bicycle-related injuries far surpassed the increase from any other type of motor vehicle-related crash in any age group. The birth cohorts born between 1944 and 1953, who were aged 35–44 in 1988, had experienced a fourfold increase in bicyclist death

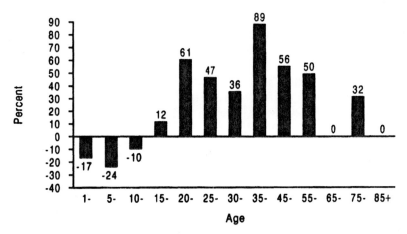

Figure 21-1. Percentage Change in Bicyclist Death Rates by Age, 1984–1986 Compared with 1977–1979

rates in the 1970s, which was also the greatest increase in motor vehicle-related death rates for any group at that time (Baker et al. 1984). These increases probably reflect increased bicycling by adults, but there are no good measures available to reliably assess the extent to which exposure has increased.

PREVENTIVE MEASURES

The use of helmets is the most practical means to reduce bicycle-related head injuries. Evidence supporting their efficacy includes biomechanical laboratory studies, case reports, studies of injury frequency in helmeted versus unhelmeted bicyclists, and comparisons with analogous cases involving motorcycle helmet use. In addition, decreases in the proportion of head injuries among hospitalized bicyclists in Australia were reported during a period of increasing bicycle helmet use (Brown and Farley 1989; Wood and Milne 1988).

Bicyclists wearing helmets were found in one study to have an 85 percent reduction in the risk of head injury (Thompson et al. 1989). Although helmet use is increasing, most bicyclists do not wear helmets. Helmet use by children has been reported as less than 5 percent in several studies, but wearing rates increase with age (Wasserman et al. 1988).

A review of bicyclist deaths in Dade County, Florida, indicated that the head or neck is the most seriously injured part of the body in five out of six fatally injured bicyclists (Fife et al. 1983). Typically, bicyclists who die with serious head injuries do not have other life-threatening or potentially disabling injuries. Thus, if bicyclists used helmets, many fatalities and serious head injuries would not occur.

The primary means to increase bicycle helmet usage in the past have been educational campaigns. One intensive campaign in Seattle included physician education of parents about helmets; extensive newspaper, television, and radio advertising; numerous presentations in schools; and discount coupons for helmets (Bergman et al. 1990). Despite the intensity of the efforts, observed helmet use rose from 6 percent to only 16 percent, leaving most child bicyclists still riding without helmets (DiGuiseppi et al. 1989).

Mandatory bicycle helmet laws are another method to increase helmet usage. With enforcement, legislation is likely to be more effective than education alone. A law mandating helmet use by child bicyclists recently went into effect in Howard County, Maryland; evaluation of the impact of the new law is not yet available. Similar legislation is being considered in several other jurisdictions. On July 1, 1990, it became a legal requirement for all bicyclists in the State of Victoria, Australia, to wear an approved helmet in all riding environments (Sullivan 1990). By mid-1991, helmet use was required in four Australian states; the law in New South Wales was implemented in two phases, with adults required to wear helmets 6 months before use was required by bicyclists under 16 years of age (Baxter and Maisey 1990).

Other promising approaches to reducing bicycle-related injuries include protective and reflective clothing, improvement in bicycle handling characteristics and visibility, and greater opportunity for cycling where the potential for collision with motor vehicles is minimized.

REFERENCES

Baker, S.P., B. O'Neill, and R. Karpf (1984). *The injury fact book*. Lexington, MA: Lexington Books.

Baxter, M., and G. Maisey (1990). *Trends in bicyclist helmet wearing in Western Australia: February/March 1990 Survey*. Perth, Western Australia: W.A. Police Department.

Bergman, A.B., F.P. Rivara, D.D. Richards, and L.W. Rogers (1990). The Seattle children's bicycle helmet campaign. *American Journal of Diseases of Children* 144:727–731.

Brown, B., and C. Farley (1989). The pertinence of promoting the use of bicycle helmets for 8- to 12-year old children. *Chronic Diseases in Canada* 10:92–94.

Centers for Disease Control (1987). Bicycle-related injuries: Data from the National Electronic Injury Surveillance System. *Morbidity and Mortality Weekly Report* 36(17):269–271.

DiGuiseppi, C.G., F.P. Rivara, T.D. Koepsell, and L. Polissar (1989). Bicycle helmet use by children: Evaluation of a community-wide helmet campaign. *Journal of the American Medical Association* 262:2256–2261.

Fife, D., J. Davis, L. Tate, J.K. Wells, D. Mohan, and A.F. Williams (1983). Fatal injuries to bicyclists: The experience of Dade County, Florida. *Journal of Trauma* 23:745–755.

Insurance Institute for Highway Safety (1990). Bicycles. In *Fatality facts 1990.* Arlington, VA: Insurance Institute for Highway Safety.

Kiburz, D., R. Jacobs, F. Reckling, and J. Mason (1986). Bicycle accidents and injuries among adult cyclists. *American Journal of Sports Medicine* 14:416–419.

Kraus, J.F., D. Fife, and C. Conroy (1987). Incidence, severity, and outcomes of brain injuries involving bicycles. *American Journal of Public Health* 77:76–78.

Selbst, S.M., D. Alexander, and R. Ruddy (1987). Bicycle-related injuries. *American Journal of Diseases of Children* 141:140–144.

Sullivan, G. (1990). Initial effects of mandatory bicycle helmet wearing legislation. Hawthorn, Victoria, Australia: VIC Roads.

Thompson, R.S., F.P. Rivara, and D.C. Thompson (1989). A case-control study of the effectiveness of bicycle safety helmets. *New England Journal of Medicine* 320:1361–1367

Thompson, D.C., R.S. Thompson, and F.P. Rivara (1990). Incidence of bicycle-related injuries in a defined population. *American Journal of Public Health* 80:1388–1390.

Waller, J.A. (1971). Bicycle ownership, use and injury patterns among elementary school children. *Pediatrics* 47:1042–1050.

Wasserman, R.C., J.A. Waller, M.J. Monty, A.B. Emery, and D.R. Robinson (1988). Bicyclists, helmets and head injuries: A rider-based study of helmet use and effectiveness. *American Journal of Public Health* 78:1220–1221.

Williams, A.F. (1976). Factors in the initiation of bicycle-motor vehicle collisions. *American Journal of Diseases of Children* 130:370–377.

Wood, T., and P. Milne (1988). Head injuries to pedal cyclists and the promotion of helmet use in Victoria, Australia. *Accident Analysis and Prevention* 20:177–185.

22

Conclusion

Injuries impose a greater burden on modern societies than any disease. Unlike many other major health problems, a variety of effective preventive measures are available that are well within the state of the art and inexpensive in relation to their potential benefits (Rice, MacKenzie, and associates 1989). These measures often are not applied. Too commonly, efforts to reduce the injury problem have utilized unproductive approaches. The results of neglect and misdirected efforts are reflected in the death rates reported in the preceding chapters.

Analyses in this book identify population subgroups at high risk of injury and death. More comprehensive discussions of ways to reduce injuries and of related public policies are presented in many of the references cited in Chapter 1 and elsewhere in the literature. Many new questions raised by the analyses in this book, however, can be answered only by additional research requiring better data or the enhancement of existing sources of data.

GAPS IN INFORMATION

A major information gain would result if computerized hospital discharge records for all injured patients included ICD E-codes detailing the cause of injury. It would then be possible to study the morbidity and incidence of serious injuries in relation to their causes, as we have done with mortality data in this book. At present, data on people hospitalized for injuries include the type of injury but too often fail to identify its cause. As a result, the potential value of NCHS's Hospital Discharge Survey and of statewide hospital-based data systems for developing and evaluating countermeasures is not realized.

Further gains would result from including relevant questions on injury causation in the National Health Interview Survey. The most recent attempt to identify products other than motor vehicles was in 1975, and almost two decades have elapsed since questions were included on the incidence of gunshot wounds (Baker 1983). Although designed to give information on injuries from consumer products, NEISS does not routinely collect identifying information, such as make and model, on the products involved in injury. When such data are collected they are not available to the public, even though comparable specifics on vehicles are available for every police-reported crash. Such data have been invaluable in promoting and evaluating improvements in automobiles.

Data for fatal injuries, while far better than those for nonfatal injuries, also leave much to be desired. For instance, the place of injury (home, nursing home, school, etc.) is not recorded on many death certificates, nor are the circumstances of falls (on one level, on stairs, from a ladder, etc.). Similarly, ICD codes for describing the specific type of firearm that caused an injury generally are not used. In many states death certificates indicate whether a fatal injury occurred at work, but this information often is lacking for a substantial portion of cases and is not reported by NCHS (Smith et al. 1991). NIOSH now collects and publishes the data, but underreporting is still a problem (see Chapter 9).

Until some of these gaps in injury information from hospital records and death certificates are filled, we will remain overly dependent on sources such as work-related injury information furnished by employers. Such sources notoriously underreport the occurrence of injuries and do not provide the detail needed for setting priorities and planning interventions (Pollack and Kleimig 1987). Similarly, incidence rates for nonfatal injuries from motor vehicle crashes and assaults based on police reports are likely to be greatly underestimated. Such incidence data are almost nonexistent for other injuries (Baker 1983; Barancik et al. 1983; Rice et al. 1989).

GAPS IN PREVENTION

Even more serious than the gaps in our information base is the discrepancy between what is already known about the etiology and prevention of injuries and the application of that knowledge. More than four decades ago, Hugh DeHaven, in his classic study of falls from heights, noted that the "structural environment is the dominant cause of injury" and that fatal injuries in aircraft and automobiles "are often sustained under moderate and controllable circumstances" (DeHaven 1942). Despite progress in making automobiles more crashworthy, the statement is still true. State-of-the-art crash protection systems such as air bags, which were sufficiently developed for application in the early 1970s, are only now being used on a large scale, and it will be the late 1990s before all new passenger vehicles will be equipped with them. Improvements in side impact protection, especially protection to prevent head injuries, are still some years away. In addition, most roads today do not provide state-of-the-art protection against foreseeable events such as cars leaving the roadway on curves. Nor have available knowledge and technology been adequately applied in the designs of trucks, aircraft, boats, tractors, cranes, forklifts, guns, and many other products associated with high injury rates.

The literature on injuries has given an inordinate amount of attention to the behavior of the people involved. Less emphasis has been placed on the relationships between high-risk groups of people and effective means of protecting them. Failure to use automobile seat belts, for example, has been shown to be especially common among those at greatest risk of being involved in crashes, such as teenagers, alcohol-impaired drivers, people traveling at night, drivers who follow other cars too closely or ignore red traffic lights, and people in low income areas (see Chapter 17). Thus, the groups at risk are often those whose behavior is the most difficult to change. If injuries among the people at greatest risk are to be reduced, the difficulty of changing their behavior must be taken into account in planning effective approaches. Virtually all available evidence indicates that, for injuries as for diseases, the most effective way to protect high-risk groups as well as the rest of the population is with measures—such as pasteurization and household fuses—that do not require individual motivation and frequent effort (Baker 1981; Barry 1975; Haddon 1974, 1980; Robertson 1983). Where correct behavior is important, for example, wearing a helmet when riding a motorcycle, making the appropriate behavior mandatory is more successful than reliance on education and training to provide the desired behavior voluntarily. Despite the overwhelming evidence in favor of legislation in this regard, many policy makers continue to advocate educational approaches that are demonstrated failures.

Some of the facts in this book document the success of measures that have protected the public against injury. Nonpoisonous domestic fuels and stringent elevator regulations, for example, have virtually eliminated hazards that once caused hundreds of deaths each year. Most of the analyses, however, reveal the need to apply equally effective countermeasures to hazards still prevalent. In doing so, particular attention should be given to protecting groups whose activities, age, income, location, and other characteristics render them especially liable to serious injury. If that task is now easier, this book will have met its objective.

REFERENCES

Baker, S.P. (1981). Childhood injuries: The community approach to prevention. *Journal of Public Health Policy* 2:235–246.

Baker, S.P. (1983). Medical data and injuries. *American Journal of Public Health* 73:733–734.

Barancik, J.I., B.F. Chatterjee, Y.C. Greene, E.M. Michenzi, and D. Fife (1983). Northeastern Ohio Trauma Study: I. Magnitude of the problem. *American Journal of Public Health* 73:746–751.

Barry, P.Z. (1975). Individual versus community orientation in the prevention of injuries. *Preventive Medicine* 4:47–56.

DeHaven, H. (1942). Mechanical analysis of survival in falls from heights of fifty to one hundred and fifty feet. *War Medicine* 2:539–546.

Haddon, W., Jr. (1974). Strategy in preventive medicine: Passive vs. active approaches to reducing human wastage. *Journal of Trauma* 14:353–354.

Haddon, W., Jr. (1980). Advances in the epidemiology of injuries as a basis for public policy. *Public Health Reports* 95:411–421.

Haddon, W., Jr. (1983). The safety of the automobile—An international perspective. Presented at the Nordic Seminar on the Safety of the Automobile, Linkoping, Sweden.

Pollack, E.S., and D.G. Kleimig (1987). *Counting injuries and illnesses in the workplace: Proposals for a better system.* Washington, DC: National Academy Press.

Rice, D.P., E.J. MacKenzie, and associates (1989). *Cost of injury in the United States: A report to Congress.* San Francisco: Institute for Health and Aging, University of California and Injury Prevention Center, The Johns Hopkins University.

Robertson, L.S. (1983). *Injuries: Causes, control strategies, and public policy.* Lexington, MA: Lexington Books.

Smith, G.S., L. Jenkins, and M. Goldstein (1991). Case finding for occupational injury fatalities. Baltimore, MD: The Johns Hopkins Injury Prevention Center.

APPENDIX

SOURCES OF DATA AND BASIS FOR COMPUTATIONS

Except where otherwise indicated, rates in figures were based on the following data:

Type of Figure	Source of Numerator	Source of Denominator
Death rates per 100,000 population for 1980-1986	Underlying cause of death, U.S. residents, 1980-1986[1]	U.S. resident population, 1980 census[2] and Census Bureau estimates for 1981-1986[3]
Death rates by year for 1930-1986	1930-1977 underlying cause of death, U.S. residents, for each year[4]; 1978-1986 from mortality tapes[1]	U.S. resident population estimates for each year as of July 1 (Census Bureau)
Death rates per 100,000 population 1980-1988 (motor vehicle-related)	Deaths in U.S. from motor vehicle crashes on public roads in 1980-1988, from FARS[5]	U.S. resident population, 1980 Census,[2] and Census Bureau estimates for 1981-1986[3]
Deaths per 1,000 injuries or per 1,000 occupants in crashes	Deaths in U.S. from motor vehicle crashes on public roads from FARS[5]	Estimates of injured persons or occupants from NASS[6]
Death rates per million vehicle miles	Deaths in U.S. from motor vehicle crashes on public roads from FARS[5]	Estimates of vehicle miles of travel from FHWA[7]

1. Mortality Detail Tapes. Annual tapes, National Center for Health Statistics.
2. Census of Population and Housing 1980: Summary Tape File C1, Bureau of the Census.
3. United States Population Estimates, by Age, Sex, and Race: 1980 to 1987. Series P-25, No. 1022, Bureau of the Census.
4. Vital Statistics of the United States. Annual volumes, National Center for Health Statistics.
5. Fatal Accident Reporting System (FARS) Annual tapes, National Highway Traffic Safety Administration.
6. National Accident Sampling System (NASS) Annual tapes, National Highway Traffic Safety Administration.
7. Highway Statistics. Annual publication, Federal Highway Administration.

COMPUTATIONAL METHODS

Death rates, unless otherwise indicated, are calculated per year and for the entire United States. They are not adjusted for age, race, or other populations characteristics (see page 30).

Sex ratios were calculated by dividing the unadjusted death rate for males by the unadjusted death rate for females.

Rural to urban ratios were calculated by dividing the death rate in rural remote areas by the death rate in central cities (see page 26).

Age-specific rates plotted at age 90 are for persons 85 and older. Where the last plotted point is at age 80, it represents age group 75-84.

Maps divide the 50 states into four strata: the 10 areas with the lowest rates, the 15 next lowest, the 15 next to the highest, and the 10 with the highest rates. On a few maps, the number in each strata differs slightly from these specifications because two or more states had the same death rate and therefore needed to be in the same stratum.

Table 1. Number of Deaths and Death Rates by Sex and Race, 69 Causes

Cause	ICD E-Code (9th Rev.)	Deaths					Deaths per 100,000 population, 1980-1986						
		1986	1987	1988 (prelim.)	Male (1986)	Female (1986)	Male	Female	Total	White	Black	Native Amer	Asian
Transportation													
1. Motor Vehicle-Train	810	574	554	638	388	185	0.38	0.14	0.26	0.27	0.19	0.32	0.06
2. Motor Vehicle Occupant	810-819(.0,.1,.9)	35,343	36,184	37,063	24,320	11,023	21.41	8.69	14.88	15.50	10.80	28.95	7.70
3. Motorcyclist	810-819(.2,.3)	3,494	3,089	2,837	3,205	289	2.84	0.25	1.51	1.63	0.88	1.40	0.37
4. Bicyclist	810-819(.6)	886	922	859	754	132	0.61	0.12	0.36	0.35	0.39	0.33	0.25
5. Pedestrian	810-819(.7)	7,039	7,062	7,219	4,946	2,093	4.61	1.86	3.19	2.91	4.80	11.25	2.50
6. Motor Vehicle-Traffic (Total)	810-819	46,867	47,297	48,024	33,315	13,552	29.50	10.83	19.96	20.42	16.68	41.97	10.82
7. Pedestrian-Nontraffic	822.7	381	379	380	248	132	0.26	0.13	0.20	0.20	0.16	0.79	0.13
8. Pedestrian-Train	805.2	465	486	470	413	52	0.33	0.05	0.18	0.16	0.30	0.85	0.08
9. Aircraft	840-845	1,148	1,263	1,012	960	188	1.02	0.20	0.60	0.68	0.08	0.52	0.19
Drowning													
10. Boat-Related	830,832	923	740	767	848	75	0.84	0.06	0.44	0.43	0.54	1.14	0.21
11. Non-Boat	910	4,777	4,360	4,199	3,856	921	3.53	0.77	2.16	1.91	3.59	5.78	1.89
12. Drowning (Total)	830,832,910	5,700	5,100	4,966	4,704	996	4.47	0.83	2.60	2.34	4.22	6.92	2.09
Poisoning													
13. Opiates	850.0	930	595	798	786	144	0.45	0.08	0.26	0.24	0.42	0.20	0.06
14. Barbiturates	851	49	30	29	33	16	0.04	0.03	0.03	0.03	0.03	0.03	0.01
15. Tranquilizers	853	92	63	83	55	37	0.05	0.03	0.04	0.04	0.04	0.04	0.01
16. Antidepressants	854.0	154	122	147	81	73	0.05	0.06	0.06	0.06	0.05	0.10	0.00
17. Alcohol	860	352	347	334	280	72	0.24	0.07	0.15	0.12	0.38	0.59	0.02
18. Solids/Liquids (Total)	850-866	4,731	4,415	5,353	3,341	1,390	2.18	1.00	1.57	1.49	2.34	2.28	0.37
19. Motor Vehicle Exhaust	868.2	475	402	372	386	89	0.38	0.10	0.24	0.24	0.24	0.26	0.03
20. Gas/Vapor (Total)	867-869	1,009	900	873	764	245	0.76	0.25	0.50	0.49	0.61	0.70	0.07
Falls													
21. Stairs	880	1,137	1,135	1,093	654	483	0.61	0.44	0.52	0.55	0.43	0.29	0.12
22. Ladder/Scaffold	881	325	354	364	311	14	0.29	0.01	0.15	0.16	0.09	0.10	0.07
23. Building/Structure	882	650	685	672	540	110	0.51	0.08	0.29	0.28	0.40	0.40	0.20
24. Different Level	884	1,003	1,086	1,089	661	342	0.61	0.30	0.45	0.47	0.31	0.56	0.23
25. Same Level	885	399	400	426	195	194	0.17	0.18	0.17	0.18	0.07	0.10	0.04
26. Other/Unspecified	883,886-888	7,940	8,071	8,452	3,682	4,258	3.45	3.79	3.63	3.87	2.35	2.25	1.06
27. Fall (Total)	880-888	11,444	11,733	12,096	6,043	5,401	5.64	4.80	5.21	5.52	3.66	3.70	1.72
Fires and Burns													
28. Housefires	890	3,971	3,909	4,088	2,391	1,560	2.20	1.38	1.76	1.41	4.55	3.20	0.45
29. Clothing Ignition	893	179	200	205	90	89	0.11	0.11	0.11	0.10	0.20	0.10	0.01
30. Fires/Burns Excl. Scalds	890-899	4,835	4,710	4,965	2,984	1,851	2.61	1.67	2.23	1.81	5.37	3.78	0.61
31. Fires/Burns (Total)	890-899,924	4,969	4,847	5,087	3,055	1,914	2.89	1.74	2.30	1.87	5.52	3.62	0.65

Table 1 (cont.) Number of Deaths and Death Rates by Sex and Race, 69 Causes

Cause	ICD E-Code (9th Rev.)	Deaths					Deaths per 100,000 population, 1980-1986						
		1986	1987	1988 (prelim.)	Male (1986)	Female (1986)	Male	Female	Total	White	Black	Native Amer	Asian
Other Unintentional													
32. Firearm	922	1,452	1,440	1,501	1,254	198	1.30	0.20	0.73	0.71	0.93	2.33	0.16
33. Excessive Heat	900	364	338	454	220	144	0.25	0.18	0.22	0.15	0.70	0.31	0.01
34. Excessive Cold	901	619	531	846	430	189	0.51	0.19	0.34	0.25	0.95	2.61	0.04
35. Exposure/Neglect	904	207	169	199	115	92	0.14	0.09	0.12	0.10	0.16	1.41	0.02
36. Lightning	907	78	99	82	69	9	0.07	0.01	0.04	0.04	0.03	0.18	0.01
37. Natural Disaster	908-909	70	116	66	46	24	0.08	0.05	0.06	0.08	0.05	0.10	0.02
38. Aspiration-Food	911	1,709	1,569	1,575	966	743	0.93	0.64	0.78	0.77	0.90	1.10	0.34
39. Aspiration-Nonfood	912	1,983	2,119	2,230	1,037	946	0.77	0.60	0.68	0.65	0.99	0.83	0.25
40. Suffocation	913	941	1,009	956	728	213	0.60	0.18	0.38	0.36	0.41	0.85	0.18
41. Struck by Falling Object	916	888	902	835	851	37	0.80	0.05	0.42	0.42	0.41	0.48	0.08
42. Collision with Object/Person	917	243	193	239	208	35	0.20	0.03	0.11	0.12	0.11	0.17	0.06
43. Caught/Crushed	918	112	122	133	95	17	0.09	0.01	0.05	0.05	0.05	0.05	0.04
44. Machinery	919	1,202	1,253	1,176	1,141	61	1.13	0.05	0.57	0.62	0.34	0.49	0.13
45. Cutting/Piercing	920	118	87	119	105	13	0.09	0.02	0.05	0.05	0.10	0.12	0.03
46. Explosion	923	242	216	193	203	39	0.22	0.03	0.12	0.12	0.14	0.16	0.06
47. Electric Current	925	854	760	714	805	49	0.77	0.04	0.40	0.42	0.27	0.27	0.08
48. Unintentional Excl. Traffic	800-807,820-949	48,410	47,723	49,076	32,255	16,155	29.27	13.55	21.20	20.57	26.76	35.19	8.08
49. Unintentional (Total)	800-949	95,277	95,020	97,100	65,570	29,707	58.77	24.48	41.15	40.99	43.84	77.16	18.90
Suicide													
50. Firearm	955	18,160	18,144	18,181	15,525	2,635	12.42	2.18	7.16	7.60	3.47	7.21	1.76
51. Poison Solids/Liquids	950	3,070	3,106	3,133	1,383	1,687	1.14	1.42	1.28	1.40	0.50	1.15	0.79
52. Motor Vehicle Exhaust	952.0	2,450	2,684	2,247	1,757	693	1.34	0.52	0.82	1.06	0.12	0.22	0.18
53. Hanging	953	4,606	4,235	4,375	3,761	845	2.93	0.63	1.75	1.81	1.08	3.71	2.39
54. Drowning	954	493	454	401	282	211	0.26	0.18	0.22	0.21	0.28	0.12	0.19
55. Cutting/Piercing	956	432	433	461	328	104	0.28	0.08	0.18	0.19	0.09	0.20	0.20
56. Jumping	957	680	642	625	471	209	0.44	0.21	0.32	0.32	0.34	0.09	0.57
57. Non-Firearm (Total)	950-954,956-959	12,744	12,652	12,226	8,701	4,043	6.99	3.27	5.08	5.42	2.62	5.90	4.56
58. Suicide (Total)	950-959	30,904	30,796	30,407	24,226	6,678	19.42	5.45	12.24	13.23	6.09	13.11	6.31
Homicide													
59. Firearm	965	13,045	12,665	13,666	10,665	2,380	9.60	1.98	5.69	3.58	21.06	5.69	2.72
60. Cutting/Stabbing	966	4,342	4,099	3,939	3,308	1,034	2.89	0.77	1.60	1.09	6.86	4.40	0.91
61. Strangulation	963	1,006	1,015	928	321	685	0.28	0.52	0.40	0.31	1.00	0.57	0.35
62. Other	960-962,964,967-969	3,069	3,033	3,251	2,038	1,031	1.69	0.85	1.25	0.93	3.41	3.35	0.84
63. Non-Firearm (Total)	960-964,966-969	8,417	8,147	8,118	5,667	2,750	4.85	2.14	3.46	2.33	11.28	8.32	2.11
64. Homicide (Total)	960-969	21,462	20,812	21,784	16,332	5,130	14.46	4.12	9.15	5.91	32.36	14.01	4.83
65. Legal Intervention-Firearm	970	247	257	232	241	6	0.23	0.00	0.11	0.08	0.36	0.17	0.04
66. Undetermined-Firearm	985	496	413	443	419	77	0.40	0.06	0.23	0.23	0.28	0.71	0.07
67. Undet-Poison Solids/Liquids	980	1,033	1,146	1,285	648	385	0.45	0.29	0.37	0.35	0.49	0.63	0.18
68. Undetermined (Total)	980-989	3,108	3,011	3,018	2,258	850	2.01	0.77	1.37	1.20	2.50	3.52	0.78
69. Injuries (Total)	800-999	151,032	149,942	153,275	106,661	42,371	94.91	34.81	64.04	61.42	84.96	107.98	30.96

Table 2. Number of Deaths of Males by Age, 69 Causes, 1986

Cause	0	1-	5-	10-	15-	20-	25-	30-	35-	45-	55-	65-	75-	85+
Transportation														
1. Motor Vehicle-Train	2	4	6	11	65	68	55	38	47	29	31	15	12	6
2. Motor Vehicle Occupant	76	233	203	365	3,914	4,792	3,378	2,408	2,974	1,752	1,604	1,294	1,048	268
3. Motorcyclist	1	1	8	56	529	961	690	428	349	105	47	22	5	0
4. Bicyclist	0	17	105	192	131	69	52	46	42	29	23	25	18	4
5. Pedestrian	10	227	317	168	340	535	513	388	596	476	464	370	376	139
6. Motor Vehicle-Traffic (Total)	87	483	641	793	4,931	6,369	4,644	3,277	3,965	2,371	2,140	1,713	1,448	411
7. Pedestrian-Nontraffic	7	71	13	6	3	14	22	15	27	22	19	14	14	2
8. Pedestrian-Train	0	2	3	6	48	71	64	51	76	38	17	15	11	3
9. Aircraft	1	6	7	9	20	78	119	137	237	180	120	33	2	1
Drowning														
10. Boat-Related	0	6	11	21	61	105	121	81	155	105	97	63	19	3
11. Non-Boat	47	433	229	246	548	524	436	320	369	219	167	143	101	33
12. Drowning (Total)	47	439	240	267	609	629	557	401	524	324	264	206	120	36
Poisoning														
13. Opiates	0	2	0	0	9	54	169	231	249	52	14	1	2	0
14. Barbiturates	0	0	0	0	1	3	7	4	7	4	5	0	2	0
15. Tranquilizers	0	3	0	0	1	2	8	12	11	8	5	4	1	0
16. Antidepressants	0	1	1	1	1	5	8	13	26	13	9	3	0	0
17. Alcohol	1	0	1	2	6	7	18	27	75	60	56	20	5	1
18. Solids/Liquids (Total)	8	29	7	14	83	258	651	747	850	257	180	123	92	37
19. Motor Vehicle Exhaust	1	4	1	2	39	45	50	50	65	46	29	23	22	9
20. Gas/Vapor (Total)	3	11	7	7	71	76	92	78	119	90	76	65	50	19
Falls														
21. Stairs	1	2	0	0	3	7	8	20	40	55	94	165	158	101
22. Ladder/Scaffold	0	0	0	1	6	14	10	25	34	41	64	57	45	14
23. Building/Structure	3	20	2	2	33	70	71	56	78	67	47	46	36	11
24. Different Level	11	12	8	13	44	57	52	46	68	62	73	65	92	58
25. Same Level	0	3	1	2	6	4	1	2	10	8	21	39	57	41
26. Other/Unspecified	10	15	8	11	38	61	68	85	189	228	377	531	1,001	1,057
27. Fall (Total)	25	52	19	29	130	213	210	234	417	461	676	903	1,389	1,282
Fires and Burns														
28. Housefires	49	357	155	83	76	126	173	156	233	206	231	247	195	101
29. Clothing Ignition	0	2	0	0	0	2	2	0	5	6	11	23	23	16
30. Fires/Burns Excl. Scalds	54	369	168	87	89	161	216	193	301	269	319	333	282	135
31. Fires/Burns (Total)	59	376	169	87	90	167	218	195	307	272	328	345	292	142

Table 2 (cont.) Number of Deaths of Males by Age, 69 Causes, 1986

Cause	0	1-	5-	10-	15-	20-	25-	30-	35-	45-	55-	65-	75-	85+
Other Unintentional														
32. Firearm	2	20	40	125	210	183	148	116	143	93	73	56	33	9
33. Excessive Heat	1	4	0	1	11	11	8	13	29	28	36	28	40	12
34. Excessive Cold	0	1	0	1	12	16	14	18	47	64	69	85	64	36
35. Exposure/Neglect	4	1	0	0	0	3	3	2	7	9	15	14	35	15
36. Lightning	0	0	2	3	7	19	4	7	8	5	10	2	2	0
37. Natural Disaster	0	0	0	4	7	3	5	2	6	5	6	4	3	1
38. Aspiration-Food	48	38	6	10	7	27	24	38	86	80	127	181	173	121
39. Aspiration-Nonfood	48	35	8	8	12	6	20	14	33	58	106	193	257	239
40. Suffocation	109	36	24	63	58	76	78	74	85	39	39	30	8	11
41. Struck by Falling Object	0	4	11	8	42	74	84	98	146	156	105	78	24	3
42. Collision with Object/Person	0	4	3	10	20	20	35	12	32	21	21	17	8	5
43. Caught/Crushed	2	3	2	4	5	8	17	14	11	12	8	6	3	0
44. Machinery	1	25	16	23	54	94	95	96	164	140	214	132	69	16
45. Cutting/Piercing	0	3	1	1	5	9	10	13	16	17	11	10	6	3
46. Explosion	0	3	2	4	8	12	28	21	39	28	36	11	12	1
47. Electric Current	2	10	10	18	81	126	136	111	142	79	52	26	11	0
48. Unintentional Excl. Traffic	405	1,261	663	817	1,749	2,417	2,871	2,719	3,967	2,858	3,208	3,381	3,460	2,375
49. Unintentional (Total)	492	1,744	1,304	1,610	6,680	8,788	7,515	5,996	7,932	5,229	5,348	5,094	4,908	2,786
Suicide														
50. Firearm	0	0	1	114	896	1,683	1,584	1,465	2,198	1,760	1,954	2,052	1,408	306
51. Poison Solids/Liquids	0	0	0	3	54	114	202	214	339	171	128	95	45	18
52. Motor Vehicle Exhaust	0	0	0	0	108	185	223	234	372	238	172	128	78	19
53. Hanging	0	0	2	77	324	561	569	477	527	317	330	273	205	95
54. Drowning	0	0	0	0	5	24	36	39	45	31	31	27	31	13
55. Cutting/Piercing	0	0	0	1	3	19	50	33	52	28	59	49	25	9
56. Jumping	0	0	0	1	16	56	66	66	67	56	46	39	40	16
57. Non-Firearm (Total)	0	0	2	82	556	1,041	1,241	1,150	1,544	948	834	660	448	178
58. Suicide (Total)	0	0	3	196	1,552	2,724	2,825	2,625	3,742	2,708	2,788	2,712	1,856	484
Homicide														
59. Firearm	3	29	33	111	1,044	2,093	2,077	1,676	1,932	893	442	217	70	13
60. Cutting/Stabbing	3	11	8	13	258	587	608	511	590	316	214	120	51	9
61. Strangulation	9	13	7	4	18	29	33	30	61	46	27	18	13	7
62. Other	137	170	20	19	68	154	222	209	343	212	213	129	83	21
63. Non-Firearm (Total)	149	194	35	36	364	770	863	750	994	574	454	267	147	37
64. Homicide (Total)	152	223	68	147	1,408	2,863	2,940	2,426	2,926	1,467	896	484	217	50
65. Legal Intervention-Firearm	0	0	0	0	24	44	43	46	42	21	11	7	2	0
66. Undetermined-Firearm	0	0	0	16	47	72	64	45	54	38	37	26	17	2
67. Undet-Poison Solids/Liquids	0	3	0	1	19	59	115	172	177	53	21	16	6	2
68. Undetermined (Total)	30	33	5	32	121	238	319	335	453	243	199	117	83	28
69. Injuries (Total)	674	2,000	1,380	1,985	9,785	14,657	13,649	11,431	15,107	9,670	9,248	8,414	7,067	3,349

Table 3. Death Rates per 100,000 Population for Males by Age, 69 Causes, 1980-1986

Cause	0	1-	5-	10-	15-	20-	25-	30-	35-	45-	55-	65-	75-	85+
Transportation														
1. Motor Vehicle-Train	0.08	0.09	0.07	0.07	0.75	0.74	0.54	0.39	0.35	0.33	0.31	0.32	0.46	0.52
2. Motor Vehicle Occupant	4.87	3.41	2.45	4.01	40.05	46.92	32.02	24.73	19.88	17.27	16.16	17.20	27.79	31.37
3. Motorcyclist	0.04	0.02	0.12	0.77	5.83	9.31	6.46	4.00	2.26	1.01	0.52	0.35	0.21	0.21
4. Bicyclist	0.01	0.16	1.23	1.53	1.28	0.63	0.42	0.29	0.26	0.24	0.26	0.33	0.51	0.54
5. Pedestrian	0.37	3.35	3.98	2.25	4.29	5.47	4.67	4.02	3.95	4.61	4.99	6.03	12.54	19.27
6. Motor Vehicle-Traffic (Total)	5.29	6.95	7.81	9.00	51.51	62.37	43.59	33.04	26.37	23.15	21.95	23.92	41.06	51.51
7. Pedestrian-Nontraffic	0.22	1.32	0.16	0.05	0.11	0.18	0.16	0.15	0.17	0.22	0.26	0.34	0.52	0.77
8. Pedestrian-Train	0.00	0.03	0.05	0.13	0.45	0.63	0.51	0.42	0.39	0.34	0.23	0.22	0.39	0.50
9. Aircraft	0.09	0.10	0.10	0.16	0.36	1.08	1.57	1.81	1.96	1.93	1.12	0.44	0.10	0.04
Drowning														
10. Boat-Related	0.02	0.13	0.17	0.29	0.88	1.30	1.28	1.09	1.05	1.01	0.92	0.89	0.54	0.31
11. Non-Boat	2.59	6.04	2.82	2.96	6.40	5.97	4.34	3.34	2.45	2.20	2.01	2.14	2.96	3.87
12. Drowning (Total)	2.61	6.17	2.98	3.24	7.28	7.26	5.62	4.43	3.50	3.21	2.93	3.03	3.50	4.17
Poisoning														
13. Opiates	0.00	0.01	0.00	0.00	0.08	0.50	1.22	1.52	0.88	0.31	0.07	0.02	0.01	0.06
14. Barbiturates	0.01	0.00	0.00	0.00	0.02	0.06	0.08	0.07	0.06	0.05	0.03	0.03	0.03	0.02
15. Tranquilizers	0.00	0.01	0.00	0.00	0.01	0.06	0.08	0.08	0.08	0.07	0.06	0.04	0.02	0.04
16. Antidepressants	0.01	0.03	0.01	0.00	0.02	0.05	0.08	0.09	0.12	0.07	0.06	0.04	0.02	0.02
17. Alcohol	0.02	0.01	0.00	0.01	0.07	0.12	0.21	0.30	0.41	0.58	0.55	0.29	0.07	0.02
18. Solids/Liquids (Total)	0.40	0.41	0.06	0.13	0.82	2.47	4.79	5.24	3.38	1.96	1.53	1.55	2.27	4.31
19. Motor Vehicle Exhaust	0.03	0.02	0.02	0.02	0.33	0.58	0.50	0.52	0.52	0.50	0.43	0.32	0.67	0.97
20. Gas/Vapor (Total)	0.14	0.22	0.09	0.11	0.68	1.08	0.96	0.94	0.92	0.96	0.92	0.84	1.59	2.05
Falls														
21. Stairs	0.12	0.09	0.01	0.01	0.03	0.08	0.13	0.18	0.29	0.70	1.21	2.15	4.99	12.20
22. Ladder/Scaffold	0.00	0.00	0.00	0.00	0.06	0.15	0.15	0.19	0.25	0.42	0.68	0.79	1.54	1.74
23. Building/Structure	0.08	0.25	0.06	0.09	0.36	0.69	0.64	0.58	0.51	0.63	0.66	0.76	1.26	1.87
24. Different Level	0.68	0.23	0.09	0.14	0.51	0.65	0.53	0.48	0.43	0.53	0.65	1.00	2.72	10.49
25. Same Level	0.00	0.01	0.01	0.01	0.03	0.04	0.02	0.03	0.04	0.08	0.17	0.54	1.81	6.61
26. Other/Unspecified	0.59	0.23	0.10	0.12	0.41	0.67	0.71	0.93	1.30	2.34	4.00	8.35	33.68	147.56
27. Fall (Total)	1.47	0.82	0.27	0.37	1.39	2.27	2.18	2.39	2.82	4.71	7.37	13.59	46.00	180.48
Fires and Burns														
28. Housefires	3.42	4.99	1.83	0.86	0.85	1.46	1.65	1.52	1.54	2.13	2.68	3.73	6.32	12.62
29. Clothing Ignition	0.00	0.02	0.01	0.00	0.01	0.02	0.01	0.01	0.04	0.08	0.19	0.37	1.02	2.74
30. Fires/Burns Excl. Scalds	3.58	5.33	1.95	0.94	1.03	1.80	2.04	1.97	2.04	2.85	3.71	5.17	9.67	19.17
31. Fires/Burns (Total)	3.85	5.48	1.96	0.94	1.04	1.84	2.06	2.01	2.09	2.92	3.81	5.36	10.08	20.26

Table 3 (cont.) Death Rates per 100,000 Population for Males by Age, 69 Causes, 1980-1986

Cause	0	1-	5-	10-	15-	20-	25-	30-	35-	45-	55-	65-	75-	85+
Other Unintentional														
32. Firearm	0.05	0.38	0.56	1.67	2.54	2.23	1.68	1.35	1.14	1.02	0.86	0.86	0.93	0.65
33. Excessive Heat	0.14	0.04	0.01	0.01	0.04	0.08	0.08	0.15	0.22	0.35	0.50	0.75	1.48	2.53
34. Excessive Cold	0.14	0.02	0.01	0.03	0.17	0.18	0.16	0.21	0.36	0.75	1.14	1.51	2.95	5.35
35. Exposure/Neglect	0.25	0.01	0.00	0.00	0.03	0.03	0.04	0.06	0.09	0.15	0.24	0.44	1.06	2.73
36. Lightning	0.00	0.00	0.02	0.06	0.14	0.11	0.08	0.06	0.08	0.07	0.06	0.04	0.03	0.04
37. Natural Disaster	0.04	0.04	0.05	0.05	0.05	0.07	0.09	0.08	0.09	0.09	0.09	0.12	0.12	0.12
38. Aspiration-Food	3.62	0.60	0.09	0.10	0.19	0.28	0.35	0.44	0.58	0.98	1.58	2.58	5.38	13.07
39. Aspiration-Nonfood	2.60	0.44	0.09	0.09	0.08	0.11	0.14	0.18	0.25	0.48	1.04	2.45	6.61	20.85
40. Suffocation	5.25	0.71	0.35	0.84	0.62	0.67	0.65	0.57	0.46	0.37	0.30	0.29	0.42	0.89
41. Struck by Falling Object	0.08	0.32	0.19	0.15	0.50	0.85	0.86	0.93	1.10	1.36	1.19	1.01	0.84	0.72
42. Collision with Object/Person	0.08	0.09	0.07	0.12	0.22	0.25	0.24	0.18	0.22	0.24	0.23	0.23	0.27	0.73
43. Caught/Crushed	0.10	0.07	0.06	0.03	0.06	0.12	0.11	0.10	0.10	0.12	0.11	0.08	0.09	0.08
44. Machinery	0.03	0.45	0.25	0.30	0.74	1.18	1.13	1.03	1.17	1.61	2.06	2.03	2.27	1.45
45. Cutting/Piercing	0.01	0.04	0.04	0.03	0.07	0.10	0.13	0.10	0.10	0.12	0.13	0.12	0.15	0.17
46. Explosion	0.02	0.04	0.04	0.05	0.12	0.26	0.30	0.31	0.31	0.29	0.29	0.22	0.33	0.35
47. Electric Current	0.15	0.18	0.12	0.29	0.96	1.51	1.35	1.06	0.99	0.78	0.56	0.38	0.27	0.10
48. Unintentional Excl. Traffic	23.49	19.03	8.38	10.01	20.58	27.49	27.61	26.49	25.12	28.71	34.34	48.54	107.95	305.60
49. Unintentional (Total)	28.78	25.98	16.18	19.01	72.09	89.66	71.20	59.53	51.49	51.86	56.29	72.46	149.01	357.11
Suicide														
50. Firearm	0.00	0.00	0.01	0.94	9.29	16.15	15.20	13.73	13.50	15.16	17.81	23.73	34.87	34.05
51. Poison Solids/Liquids	0.00	0.00	0.00	0.03	0.48	1.19	1.87	2.07	1.90	1.61	1.27	1.07	1.55	1.89
52. Motor Vehicle Exhaust	0.00	0.00	0.00	0.00	0.89	1.56	1.85	2.00	2.13	1.95	1.68	1.42	2.26	1.91
53. Hanging	0.00	0.00	0.03	0.73	3.09	4.90	4.64	3.90	2.99	2.81	3.17	3.51	5.83	9.55
54. Drowning	0.00	0.00	0.00	0.00	0.10	0.30	0.35	0.33	0.29	0.33	0.35	0.44	0.83	1.72
55. Cutting/Piercing	0.00	0.00	0.00	0.00	0.05	0.24	0.35	0.36	0.34	0.37	0.54	0.61	0.73	1.04
56. Jumping	0.00	0.00	0.00	0.02	0.24	0.71	0.71	0.64	0.49	0.49	0.49	0.55	1.21	2.09
57. Non-Firearm (Total)	0.00	0.00	0.03	0.79	5.26	9.68	10.72	10.27	9.07	8.38	8.19	8.19	13.17	19.31
58. Suicide (Total)	0.00	0.00	0.05	1.74	14.55	25.83	25.91	23.99	22.57	23.54	26.00	31.93	48.03	53.36
Homicide														
59. Firearm	0.33	0.40	0.38	1.07	10.20	19.28	19.86	17.23	13.70	9.56	5.63	3.51	2.43	1.76
60. Cutting/Stabbing	0.21	0.15	0.11	0.23	2.84	5.74	5.78	5.00	3.85	3.14	2.09	1.43	1.17	0.93
61. Strangulation	0.62	0.15	0.08	0.09	0.18	0.26	0.30	0.29	0.34	0.35	0.36	0.32	0.49	0.85
62. Other	5.28	1.99	0.37	0.24	0.83	1.51	1.77	1.89	2.09	2.28	2.02	1.86	2.62	3.88
63. Non-Firearm (Total)	6.10	2.29	0.56	0.55	3.85	7.51	7.85	7.18	6.28	5.77	4.47	3.61	4.29	5.66
64. Homicide (Total)	6.43	2.69	0.94	1.62	14.05	26.80	27.70	24.41	19.98	15.33	10.10	7.11	8.72	7.42
65. Legal Intervention-Firearm	0.00	0.00	0.00	0.00	0.25	0.52	0.49	0.46	0.32	0.19	0.08	0.08	0.07	0.00
66. Undetermined-Firearm	0.00	0.02	0.02	0.14	0.56	0.73	0.67	0.50	0.42	0.37	0.38	0.34	0.48	0.39
67. Undet-Poison Solids/Liquids	0.04	0.02	0.00	0.02	0.16	0.54	1.08	1.22	0.76	0.40	0.25	0.19	0.19	0.25
68. Undetermined (Total)	1.68	0.60	0.16	0.39	1.42	2.53	3.17	3.21	2.54	2.28	2.10	1.89	2.63	4.17
69. Injuries (Total)	37.08	29.27	17.32	22.76	102.36	145.56	128.52	111.66	97.05	93.24	94.63	113.51	206.50	422.32

Table 4. Number of Deaths of Females by Age, 69 Causes, 1986

Cause	0	1-	5-	10-	15-	20-	25-	30-	35-	45-	55-	65-	75-	85+
Transportation														
1. Motor Vehicle-Train	5	8	7	8	38	19	17	16	23	11	12	10	9	2
2. Motor Vehicle Occupant	72	259	177	249	1,750	1,559	1,090	845	1,192	810	954	1,069	809	187
3. Motorcyclist	0	0	3	17	54	66	59	25	46	11	5	2	0	1
4. Bicyclist	0	0	21	38	21	13	8	6	9	7	4	2	1	2
5. Pedestrian	11	120	154	107	154	118	138	108	181	173	182	257	300	86
6. Motor Vehicle-Traffic (Total)	84	379	355	415	1,980	1,758	1,295	985	1,430	1,002	1,145	1,331	1,111	277
7. Pedestrian-Nontraffic	4	47	15	3	1	4	4	5	5	5	10	13	12	4
8. Pedestrian-Train	0	1	0	2	9	8	3	11	4	5	2	3	4	0
9. Aircraft	0	4	6	5	10	21	23	24	49	23	12	5	2	0
Drowning														
10. Boat-Related	0	6	4	2	8	5	9	5	15	12	4	3	2	0
11. Non-Boat	47	215	82	54	42	48	58	41	55	51	61	61	75	30
12. Drowning (Total)	47	221	86	56	50	53	67	46	70	63	65	84	77	30
Poisoning														
13. Opiates	0	0	1	0	5	17	26	43	33	7	7	5	0	0
14. Barbiturates	0	0	0	1	0	0	2	3	5	1	2	1	1	0
15. Tranquilizers	1	1	0	0	0	3	3	5	10	5	3	3	3	0
16. Antidepressants	0	0	0	0	3	3	4	11	16	14	15	3	2	1
17. Alcohol	0	0	0	0	0	2	4	4	18	22	10	9	2	1
18. Solids/Liquids (Total)	8	14	3	2	39	93	171	195	271	138	141	120	127	67
19. Motor Vehicle Exhaust	0	1	1	2	16	9	8	7	16	5	6	8	7	3
20. Gas/Vapor (Total)	5	15	7	7	26	27	13	16	25	20	21	27	23	13
Falls														
21. Stairs	1	3	0	0	0	2	3	5	19	28	53	110	145	114
22. Ladder/Scaffold	0	0	0	0	0	0	0	0	0	1	1	5	7	0
23. Building/Structure	0	7	0	2	7	12	7	8	14	15	10	10	10	8
24. Different Level	5	9	1	1	6	11	10	11	11	8	18	36	91	124
25. Same Level	1	1	0	0	0	1	1	1	1	2	15	25	71	75
26. Other/Unspecified	3	10	2	1	7	10	14	14	55	70	161	465	1,340	2,103
27. Fall (Total)	10	30	3	4	20	36	35	39	100	124	258	651	1,664	2,424
Fires and Burns														
28. Housefires	60	272	114	55	59	73	74	75	106	86	129	178	201	95
29. Clothing Ignition	0	1	0	0	0	0	1	1	2	1	6	20	35	22
30. Fires/Burns Excl. Scalds	66	279	122	57	63	82	84	88	121	100	153	229	264	140
31. Fires/Burns (Total)	73	285	123	57	63	82	86	88	124	102	157	236	285	150

Table 4 (cont.) Number of Deaths of Females by Age, 69 Causes, 1986

Cause	0	1-	5-	10-	15-	20-	25-	30-	35-	45-	55-	65-	75-	85+
Other Unintentional														
32. Firearm	1	11	17	18	28	22	17	18	29	16	14	5	2	0
33. Excessive Heat	2	2	0	0	0	1	3	2	5	9	17	36	47	20
34. Excessive Cold	1	1	1	0	6	2	0	2	14	3	16	30	67	46
35. Exposure/Neglect	4	0	0	1	1	0	0	1	1	3	5	15	21	42
36. Lightning	0	0	1	0	2	3	0	2	0	0	0	1	0	0
37. Natural Disaster	1	3	1	2	3	1	1	1	2	3	4	1	2	0
38. Aspiration-Food	35	27	6	5	7	6	13	13	28	43	83	132	183	166
39. Aspiration-Nonfood	26	23	7	5	2	7	14	13	24	35	68	137	262	324
40. Suffocation	79	26	3	3	6	4	13	6	5	4	10	5	23	22
41. Struck by Falling Object	1	11	3	0	2	2	3	3	4	1	0	0	3	2
42. Collision with Object/Person	0	6	2	1	2	3	1	1	1	3	2	3	3	7
43. Caught/Crushed	1	2	3	1	1	1	1	1	1	0	1	0	0	4
44. Machinery	1	17	4	0	3	6	3	4	7	3	5	7	1	0
45. Cutting/Piercing	0	0	0	1	0	0	0	0	2	3	3	3	0	2
46. Explosion	1	4	2	1	2	0	3	1	2	1	7	4	4	5
47. Electric Current	2	9	2	6	5	2	5	3	8	3	4	1	1	0
48. Unintentional Excl. Traffic	333	811	324	218	328	443	541	574	933	774	1,235	2,074	3,614	3,939
49. Unintentional (Total)	417	1,190	679	633	2,308	2,201	1,836	1,559	2,363	1,776	2,380	3,405	4,725	4,216
Suicide														
50. Firearm	0	0	0	0	155	264	296	282	482	380	370	287	104	8
51. Poison Solids/Liquids	0	0	0	7	69	89	120	182	374	305	253	155	109	24
52. Motor Vehicle Exhaust	0	0	0	0	41	38	48	67	161	124	111	63	34	6
53. Hanging	0	0	1	16	44	64	74	61	114	103	114	107	112	34
54. Drowning	0	0	0	0	3	4	9	13	26	33	48	41	28	6
55. Cutting/Piercing	0	0	0	2	1	6	4	8	10	22	30	15	5	1
56. Jumping	0	0	1	0	5	20	22	22	33	20	32	28	19	9
57. Non-Firearm (Total)	0	0	2	27	189	236	308	375	789	648	624	435	323	86
58. Suicide (Total)	0	0	2	54	344	500	604	657	1,271	1,028	994	702	427	94
Homicide														
59. Firearm	5	22	20	41	208	374	427	326	447	224	127	91	51	10
60. Cutting/Stabbing	3	9	6	17	94	168	201	118	163	79	58	57	45	14
61. Strangulation	11	16	15	23	73	117	104	90	76	29	31	47	30	20
62. Other	107	112	25	17	55	92	90	82	121	72	69	71	72	36
63. Non-Firearm (Total)	121	137	46	57	222	377	395	290	360	180	158	175	147	70
64. Homicide (Total)	126	159	66	98	430	751	822	616	807	404	285	266	198	80
65. Legal Intervention-Firearm	0	0	0	0	0	0	1	0	1	1	2	1	0	0
66. Undetermined-Firearm	0	0	0	1	7	15	10	21	11	4	4	4	0	0
67. Undet-Poison Solids/Liquids	1	1	1	0	10	31	45	59	93	56	50	27	8	1
68. Undetermined (Total)	21	20	6	6	28	78	88	122	159	98	87	64	43	24
69. Injuries (Total)	564	1,369	753	791	3,110	3,530	3,351	2,954	4,561	3,307	3,748	4,438	5,393	4,414

Table 5. Death Rates per 100,000 Population for Females by Age, 69 Causes, 1980-1986

Cause	0	1-	5-	10-	15-	20-	25-	30-	35-	45-	55-	65-	75-	85+
Transportation														
1. Motor Vehicle-Train	0.13	0.08	0.04	0.08	0.34	0.21	0.16	0.15	0.14	0.11	0.11	0.12	0.13	0.08
2. Motor Vehicle Occupant	4.58	3.27	2.28	2.93	17.55	14.65	9.93	8.05	7.61	7.34	7.90	9.80	12.48	8.87
3. Motorcyclist	0.01	0.01	0.03	0.15	0.75	0.80	0.51	0.29	0.21	0.11	0.04	0.03	0.01	0.03
4. Bicyclist	0.00	0.07	0.29	0.52	0.20	0.13	0.07	0.06	0.05	0.06	0.04	0.03	0.03	0.02
5. Pedestrian	0.30	2.07	2.21	1.38	1.77	1.54	1.28	1.21	1.24	1.39	1.76	2.96	5.60	4.60
6. Motor Vehicle-Traffic (Total)	5.00	5.41	4.60	5.01	20.28	17.12	11.79	9.62	9.12	8.91	9.74	12.82	18.13	13.54
7. Pedestrian-Nontraffic	0.20	1.03	0.10	0.03	0.02	0.03	0.03	0.05	0.05	0.05	0.11	0.14	0.28	0.34
8. Pedestrian-Train	0.00	0.02	0.01	0.04	0.08	0.05	0.04	0.04	0.04	0.05	0.04	0.05	0.10	0.08
9. Aircraft	0.05	0.09	0.07	0.10	0.14	0.29	0.28	0.30	0.33	0.32	0.16	0.08	0.05	0.02
Drowning														
10. Boat-Related	0.02	0.04	0.06	0.03	0.08	0.12	0.10	0.09	0.06	0.07	0.05	0.03	0.02	0.02
11. Non-Boat	2.03	3.12	0.88	0.70	0.67	0.57	0.54	0.51	0.40	0.46	0.50	0.66	1.07	1.46
12. Drowning (Total)	2.05	3.16	0.94	0.73	0.74	0.69	0.64	0.59	0.46	0.53	0.55	0.69	1.09	1.49
Poisoning														
13. Opiates	0.01	0.01	0.00	0.00	0.03	0.12	0.20	0.25	0.11	0.07	0.04	0.02	0.01	0.02
14. Barbiturates	0.00	0.00	0.00	0.00	0.01	0.03	0.03	0.05	0.03	0.05	0.03	0.03	0.04	0.04
15. Tranquilizers	0.02	0.01	0.00	0.00	0.01	0.02	0.04	0.05	0.06	0.08	0.05	0.04	0.03	0.02
16. Antidepressants	0.02	0.02	0.01	0.00	0.02	0.03	0.07	0.09	0.11	0.16	0.10	0.05	0.02	0.02
17. Alcohol	0.01	0.00	0.00	0.00	0.02	0.03	0.04	0.05	0.11	0.21	0.16	0.09	0.03	0.02
18. Solids/Liquids (Total)	0.39	0.27	0.04	0.08	0.38	0.91	1.40	1.44	1.29	1.39	1.17	1.19	1.89	2.97
19. Motor Vehicle Exhaust	0.02	0.03	0.01	0.02	0.24	0.17	0.10	0.10	0.12	0.11	0.08	0.07	0.16	0.14
20. Gas/Vapor (Total)	0.22	0.16	0.08	0.07	0.36	0.33	0.20	0.20	0.22	0.26	0.27	0.35	0.53	0.69
Falls														
21. Stairs	0.05	0.05	0.01	0.00	0.02	0.02	0.03	0.05	0.12	0.31	0.57	1.15	3.13	6.45
22. Ladder/Scaffold	0.00	0.01	0.00	0.00	0.00	0.00	0.01	0.01	0.00	0.02	0.03	0.04	0.07	0.06
23. Building/Structure	0.03	0.18	0.03	0.02	0.05	0.07	0.05	0.05	0.05	0.08	0.08	0.12	0.28	0.43
24. Different Level	0.49	0.14	0.04	0.05	0.08	0.09	0.08	0.08	0.07	0.08	0.12	0.40	1.66	7.84
25. Same Level	0.02	0.01	0.01	0.00	0.00	0.01	0.00	0.01	0.01	0.06	0.11	0.34	1.32	4.93
26. Other/Unspecified	0.39	0.16	0.04	0.03	0.08	0.09	0.14	0.16	0.33	0.82	1.76	5.50	27.51	121.30
27. Fall (Total)	0.97	0.55	0.12	0.11	0.22	0.28	0.31	0.34	0.59	1.37	2.68	7.55	33.96	141.01
Fires and Burns														
28. Housefires	3.31	3.87	1.61	0.82	0.58	0.81	0.69	0.66	0.72	0.97	1.31	2.16	3.69	5.21
29. Clothing Ignition	0.03	0.01	0.01	0.00	0.01	0.01	0.02	0.01	0.02	0.04	0.10	0.33	0.87	1.67
30. Fires/Burns Excl. Scalds	3.58	4.06	1.68	0.86	0.64	0.91	0.79	0.76	0.85	1.17	1.65	2.91	5.29	8.01
31. Fires/Burns (Total)	3.76	4.19	1.68	0.86	0.65	0.91	0.81	0.76	0.87	1.19	1.69	3.02	5.73	8.99

Table 5 (cont.) Death Rates per 100,000 Population for Females by Age, 69 Causes, 1980-1986

Cause	0	1-	5-	10-	15-	20-	25-	30-	35-	45-	55-	65-	75-	85+
Other Unintentional														
32. Firearm	0.06	0.19	0.20	0.23	0.28	0.32	0.24	0.26	0.21	0.15	0.11	0.09	0.06	0.04
33. Excessive Heat	0.12	0.04	0.00	0.01	0.01	0.01	0.02	0.03	0.05	0.13	0.27	0.53	1.33	1.96
34. Excessive Cold	0.07	0.01	0.01	0.01	0.03	0.03	0.05	0.04	0.07	0.15	0.24	0.43	1.22	2.70
35. Exposure/Neglect	0.19	0.00	0.00	0.00	0.01	0.01	0.01	0.02	0.01	0.04	0.06	0.19	0.55	2.00
36. Lightning	0.00	0.00	0.01	0.01	0.02	0.02	0.01	0.01	0.01	0.01	0.01	0.00	0.01	0.00
37. Natural Disaster	0.06	0.04	0.04	0.02	0.03	0.04	0.04	0.03	0.04	0.05	0.06	0.07	0.12	0.09
38. Aspiration-Food	2.53	0.37	0.04	0.07	0.10	0.13	0.13	0.15	0.28	0.51	0.75	1.52	3.07	8.08
39. Aspiration-Nonfood	1.90	0.32	0.10	0.06	0.04	0.06	0.08	0.10	0.13	0.25	0.52	1.21	3.62	11.48
40. Suffocation	4.15	0.42	0.12	0.06	0.05	0.05	0.07	0.04	0.04	0.08	0.13	0.16	0.29	0.68
41. Struck by Falling Object	0.06	0.22	0.10	0.03	0.02	0.03	0.04	0.04	0.03	0.04	0.05	0.05	0.06	0.07
42. Collision with Object/Person	0.07	0.08	0.03	0.01	0.03	0.01	0.01	0.02	0.02	0.03	0.03	0.03	0.11	0.35
43. Caught/Crushed	0.05	0.03	0.02	0.00	0.00	0.01	0.00	0.01	0.01	0.01	0.01	0.01	0.02	0.09
44. Machinery	0.01	0.14	0.07	0.04	0.03	0.03	0.04	0.04	0.05	0.05	0.06	0.05	0.04	0.05
45. Cutting/Piercing	0.01	0.02	0.02	0.01	0.01	0.01	0.01	0.01	0.01	0.02	0.02	0.02	0.05	0.09
46. Explosion	0.03	0.03	0.02	0.01	0.02	0.02	0.03	0.03	0.03	0.04	0.05	0.05	0.09	0.12
47. Electric Current	0.11	0.13	0.05	0.05	0.06	0.05	0.04	0.04	0.04	0.02	0.03	0.02	0.02	0.02
48. Unintentional Excl. Traffic	18.88	12.25	4.25	3.08	3.95	4.98	5.24	5.31	5.77	8.15	11.57	22.89	66.31	209.07
49. Unintentional (Total)	23.88	17.66	9.05	8.09	24.23	22.10	17.03	14.93	14.89	17.06	21.32	35.71	84.45	222.61
Suicide														
50. Firearm	0.00	0.00	0.00	0.30	1.79	2.80	2.96	2.82	3.13	3.44	3.12	2.38	1.42	0.61
51. Poison Solids/Liquids	0.00	0.00	0.01	0.11	0.64	1.01	1.52	1.96	2.31	2.57	2.24	1.69	1.78	1.25
52. Motor Vehicle Exhaust	0.00	0.00	0.00	0.01	0.28	0.33	0.48	0.62	0.98	1.15	0.85	0.56	0.41	0.16
53. Hanging	0.00	0.00	0.00	0.13	0.40	0.57	0.65	0.63	0.65	0.88	0.99	1.13	1.38	1.39
54. Drowning	0.00	0.00	0.00	0.00	0.03	0.07	0.10	0.14	0.17	0.31	0.39	0.47	0.48	0.44
55. Cutting/Piercing	0.00	0.00	0.00	0.00	0.01	0.04	0.04	0.08	0.09	0.16	0.19	0.16	0.14	0.10
56. Jumping	0.00	0.00	0.00	0.00	0.11	0.21	0.25	0.25	0.25	0.24	0.30	0.36	0.43	0.52
57. Non-Firearm (Total)	0.00	0.00	0.01	0.27	1.63	2.41	3.29	3.97	4.81	5.72	5.30	4.63	4.83	4.01
58. Suicide (Total)	0.00	0.00	0.01	0.57	3.42	5.21	6.25	6.79	7.94	9.16	8.42	7.01	6.25	4.62
Homicide														
59. Firearm	0.26	0.30	0.29	0.49	2.09	3.65	3.76	3.26	2.95	2.16	1.32	0.95	0.80	0.51
60. Cutting/Stabbing	0.14	0.13	0.10	0.22	0.91	1.56	1.50	1.06	0.92	0.66	0.53	0.53	0.71	0.66
61. Strangulation	0.57	0.16	0.18	0.25	0.77	1.05	0.87	0.65	0.43	0.30	0.29	0.40	0.73	0.90
62. Other	4.91	1.73	0.35	0.27	0.67	0.95	0.90	0.79	0.72	0.61	0.56	0.75	1.33	1.88
63. Non-Firearm (Total)	5.62	2.02	0.64	0.73	2.35	3.56	3.27	2.51	2.06	1.57	1.37	1.68	2.77	3.33
64. Homicide (Total)	5.88	2.32	0.92	1.22	4.44	7.21	7.04	5.77	5.02	3.73	2.69	2.63	3.57	3.84
65. Legal Intervention-Firearm	0.00	0.00	0.00	0.00	0.00	0.01	0.01	0.00	0.01	0.00	0.00	0.00	0.00	0.01
66. Undetermined-Firearm	0.02	0.00	0.01	0.02	0.10	0.19	0.13	0.14	0.10	0.08	0.06	0.03	0.01	0.02
67. Undet-Poison Solids/Liquids	0.03	0.02	0.01	0.02	0.14	0.31	0.39	0.43	0.51	0.54	0.37	0.24	0.19	0.14
68. Undetermined (Total)	1.57	0.44	0.12	0.10	0.43	0.84	0.91	0.94	1.01	1.06	0.87	0.75	0.97	1.51
69. Injuries (Total)	31.33	20.42	10.11	9.99	32.53	35.36	31.23	28.43	28.86	31.01	33.30	46.11	95.24	232.59

Table 6. Number of Deaths by Age, 69 Causes, 1986

Cause	0	1-	5-	10-	15-	20-	25-	30-	35-	45-	55-	65-	75-	85+
Transportation														
1. Motor Vehicle-Train	7	12	13	19	103	87	72	54	70	40	43	25	21	8
2. Motor Vehicle Occupant	148	492	380	614	5,664	6,351	4,468	3,253	4,166	2,562	2,558	2,363	1,857	455
3. Motorcyclist	1	1	11	73	583	1,027	749	453	395	116	52	24	5	1
4. Bicyclist	0	17	126	230	152	82	60	52	51	36	27	27	19	6
5. Pedestrian	21	347	471	275	494	653	651	496	777	649	646	627	676	225
6. Motor Vehicle-Traffic (Total)	171	862	996	1,208	6,911	8,127	5,939	4,262	5,395	3,373	3,285	3,044	2,559	688
7. Pedestrian-Nontraffic	11	118	28	9	4	18	26	20	32	27	29	27	26	6
8. Pedestrian-Train	0	3	3	8	57	79	67	62	80	43	19	18	15	3
9. Aircraft	1	10	13	14	30	99	142	161	286	203	132	38	4	1
Drowning														
10. Boat-Related	0	12	15	23	69	110	130	86	170	117	101	66	21	3
11. Non-Boat	94	648	311	300	590	572	494	361	424	270	228	204	176	63
12. Drowning (Total)	94	660	326	323	659	682	624	447	594	387	329	270	197	66
Poisoning														
13. Opiates	0	2	1	0	14	71	195	274	282	59	21	6	2	0
14. Barbiturates	0	0	0	1	1	3	9	7	12	5	7	1	3	0
15. Tranquilizers	1	4	0	0	1	5	11	17	21	13	8	7	4	0
16. Antidepressants	0	2	1	1	4	8	12	24	42	27	24	6	2	1
17. Alcohol	1	0	1	2	6	9	22	31	93	82	66	29	7	2
18. Solids/Liquids (Total)	16	43	10	16	122	351	822	942	1,121	395	321	243	219	104
19. Motor Vehicle Exhaust	1	5	2	4	55	54	58	57	81	51	35	31	29	12
20. Gas/Vapor (Total)	8	26	14	14	97	103	105	94	144	110	97	92	73	32
Falls														
21. Stairs	2	5	0	0	3	9	11	25	59	83	147	275	303	215
22. Ladder/Scaffold	0	0	0	1	6	14	10	25	34	42	65	62	52	14
23. Building/Structure	3	27	2	4	40	82	78	64	90	82	57	56	46	19
24. Different Level	16	21	9	14	50	68	62	57	79	70	91	101	183	182
25. Same Level	1	4	1	2	6	5	2	3	11	10	36	64	128	116
26. Other/Unspecified	13	25	10	12	45	71	82	99	244	298	538	996	2,341	3,160
27. Fall (Total)	35	82	22	33	150	249	245	273	517	585	934	1,554	3,053	3,706
Fires and Burns														
28. Housefires	109	629	269	138	135	199	247	231	339	292	360	425	396	196
29. Clothing Ignition	0	3	0	0	0	2	3	1	7	7	17	43	58	38
30. Fires/Burns Excl.Scalds	120	648	290	144	152	243	300	281	422	369	472	562	546	275
31. Fires/Burns (Total)	132	661	292	144	153	249	304	283	431	374	485	581	577	292

Table 6 (cont.) Number of Deaths by Age, 69 Causes, 1986

Cause	0	1-	5-	10-	15-	20-	25-	30-	35-	45-	55-	65-	75-	85+
Other Unintentional														
32. Firearm	3	31	57	143	238	205	165	134	172	109	87	61	35	9
33. Excessive Heat	3	6	0	1	1	12	11	15	34	37	53	64	87	32
34. Excessive Cold	1	2	1	1	18	18	14	20	61	67	85	115	131	82
35. Exposure/Neglect	8	1	0	1	1	3	3	3	8	10	20	29	56	57
36. Lightning	0	0	3	3	9	22	4	9	8	5	10	3	2	0
37. Natural Disaster	1	3	0	6	10	4	6	3	8	8	10	5	5	1
38. Aspiration-Food	83	65	7	15	14	33	37	51	114	123	210	313	356	287
39. Aspiration-Nonfood	74	58	14	13	14	13	34	27	57	93	174	330	519	563
40. Suffocation	188	62	31	66	64	80	89	80	90	43	49	35	31	33
41. Struck by Falling Object	1	34	14	9	44	76	87	101	150	157	107	76	27	5
42. Collision with Object/Person	0	10	5	11	22	23	36	13	33	24	23	20	11	12
43. Caught/Crushed	3	5	5	5	6	9	18	15	12	12	9	6	3	4
44. Machinery	2	42	20	23	57	100	98	100	171	143	219	139	70	16
45. Cutting/Piercing	0	3	1	2	5	9	10	14	18	18	14	13	6	5
46. Explosion	1	7	4	5	10	12	31	24	41	27	43	15	16	6
47. Electric Current	4	19	11	24	86	128	141	113	150	82	56	27	12	0
48. Unintentional Excl. Traffic	738	2,072	987	1,035	2,077	2,860	3,412	3,293	4,900	3,632	4,443	5,455	7,074	6,314
49. Unintentional (Total)	909	2,934	1,963	2,243	8,988	10,987	9,351	7,555	10,295	7,005	7,728	8,499	9,633	7,002
Suicide														
50. Firearm	0	0	1	141	1,151	1,947	1,880	1,747	2,680	2,140	2,324	2,319	1,512	314
51. Poison Solids/Liquids	0	0	0	10	123	203	322	396	713	476	381	250	154	42
52. Motor Vehicle Exhaust	0	0	0	0	149	223	271	301	533	362	283	191	112	25
53. Hanging	0	0	3	93	368	625	643	538	641	420	444	380	317	129
54. Drowning	0	0	0	0	8	28	45	52	71	64	79	68	59	19
55. Cutting/Piercing	0	0	0	2	4	25	54	41	62	50	89	64	30	10
56. Jumping	0	0	1	1	21	76	88	88	100	76	78	65	59	25
57. Non-Firearm (Total)	0	0	4	109	745	1,277	1,549	1,535	2,333	1,596	1,458	1,095	771	264
58. Suicide (Total)	0	0	5	250	1,896	3,224	3,429	3,282	5,013	3,736	3,782	3,414	2,283	578
Homicide														
59. Firearm	8	51	53	152	1,252	2,467	2,504	2,002	2,379	1,117	569	308	121	23
60. Cutting/Stabbing	6	20	14	30	352	755	809	629	753	395	272	177	96	23
61. Strangulation	20	29	22	27	91	146	137	120	137	75	58	65	43	27
62. Other	244	282	45	36	143	246	312	291	464	284	282	200	155	57
63. Non-Firearm (Total)	270	331	81	93	586	1,147	1,258	1,040	1,354	754	612	442	294	107
64. Homicide (Total)	278	382	134	245	1,838	3,614	3,762	3,042	3,733	1,871	1,181	750	415	130
65. Legal Intervention-Firearm	0	0	0	0	24	44	44	46	43	22	13	8	2	0
66. Undetermined-Firearm	0	0	0	17	54	87	74	66	65	42	41	30	17	2
67. Undet-Poison Solids/Liquids	1	4	1	1	29	90	160	231	270	109	71	43	14	3
68. Undetermined (Total)	51	53	11	38	149	316	407	457	612	341	286	181	126	52
69. Injuries (Total)	1,238	3,369	2,133	2,776	12,895	18,187	17,000	14,365	19,708	12,977	12,996	12,852	12,460	7,763

Table 7. Death Rates per 100,000 Population by Age, 69 Causes, 1980-1986

Cause	0	1-	5-	10-	15-	20-	25-	30-	35-	45-	55-	65-	75-	85+
Transportation														
1. Motor Vehicle-Train	0.10	0.08	0.06	0.08	0.55	0.48	0.35	0.27	0.24	0.22	0.20	0.21	0.25	0.21
2. Motor Vehicle Occupant	4.78	3.34	2.35	3.48	29.00	30.81	20.96	16.34	13.64	12.15	11.78	13.03	18.17	15.43
3. Motorcyclist	0.02	0.02	0.08	0.47	3.33	5.06	3.48	2.13	1.22	0.55	0.26	0.17	0.09	0.08
4. Bicyclist	0.00	0.11	0.77	1.24	0.75	0.38	0.24	0.17	0.15	0.15	0.15	0.16	0.21	0.20
5. Pedestrian	0.34	2.73	3.12	1.83	3.05	3.50	2.97	2.61	2.57	2.95	3.27	4.30	8.18	8.88
6. Motor Vehicle-Traffic (Total)	5.15	6.20	6.34	7.05	36.17	39.78	27.68	21.25	17.50	15.81	15.47	17.67	26.66	24.61
7. Pedestrian-Nontraffic	0.21	1.18	0.13	0.04	0.07	0.11	0.10	0.10	0.11	0.13	0.18	0.22	0.37	0.47
8. Pedestrian-Train	0.00	0.02	0.03	0.09	0.27	0.34	0.28	0.23	0.21	0.19	0.13	0.12	0.21	0.20
9. Aircraft	0.07	0.10	0.09	0.13	0.25	0.69	0.93	1.05	1.13	1.10	0.61	0.24	0.07	0.03
Drowning														
10. Boat-Related	0.02	0.09	0.12	0.16	0.48	0.71	0.69	0.59	0.55	0.52	0.46	0.41	0.21	0.11
11. Non-Boat	2.32	4.61	1.87	1.85	3.59	3.28	2.44	1.91	1.41	1.30	1.21	1.31	1.77	2.16
12. Drowning (Total)	2.34	4.70	1.99	2.01	4.07	3.98	3.13	2.50	1.95	1.83	1.67	1.71	1.98	2.27
Poisoning														
13. Opiates	0.00	0.01	0.00	0.00	0.05	0.31	0.71	0.88	0.49	0.19	0.05	0.02	0.01	0.03
14. Barbiturates	0.00	0.00	0.00	0.00	0.02	0.05	0.06	0.06	0.04	0.05	0.03	0.03	0.04	0.03
15. Tranquilizers	0.01	0.01	0.00	0.00	0.01	0.04	0.06	0.06	0.07	0.07	0.05	0.04	0.03	0.03
16. Antidepressants	0.01	0.02	0.01	0.00	0.02	0.04	0.07	0.09	0.11	0.11	0.08	0.05	0.02	0.02
17. Alcohol	0.01	0.01	0.00	0.01	0.05	0.08	0.13	0.17	0.26	0.39	0.35	0.18	0.04	0.02
18. Solids/Liquids (Total)	0.39	0.34	0.05	0.10	0.60	1.69	3.09	3.32	2.32	1.56	1.34	1.35	2.03	3.36
19. Motor Vehicle Exhaust	0.02	0.02	0.01	0.02	0.28	0.37	0.30	0.31	0.32	0.30	0.25	0.18	0.35	0.38
20. Gas/Vapor (Total)	0.18	0.19	0.09	0.09	0.53	0.71	0.58	0.57	0.56	0.60	0.58	0.56	0.93	1.09
Falls														
21. Stairs	0.09	0.07	0.01	0.01	0.02	0.05	0.08	0.12	0.21	0.50	0.87	1.59	3.82	8.12
22. Ladder/Scaffold	0.00	0.00	0.00	0.00	0.03	0.08	0.08	0.10	0.12	0.21	0.33	0.37	0.62	0.55
23. Building/Structure	0.05	0.22	0.04	0.05	0.21	0.39	0.34	0.31	0.28	0.35	0.36	0.40	0.64	0.85
24. Different Level	0.59	0.19	0.06	0.10	0.30	0.37	0.31	0.27	0.24	0.30	0.37	0.67	2.06	8.62
25. Same Level	0.01	0.01	0.01	0.01	0.02	0.02	0.01	0.02	0.03	0.07	0.14	0.43	1.50	5.42
26. Other/Unspecified	0.50	0.20	0.07	0.08	0.24	0.38	0.42	0.54	0.81	1.56	2.81	6.74	29.80	128.96
27. Fall (Total)	1.23	0.68	0.20	0.24	0.82	1.28	1.24	1.36	1.69	2.98	4.88	10.19	38.45	152.51
Fires and Burns														
28. Housefires	3.37	4.44	1.72	0.84	0.71	1.13	1.17	1.09	1.12	1.54	1.95	2.85	4.67	7.37
29. Clothing Ignition	0.02	0.02	0.01	0.00	0.01	0.01	0.02	0.01	0.03	0.06	0.14	0.35	0.92	1.98
30. Fires/Burns Excl. Scalds	3.58	4.71	1.82	0.90	0.84	1.36	1.42	1.36	1.44	1.98	2.62	3.90	6.92	11.26
31. Fires/Burns (Total)	3.81	4.85	1.82	0.90	0.84	1.37	1.43	1.38	1.47	2.03	2.66	4.04	7.34	12.27

Table 7 (cont.) Death rates per 100,000 Population by Age, 69 Causes, 1980-1986

Cause	0	1-	5-	10-	15-	20-	25-	30-	35-	45-	55-	65-	75-	85+
Other Unintentional														
32. Firearm	0.05	0.29	0.39	0.97	1.43	1.28	0.96	0.80	0.67	0.57	0.46	0.42	0.39	0.28
33. Excessive Heat	0.13	0.04	0.00	0.01	0.03	0.04	0.05	0.09	0.13	0.23	0.38	0.63	1.38	2.13
34. Excessive Cold	0.11	0.02	0.01	0.02	0.10	0.10	0.11	0.13	0.21	0.44	0.66	0.90	1.87	3.48
35. Exposure/Neglect	0.22	0.01	0.00	0.00	0.02	0.02	0.03	0.04	0.05	0.10	0.14	0.30	0.74	2.21
36. Lightning	0.00	0.00	0.01	0.04	0.08	0.06	0.05	0.04	0.05	0.04	0.03	0.02	0.02	0.01
37. Natural Disaster	0.05	0.04	0.04	0.04	0.04	0.06	0.07	0.06	0.06	0.07	0.07	0.09	0.12	0.10
38. Aspiration-Food	3.09	0.49	0.07	0.08	0.15	0.21	0.24	0.29	0.43	0.74	1.14	1.98	3.93	9.53
39. Aspiration-Nonfood	2.26	0.38	0.10	0.08	0.06	0.09	0.11	0.14	0.19	0.36	0.77	1.75	4.74	14.22
40. Suffocation	4.72	0.57	0.24	0.46	0.34	0.36	0.36	0.30	0.25	0.22	0.21	0.22	0.34	0.74
41. Struck by Falling Object	0.07	0.27	0.14	0.09	0.26	0.44	0.45	0.48	0.55	0.68	0.59	0.47	0.35	0.26
42. Collision with Object/Person	0.07	0.09	0.05	0.07	0.13	0.13	0.13	0.10	0.11	0.13	0.12	0.12	0.17	0.46
43. Caught/Crushed	0.07	0.05	0.04	0.02	0.03	0.06	0.06	0.05	0.05	0.06	0.05	0.04	0.05	0.08
44. Machinery	0.02	0.30	0.16	0.17	0.39	0.61	0.58	0.53	0.60	0.81	0.99	0.92	0.87	0.46
45. Cutting/Piercing	0.01	0.03	0.03	0.02	0.04	0.05	0.07	0.05	0.06	0.07	0.07	0.07	0.09	0.11
46. Explosion	0.03	0.04	0.03	0.03	0.07	0.14	0.16	0.17	0.17	0.16	0.16	0.12	0.18	0.19
47. Electric Current	0.13	0.16	0.08	0.17	0.52	0.78	0.70	0.55	0.51	0.39	0.28	0.18	0.11	0.05
48. Unintentional Excl. Traffic	21.23	15.71	6.36	6.63	12.41	16.25	16.41	15.83	15.28	18.11	22.25	34.11	81.80	237.22
49. Unintentional (Total)	26.38	21.91	12.70	13.58	48.58	56.04	44.09	37.06	32.66	33.92	37.72	51.78	108.46	261.82
Suicide														
50. Firearm	0.00	0.00	0.01	0.63	5.61	9.49	9.08	8.24	8.23	9.12	10.01	11.71	13.86	10.36
51. Poison Solids/Liquids	0.00	0.00	0.00	0.07	0.56	1.10	1.69	2.01	2.11	2.10	1.78	1.42	1.69	1.44
52. Motor Vehicle Exhaust	0.00	0.00	0.00	0.01	0.59	0.95	1.16	1.31	1.55	1.54	1.24	0.93	1.10	0.67
53. Hanging	0.00	0.00	0.01	0.44	1.77	2.74	2.64	2.25	1.80	1.82	2.01	2.17	3.03	3.77
54. Drowning	0.00	0.00	0.00	0.00	0.06	0.18	0.23	0.24	0.23	0.32	0.37	0.46	0.62	0.81
55. Cutting/Piercing	0.00	0.00	0.00	0.00	0.03	0.14	0.20	0.22	0.21	0.26	0.35	0.36	0.36	0.38
56. Jumping	0.00	0.00	0.00	0.01	0.17	0.46	0.48	0.44	0.36	0.36	0.39	0.45	0.72	0.98
57. Non-Firearm (Total)	0.00	0.00	0.02	0.54	3.47	6.05	7.00	7.10	6.90	7.01	6.65	6.19	7.93	8.47
58. Suicide (Total)	0.00	0.00	0.03	1.17	9.08	15.54	16.07	15.34	15.13	16.13	16.66	17.90	21.79	18.83
Homicide														
59. Firearm	0.30	0.35	0.34	0.79	6.22	11.48	11.80	10.20	8.24	5.75	3.34	2.07	1.41	0.87
60. Cutting/Stabbing	0.17	0.14	0.10	0.22	1.89	3.66	3.64	3.02	2.36	1.86	1.26	0.92	0.89	0.74
61. Strangulation	0.59	0.15	0.13	0.16	0.47	0.65	0.59	0.47	0.38	0.33	0.33	0.37	0.64	0.81
62. Other	5.10	1.86	0.36	0.25	0.75	1.23	1.33	1.34	1.39	1.42	1.24	1.23	1.81	2.46
63. Non-Firearm (Total)	5.86	2.16	0.60	0.64	3.11	5.54	5.56	4.83	4.13	3.61	2.83	2.52	3.33	4.01
64. Homicide (Total)	6.16	2.51	0.93	1.42	9.33	17.02	17.36	15.03	12.37	9.35	6.17	4.59	4.74	4.89
65. Legal Intervention-Firearm	0.00	0.00	0.00	0.00	0.13	0.26	0.25	0.23	0.16	0.09	0.04	0.04	0.03	0.01
66. Undetermined-Firearm	0.01	0.01	0.01	0.08	0.33	0.46	0.40	0.32	0.26	0.22	0.21	0.17	0.18	0.12
67. Undet-Poison Solids/Liquids	0.04	0.02	0.01	0.02	0.15	0.42	0.73	0.82	0.63	0.48	0.32	0.22	0.19	0.17
68. Undetermined (Total)	1.73	0.52	0.14	0.25	0.93	1.69	2.04	2.07	1.81	1.55	1.45	1.25	1.58	2.29
69. Injuries (Total)	34.27	24.94	13.80	16.52	68.05	90.56	79.83	69.76	62.38	61.16	62.06	75.57	136.61	287.90

Table 8. Death Rates per 100,000 Population by Per Capita Income of Area of Residence and Place of Residence, 69 Causes, 1980-1986

Cause	Per Capita Income ($000)						Central Cities	Metro >1 m.	Metro <1 m.	Non-Metro	Rural Remote
	<6	6-7	8-9	10-11	12-13	14+					
Transportation											
1. Motor Vehicle-Train	0.45	0.39	0.31	0.14	0.13	0.09	0.12	0.20	0.25	0.47	0.45
2. Motor Vehicle Occupant	24.41	20.77	15.52	11.69	10.52	9.06	10.84	12.41	15.02	21.96	26.43
3. Motorcyclist	1.19	1.36	1.60	1.74	1.55	0.91	1.73	1.44	1.56	1.46	1.27
4. Bicyclist	0.33	0.35	0.39	0.36	0.32	0.23	0.37	0.35	0.38	0.35	0.30
5. Pedestrian	4.18	3.74	3.07	3.30	2.77	2.19	4.18	2.72	3.01	3.02	2.74
6. Motor Vehicle-Traffic (Total)	30.15	26.26	20.60	17.10	15.17	12.40	17.13	16.94	19.98	26.81	30.77
7. Pedestrian-Nontraffic	0.41	0.28	0.20	0.15	0.13	0.09	0.16	0.12	0.20	0.29	0.45
8. Pedestrian-Train	0.25	0.26	0.15	0.18	0.18	0.21	0.23	0.19	0.16	0.18	0.17
9. Aircraft	0.52	0.64	0.60	0.58	0.77	0.69	0.54	0.54	0.63	0.70	1.12
Drowning											
10. Boat-Related	0.63	0.62	0.47	0.32	0.32	0.26	0.27	0.33	0.46	0.69	0.93
11. Non-Boat	3.89	2.72	2.13	1.98	1.62	1.10	2.22	1.57	2.14	2.65	3.22
12. Drowning (Total)	4.51	3.34	2.61	2.30	1.94	1.36	2.48	1.90	2.61	3.34	4.16
Poisoning											
13. Opiates	0.06	0.11	0.14	0.50	0.55	0.28	0.62	0.24	0.13	0.07	0.04
14. Barbiturates	0.02	0.03	0.03	0.05	0.04	0.02	0.06	0.03	0.03	0.02	0.02
15. Tranquilizers	0.05	0.03	0.04	0.04	0.06	0.05	0.06	0.04	0.04	0.03	0.02
16. Antidepressants	0.05	0.05	0.06	0.07	0.07	0.04	0.08	0.05	0.05	0.05	0.05
17. Alcohol	0.24	0.19	0.11	0.16	0.13	0.10	0.14	0.08	0.15	0.18	0.22
18. Solids/Liquids (Total)	1.29	1.32	1.29	2.12	2.23	1.40	2.56	1.38	1.29	1.12	1.19
19. Motor Vehicle Exhaust	0.26	0.25	0.27	0.23	0.18	0.13	0.23	0.22	0.24	0.28	0.27
20. Gas/Vapor (Total)	0.59	0.60	0.53	0.47	0.35	0.41	0.45	0.43	0.50	0.64	0.79
Falls											
21. Stairs	0.30	0.55	0.50	0.55	0.60	0.64	0.67	0.54	0.47	0.44	0.54
22. Ladder/Scaffold	0.10	0.15	0.15	0.15	0.12	0.13	0.17	0.14	0.14	0.14	0.16
23. Building/Structure	0.22	0.40	0.26	0.30	0.23	0.21	0.45	0.20	0.25	0.26	0.26
24. Different Level	0.47	0.58	0.42	0.43	0.45	0.38	0.55	0.38	0.42	0.46	0.54
25. Same Level	0.17	0.19	0.20	0.16	0.15	0.12	0.17	0.15	0.17	0.21	0.33
26. Other/Unspecified	3.55	4.53	3.64	3.19	3.71	2.97	4.17	2.92	3.30	4.16	4.74
27. Fall (Total)	4.81	6.41	5.17	4.78	5.26	4.44	6.19	4.32	4.75	5.67	6.56
Fires and Burns											
28. Housefires	3.54	2.67	1.74	1.39	0.96	0.76	1.68	1.16	1.72	2.43	3.19
29. Clothing Ignition	0.21	0.15	0.10	0.10	0.08	0.04	0.11	0.07	0.10	0.14	0.19
30. Fires/Burns Excl. Scalds	4.37	3.35	2.14	1.76	1.29	1.04	2.16	1.47	2.13	3.01	4.03
31. Fires/Burns (Total)	4.44	3.43	2.21	1.83	1.35	1.09	2.26	1.52	2.19	3.07	4.12

Table 8 (cont.)   Death Rates per 100,000 Population by Per Capita Income of Area of Residence and Place of Residence, 69 Causes, 1980-1986

Cause	Per Capita Income ($000) <6	6-7	8-9	10-11	12-13	14+	Central Cities	Metro >1 m.	Metro <1 m.	Non-Metro	Rural Remote
Other Unintentional											
32. Firearm	2.17	1.29	0.65	0.50	0.32	0.32	0.52	0.41	0.68	1.28	2.14
33. Excessive Heat	0.57	0.33	0.23	0.13	0.16	0.07	0.19	0.14	0.22	0.32	0.29
34. Excessive Cold	0.78	0.55	0.32	0.25	0.18	0.15	0.30	0.16	0.30	0.54	1.03
35. Exposure/Neglect	0.44	0.20	0.11	0.06	0.07	0.05	0.07	0.06	0.10	0.24	0.31
36. Lightning	0.11	0.05	0.04	0.03	0.02	0.02	0.02	0.03	0.04	0.06	0.05
37. Natural Disaster	0.20	0.11	0.05	0.04	0.02	0.04	0.03	0.03	0.05	0.12	0.35
38. Aspiration-Food	0.99	1.01	0.79	0.68	0.68	0.59	0.78	0.59	0.60	0.95	1.07
39. Aspiration-Nonfood	1.09	0.93	0.68	0.53	0.53	0.49	0.60	0.49	0.71	0.88	0.94
40. Suffocation	0.46	0.51	0.37	0.34	0.37	0.29	0.41	0.33	0.36	0.45	0.64
41. Struck by Falling Object	1.13	0.75	0.38	0.25	0.17	0.32	0.22	0.29	0.37	0.78	1.21
42. Collision with Object/Person	0.16	0.17	0.12	0.09	0.09	0.07	0.10	0.09	0.11	0.16	0.21
43. Caught/Crushed	0.06	0.07	0.05	0.04	0.03	0.04	0.04	0.04	0.05	0.07	0.09
44. Machinery	1.38	1.15	0.55	0.28	0.22	0.14	0.22	0.32	0.49	1.22	2.33
45. Cutting/Piercing	0.10	0.09	0.05	0.05	0.03	0.03	0.06	0.04	0.04	0.08	0.09
46. Explosion	0.29	0.18	0.12	0.10	0.06	0.06	0.10	0.09	0.10	0.20	0.32
47. Electric Current	0.64	0.57	0.42	0.31	0.26	0.16	0.28	0.30	0.40	0.60	0.73
48. Unintentional Excl. Traffic	31.21	28.07	20.54	18.77	17.86	15.06	21.89	16.28	19.96	26.43	34.78
49. Unintentional (Total)	61.35	54.33	41.14	35.87	33.04	27.46	39.01	33.22	39.95	53.24	65.55
Suicide											
50. Firearm	8.61	8.72	7.61	6.51	5.32	4.11	6.64	5.69	7.47	8.84	10.25
51. Poison Solids/Liquids	0.60	0.89	1.22	1.65	1.96	1.17	1.91	1.32	1.19	0.82	0.71
52. Motor Vehicle Exhaust	0.27	0.55	1.05	1.06	1.32	1.15	0.94	1.20	1.03	0.69	0.61
53. Hanging	1.11	1.58	1.72	1.97	2.13	1.97	2.27	1.83	1.63	1.42	1.31
54. Drowning	0.11	0.21	0.23	0.24	0.23	0.19	0.28	0.21	0.21	0.18	0.18
55. Cutting/Piercing	0.08	0.15	0.16	0.22	0.25	0.22	0.27	0.18	0.16	0.12	0.11
56. Jumping	0.05	0.37	0.21	0.42	0.47	0.47	0.76	0.26	0.19	0.07	0.06
57. Non-Firearm (Total)	2.40	4.14	4.98	6.02	6.84	5.74	6.90	5.48	4.79	3.67	3.31
58. Suicide (Total)	11.01	12.86	12.59	12.53	12.16	9.85	13.54	11.16	12.26	12.51	13.57
Homicide											
59. Firearm	7.06	6.60	5.15	6.77	3.20	2.34	10.66	2.98	4.46	4.08	4.40
60. Cutting/Stabbing	1.80	2.09	1.54	2.23	1.31	0.82	3.62	0.95	1.43	1.05	0.88
61. Strangulation	0.20	0.39	0.38	0.50	0.37	0.24	0.78	0.28	0.30	0.23	0.15
62. Other	1.30	1.32	1.18	1.50	0.98	0.62	2.19	0.77	1.10	0.88	0.85
63. Non-Firearm (Total)	3.29	3.80	3.10	4.23	2.66	1.68	6.58	1.99	2.83	2.16	1.88
64. Homicide (Total)	10.35	10.40	8.25	11.00	5.85	4.02	17.27	4.97	7.29	6.24	6.27
65. Legal Intervention-Firearm	0.12	0.12	0.11	0.13	0.08	0.06	0.20	0.06	0.10	0.08	0.09
66. Undetermined-Firearm	0.66	0.39	0.20	0.17	0.16	0.15	0.20	0.14	0.21	0.37	0.74
67. Undet-Poison Solids/Liquids	0.23	0.31	0.37	0.41	0.46	0.40	0.60	0.39	0.30	0.21	0.23
68. Undetermined (Total)	1.55	2.03	1.13	1.38	1.17	1.25	2.41	1.02	1.00	1.08	1.72
69. Injuries (Total)	84.40	79.76	63.23	60.93	52.32	42.64	72.44	50.45	60.62	73.16	87.21

313

Table 9. Death Rates per 100,000 Population by State of Residence, 69 Causes, 1980-1986

Cause	AL	AK	AZ	AR	CA	CO	CT	DE	DC	FL	GA	HI	ID	IL	IN	IA	KS
Transportation																	
1. Motor Vehicle-Train	0.29	0.24	0.12	0.74	0.12	0.22	0.05	0.14	0.02	0.20	0.26	0.00	0.52	0.38	0.69	0.35	0.73
2. Motor Vehicle Occupant	21.64	17.42	19.01	20.87	13.94	16.65	10.94	15.79	5.37	16.69	19.81	9.57	22.80	11.51	16.13	14.33	18.11
3. Motorcyclist	1.11	0.87	2.31	0.48	2.57	1.84	1.88	1.50	0.57	2.17	0.76	1.38	0.89	1.02	0.97	2.22	2.00
4. Bicyclist	0.30	0.48	0.59	0.17	0.43	0.31	0.25	0.14	0.14	0.88	0.25	0.27	0.33	0.28	0.31	0.31	0.24
5. Pedestrian	3.11	3.41	5.47	2.72	3.54	2.73	2.38	2.96	3.71	5.55	3.75	2.72	2.25	2.85	2.10	1.46	1.82
6. Motor Vehicle-Traffic (Total)	26.18	22.27	27.40	24.27	20.48	21.54	15.45	20.69	9.78	25.31	24.58	13.34	26.28	15.67	19.53	18.33	22.19
7. Pedestrian-Nontraffic	0.25	0.12	0.41	0.29	0.24	0.10	0.07	0.07	0.05	0.29	0.29	0.22	0.49	0.10	0.17	0.23	0.32
8. Pedestrian-Train	0.23	0.09	0.25	0.24	0.17	0.14	0.19	0.16	0.18	0.20	0.26	0.00	0.15	0.29	0.20	0.09	0.12
9. Aircraft	0.47	8.98	1.20	0.78	0.90	1.36	0.39	0.33	0.25	0.99	0.56	1.10	1.97	0.34	0.35	0.48	0.76
Drowning																	
10. Boat-Related	0.62	6.36	0.25	0.75	0.32	0.40	0.18	0.45	0.14	0.64	0.55	0.18	0.86	0.30	0.25	0.26	0.37
11. Non-Boat	2.88	9.25	3.27	3.15	2.49	1.60	1.42	1.76	1.45	3.48	2.61	3.40	3.08	1.58	1.55	1.36	1.73
12. Drowning (Total)	3.49	15.61	3.52	3.90	2.81	2.00	1.60	2.21	1.59	4.13	3.16	3.58	3.93	1.88	1.80	1.62	2.10
Poisoning																	
13. Opiates	0.04	0.12	0.28	0.06	1.32	0.25	0.03	0.21	0.11	0.08	0.07	0.08	0.09	0.47	0.03	0.04	0.03
14. Barbiturates	0.01	0.03	0.03	0.02	0.10	0.03	0.00	0.00	0.05	0.03	0.05	0.00	0.04	0.03	0.02	0.01	0.01
15. Tranquilizers	0.02	0.15	0.03	0.04	0.08	0.03	0.00	0.00	0.02	0.03	0.08	0.00	0.03	0.03	0.04	0.02	0.04
16. Antidepressants	0.04	0.06	0.05	0.04	0.16	0.08	0.00	0.02	0.00	0.05	0.08	0.00	0.03	0.06	0.02	0.07	0.04
17. Alcohol	0.17	0.21	0.09	0.10	0.15	0.23	0.07	0.02	0.05	0.08	0.42	0.01	0.09	0.12	0.04	0.02	0.09
18. Solids/Liquids (Total)	1.07	2.56	1.65	0.96	4.10	1.76	0.54	0.96	1.27	1.43	1.68	0.64	1.09	1.62	0.73	0.75	0.94
19. Motor Vehicle Exhaust	0.28	0.24	0.09	0.12	0.05	0.34	0.11	0.19	0.09	0.11	0.19	0.00	0.38	0.61	0.36	0.53	0.28
20. Gas/Vapor (Total)	0.58	2.02	0.35	0.41	0.22	0.77	0.83	0.33	0.32	0.31	0.45	0.03	0.65	0.84	0.69	0.76	0.63
Falls																	
21. Stairs	0.28	0.24	0.11	0.15	0.25	0.45	0.75	0.47	1.18	0.21	0.33	0.20	0.49	0.72	0.47	0.70	0.39
22. Ladder/Scaffold	0.12	0.12	0.12	0.11	0.14	0.10	0.18	0.09	0.20	0.20	0.11	0.14	0.15	0.19	0.14	0.14	0.15
23. Building/Structure	0.28	0.15	0.17	0.18	0.28	0.32	0.19	0.19	0.32	0.30	0.26	0.45	0.17	0.40	0.22	0.26	0.39
24. Different Level	0.42	0.69	0.66	0.56	0.49	0.86	0.40	0.28	0.36	0.43	0.59	0.67	0.57	0.30	0.31	0.52	0.47
25. Same Level	0.12	0.06	0.10	0.25	0.15	0.19	0.11	0.19	0.02	0.24	0.26	0.11	0.38	0.09	0.14	0.50	0.38
26. Other/Unspecified	3.81	1.87	4.48	3.54	3.04	3.68	3.75	2.79	6.34	3.53	3.89	2.28	3.57	3.18	4.07	4.91	4.18
27. Fall (Total)	5.03	3.13	5.65	4.79	4.35	5.60	5.39	4.01	8.43	4.91	5.44	3.84	5.33	4.68	5.36	7.04	5.96
Fires and Burns																	
28. Housefires	2.98	2.92	0.97	3.23	0.95	0.67	0.96	2.18	2.61	1.48	3.09	0.34	1.29	1.84	1.92	1.23	1.75
29. Clothing Ignition	0.24	0.12	0.07	0.12	0.08	0.04	0.08	0.12	0.11	0.06	0.21	0.00	0.06	0.10	0.14	0.07	0.12
30. Fires/Burns Excl. Scalds	3.76	3.74	1.28	3.68	1.30	0.97	1.31	2.53	3.21	1.82	3.76	0.49	1.67	2.23	2.40	1.56	2.15
31. Fires/Burns (Total)	3.86	3.80	1.32	3.73	1.36	1.04	1.36	2.56	3.36	1.87	3.86	0.54	1.78	2.31	2.45	1.62	2.21

Table 9 (cont.) Death Rates per 100,000 Population by State of Residence, 69 Causes, 1980-1986

Cause	AL	AK	AZ	AR	CA	CO	CT	DE	DC	FL	GA	HI	ID	IL	IN	IA	KS
Other Unintentional																	
32. Firearm	1.75	7.35	0.71	1.07	0.57	0.66	0.84	0.38	0.25	0.57	1.11	0.34	1.20	0.32	0.68	0.44	0.89
33. Excessive Heat	0.71	0.06	0.60	1.27	0.14	0.04	0.09	0.05	0.30	0.12	0.54	0.01	0.06	0.24	0.19	0.26	0.79
34. Excessive Cold	0.56	2.47	0.34	0.47	0.10	0.35	0.25	0.42	1.52	0.17	0.50	0.01	0.58	0.40	0.28	0.36	0.40
35. Exposure/Neglect	0.15	0.15	0.34	0.11	0.06	0.14	0.08	0.05	0.07	0.06	0.10	0.04	0.22	0.06	0.11	0.12	0.21
36. Lightning	0.07	0.00	0.13	0.12	0.01	0.08	0.01	0.05	0.09	0.08	0.03	0.00	0.03	0.03	0.03	0.01	0.05
37. Natural Disaster	0.07	0.27	0.11	0.25	0.04	0.11	0.03	0.05	0.02	0.01	0.01	0.04	0.10	0.04	0.01	0.07	0.06
38. Aspiration-Food	0.71	1.93	0.72	0.87	0.91	0.66	0.64	0.52	0.93	0.75	1.03	0.68	0.89	0.72	0.79	0.76	1.24
39. Aspiration-Nonfood	1.03	0.54	0.49	1.19	0.23	0.74	0.85	0.45	1.34	0.59	0.55	0.70	0.48	0.57	0.48	0.84	0.72
40. Suffocation	0.36	1.27	0.46	0.39	0.38	0.57	0.35	0.23	0.39	0.39	0.36	0.24	0.55	0.34	0.42	0.50	0.59
41. Struck by Falling Object	0.75	1.02	0.30	0.75	0.20	0.37	0.19	0.33	0.14	0.30	0.65	0.17	1.16	0.30	0.48	0.50	0.83
42. Collision with Object/Person	0.12	0.12	0.10	0.12	0.10	0.15	0.06	0.07	0.05	0.14	0.14	0.11	0.22	0.07	0.09	0.17	0.13
43. Caught/Crushed	0.05	0.12	0.06	0.02	0.03	0.09	0.01	0.05	0.00	0.03	0.05	0.03	0.16	0.05	0.07	0.07	0.05
44. Machinery	0.84	0.48	0.40	0.96	0.30	0.55	0.17	0.23	0.11	0.39	0.67	0.27	1.51	0.43	0.63	1.35	0.89
45. Cutting/Piercing	0.09	0.06	0.04	0.08	0.04	0.04	0.03	0.02	0.05	0.05	0.08	0.00	0.10	0.10	0.04	0.04	0.08
46. Explosion	0.10	0.30	0.14	0.17	0.08	0.17	0.05	0.02	0.00	0.08	0.17	0.11	0.17	0.11	0.10	0.14	0.17
47. Electric Current	0.60	0.42	0.45	0.72	0.24	0.39	0.16	0.52	0.11	0.54	0.48	0.27	0.58	0.39	0.53	0.40	0.68
48. Unintentional Excl. Traffic	26.26	61.36	22.98	26.83	20.41	21.01	17.80	16.77	26.30	21.28	24.73	15.55	27.09	18.94	19.19	21.27	23.60
49. Unintentional (Total)	52.44	83.63	50.37	51.10	40.89	42.55	33.24	37.46	36.08	46.59	49.31	29.50	53.37	34.61	38.72	39.60	45.78
Suicide																	
50. Firearm	8.82	10.22	11.57	9.90	7.56	10.21	3.65	5.37	3.23	9.97	9.64	3.13	10.26	4.40	6.86	6.28	7.75
51. Poison Solids/Liquids	0.55	0.90	2.24	0.63	2.54	1.61	0.44	1.50	1.05	2.01	0.78	1.38	0.91	1.08	0.88	0.87	0.90
52. Motor Vehicle Exhaust	0.28	0.54	0.66	0.40	0.73	2.55	1.20	1.60	0.14	0.77	0.48	0.31	1.67	1.55	1.33	1.81	0.90
53. Hanging	0.89	1.27	1.85	0.97	2.23	1.89	2.24	1.78	2.25	1.77	1.03	2.79	1.55	1.98	1.52	1.68	1.42
54. Drowning	0.15	0.06	0.14	0.17	0.20	0.09	0.14	0.70	0.59	0.45	0.11	0.21	0.09	0.21	0.15	0.21	0.15
55. Cutting/Piercing	0.06	0.18	0.26	0.10	0.31	0.20	0.18	0.26	0.23	0.26	0.11	0.41	0.16	0.18	0.12	0.13	0.08
56. Jumping	0.07	0.12	0.14	0.06	0.54	0.27	0.29	0.30	1.52	0.37	0.14	1.37	0.07	0.29	0.09	0.06	0.11
57. Non-Firearm (Total)	2.27	3.38	5.75	2.52	6.99	7.01	5.18	6.40	6.25	6.12	2.83	6.69	4.74	5.71	4.55	5.10	4.24
58. Suicide (Total)	11.09	13.59	17.32	12.42	14.55	17.22	8.82	11.78	9.48	16.09	12.47	9.82	15.00	10.11	11.42	11.38	11.99
Homicide																	
59. Firearm	8.56	6.81	4.87	6.85	6.87	3.65	2.58	2.86	16.07	8.72	8.55	1.76	1.97	6.37	4.11	1.35	3.44
60. Cutting/Stabbing	2.22	1.72	1.85	1.27	2.59	1.41	1.05	1.43	7.12	2.13	2.17	1.10	2.22	2.22	0.92	0.48	0.97
61. Strangulation	0.31	0.42	0.47	0.26	0.62	0.36	0.32	0.28	1.02	0.60	0.58	0.39	0.15	0.44	0.21	0.14	0.30
62. Other	1.26	1.05	1.82	1.32	1.64	1.10	0.70	1.10	3.84	1.72	1.51	1.17	0.61	1.52	0.85	0.42	0.81
63. Non-Firearm (Total)	3.78	3.19	4.13	2.85	4.84	2.87	2.08	2.82	11.98	4.45	4.25	2.67	1.23	4.18	1.98	1.04	2.08
64. Homicide (Total)	12.34	10.00	9.00	9.70	11.72	6.52	4.66	5.68	28.05	13.17	12.80	4.43	3.21	10.55	6.09	2.39	5.52
65. Legal Intervention-Firearm	0.08	0.12	0.20	0.12	0.13	0.11	0.09	0.09	0.61	0.10	0.12	0.01	0.07	0.07	0.13	0.04	0.11
66. Undetermined-Firearm	0.94	2.92	0.16	0.28	0.14	0.30	0.08	0.21	0.11	0.24	0.47	0.31	0.38	0.33	0.24	0.18	0.24
67. Undet-Poison Solid/Liquids	0.24	0.51	0.36	0.23	0.34	0.61	0.15	0.40	4.61	0.28	0.23	1.15	0.25	0.49	0.33	0.16	0.30
68. Undetermined (Total)	1.84	5.61	1.11	1.10	0.96	1.77	0.73	1.36	8.59	1.09	1.41	2.72	1.07	2.71	1.22	0.98	0.94
69. Injuries (Total)	77.82	112.95	78.01	74.45	68.27	68.17	47.55	56.37	82.86	77.07	76.14	46.49	72.74	58.06	57.58	54.40	64.35

Table 9 (cont.) Death Rates per 100,000 Population by State of Residence, 69 Causes, 1980-1986

Cause	KY	LA	ME	MD	MA	MI	MN	MS	MO	MT	NE	NV	NH	NJ	NM	NY	NC
Transportation																	
1. Motor Vehicle-Train	0.19	0.47	0.17	0.07	0.02	0.31	0.30	0.44	0.37	0.63	0.82	0.13	0.04	0.06	0.17	0.06	0.28
2. Motor Vehicle Occupant	18.04	19.36	13.76	12.10	9.41	12.94	12.37	22.96	16.42	25.10	15.27	20.37	13.23	9.39	24.54	8.44	18.24
3. Motorcyclist	0.68	0.70	2.19	1.58	1.36	1.39	1.74	1.28	1.21	2.48	1.78	2.42	2.00	0.88	3.34	0.81	1.36
4. Bicyclist	0.23	0.47	0.19	0.23	0.25	0.50	0.35	0.33	0.16	0.42	0.22	0.64	0.43	0.33	0.48	0.34	0.47
5. Pedestrian	2.60	3.24	2.47	3.06	2.90	2.94	2.11	3.14	2.44	2.36	1.74	3.75	2.09	3.66	6.85	3.64	3.99
6. Motor Vehicle-Traffic (Total)	21.55	23.81	18.66	16.99	13.95	17.78	16.58	27.74	20.26	30.41	19.01	27.21	17.75	14.26	35.23	13.25	24.07
7. Pedestrian-Nontraffic	0.25	0.24	0.17	0.09	0.04	0.19	0.14	0.31	0.21	0.30	0.22	0.26	0.18	0.08	0.30	0.09	0.22
8. Pedestrian-Train	0.19	0.10	0.06	0.12	0.06	0.03	0.12	0.14	0.15	0.35	0.16	0.18	0.04	0.27	0.21	0.31	0.21
9. Aircraft	0.32	0.76	0.50	0.39	0.20	0.38	0.78	0.46	0.42	2.22	0.62	2.28	0.50	0.23	1.41	0.23	0.55
Drowning																	
10. Boat-Related	0.56	1.43	1.25	0.34	0.32	0.38	0.46	1.00	0.36	1.06	0.32	0.34	0.55	0.23	0.36	0.22	0.49
11. Non-Boat	2.45	3.91	1.61	1.73	1.33	1.72	1.50	3.52	2.06	2.81	1.41	3.14	1.52	1.41	3.35	1.36	2.57
12. Drowning (Total)	3.01	5.34	2.85	2.07	1.66	2.10	1.97	4.52	2.43	3.87	1.73	3.48	2.07	1.64	3.71	1.58	3.07
Poisoning																	
13. Opiates	0.05	0.05	0.01	0.06	0.12	0.04	0.08	0.02	0.12	0.04	0.03	0.46	0.03	0.14	0.20	0.12	0.15
14. Barbiturates	0.02	0.04	0.00	0.01	0.06	0.01	0.01	0.02	0.02	0.02	0.01	0.11	0.00	0.02	0.01	0.02	0.02
15. Tranquilizers	0.07	0.03	0.01	0.01	0.06	0.03	0.02	0.04	0.06	0.02	0.02	0.06	0.01	0.02	0.09	0.02	0.02
16. Antidepressants	0.10	0.05	0.02	0.02	0.05	0.04	0.03	0.05	0.05	0.02	0.09	0.08	0.06	0.02	0.05	0.03	0.03
17. Alcohol	0.12	0.05	0.02	0.02	0.05	0.05	0.19	0.14	0.08	0.12	0.04	0.16	0.09	0.00	0.00	0.02	1.27
18. Solids/Liquids (Total)	1.29	1.12	0.83	0.79	1.21	0.99	0.96	1.32	1.17	0.79	0.85	2.45	0.72	1.35	1.02	0.88	2.29
19. Motor Vehicle Exhaust	0.28	0.13	0.21	0.12	0.22	0.42	0.50	0.17	0.32	0.39	0.77	0.10	0.13	0.12	0.26	0.17	0.20
20. Gas/Vapor (Total)	0.69	0.43	0.32	0.28	0.44	0.69	0.83	0.45	0.64	0.81	1.14	0.53	0.34	0.42	0.67	0.37	0.41
Falls																	
21. Stairs	0.57	0.08	0.91	0.84	1.06	0.65	0.71	0.12	0.57	0.79	0.75	0.26	0.75	0.70	0.13	0.67	0.28
22. Ladder/Scaffold	0.13	0.19	0.19	0.10	0.14	0.15	0.12	0.09	0.11	0.16	0.18	0.13	0.16	0.15	0.08	0.15	0.15
23. Building/Structure	0.26	0.22	0.27	0.26	0.29	0.21	0.19	0.19	0.21	0.30	0.27	0.21	0.46	0.35	0.13	0.54	0.23
24. Different Level	0.55	0.27	0.46	0.32	0.58	0.22	0.45	0.23	0.45	0.97	0.49	0.71	0.24	0.34	1.10	0.61	0.30
25. Same Level	0.17	0.05	0.16	0.12	0.25	0.10	0.22	0.07	0.21	0.44	0.53	0.13	0.13	0.15	0.06	0.08	0.05
26. Other/Unspecified	4.01	3.09	3.24	3.13	4.65	3.51	5.32	3.37	5.29	4.27	5.11	2.45	3.48	3.38	3.50	4.02	3.52
27. Fall (Total)	5.68	3.80	5.23	4.77	6.97	4.86	7.02	4.07	6.84	6.93	7.33	3.88	5.22	5.06	5.01	6.08	4.53
Fires and Burns																	
28. Housefires	2.29	2.77	2.17	1.96	1.41	1.99	1.38	4.20	2.07	1.53	1.14	1.25	1.33	1.69	1.15	1.53	2.69
29. Clothing Ignition	0.17	0.11	0.19	0.09	0.14	0.06	0.06	0.32	0.13	0.07	0.11	0.06	0.10	0.07	0.04	0.07	0.11
30. Fires/Burns Excl. Scalds	2.80	3.46	2.67	2.34	1.85	2.32	1.70	5.30	2.57	1.78	1.61	1.81	1.63	2.26	1.49	2.04	3.31
31. Fires/Burns (Total)	2.86	3.53	2.69	2.41	1.91	2.39	1.75	5.46	2.65	1.86	1.69	1.86	1.69	2.34	1.59	2.12	3.37

Table 9 (cont.) Death Rates per 100,000 Population by State of Residence, 69 Causes, 1980-1986

Cause	KY	LA	ME	MD	MA	MI	MN	MS	MO	MT	NE	NV	NH	NJ	NM	NY	NC
Other Unintentional																	
32. Firearm	1.53	1.58	0.30	0.21	0.29	0.44	0.40	2.81	1.06	1.32	0.62	0.95	0.47	0.34	0.79	0.45	0.69
33. Excessive Heat	0.35	0.28	0.08	0.07	0.06	0.04	0.07	1.07	1.10	0.04	0.20	0.09	0.09	0.09	0.07	0.05	0.18
34. Excessive Cold	0.39	0.24	0.36	0.28	0.22	0.38	0.44	0.48	0.36	1.30	0.41	0.29	0.37	0.28	0.61	0.24	0.77
35. Exposure/Neglect	0.20	0.11	0.14	0.05	0.14	0.13	0.20	0.38	0.12	0.23	0.16	0.21	0.15	0.08	1.21	0.06	0.21
36. Lightning	0.09	0.07	0.02	0.03	0.01	0.04	0.03	0.12	0.04	0.05	0.05	0.03	0.03	0.02	0.09	0.02	0.06
37. Natural Disaster	0.03	0.03	0.04	0.02	0.02	0.02	0.02	0.15	0.10	0.19	0.10	0.14	0.01	0.01	0.04	0.01	0.12
38. Aspiration-Food	1.03	1.15	0.55	0.61	0.86	0.60	0.48	1.30	0.80	0.77	0.88	0.77	0.49	0.65	0.49	0.84	0.66
39. Aspiration-Nonfood	0.87	1.07	0.82	1.04	1.18	0.55	0.79	1.36	1.13	0.51	0.78	0.46	0.56	0.60	0.57	0.53	1.09
40. Suffocation	0.40	0.34	0.39	0.21	0.39	0.34	0.54	0.44	0.37	0.65	0.56	0.42	0.21	0.26	0.30	0.46	0.37
41. Struck by Falling Object	0.84	0.55	0.51	0.28	0.19	0.33	0.44	0.84	0.65	0.91	0.51	0.32	0.61	0.18	0.55	0.21	0.55
42. Collision with Object/Person	0.12	0.19	0.12	0.07	0.07	0.08	0.11	0.15	0.09	0.35	0.10	0.19	0.12	0.09	0.27	0.11	0.15
43. Caught/Crushed	0.10	0.04	0.04	0.06	0.03	0.03	0.05	0.05	0.03	0.02	0.09	0.10	0.03	0.05	0.05	0.04	0.02
44. Machinery	1.18	0.95	0.57	0.44	0.14	0.46	0.95	1.02	0.82	1.25	1.43	0.37	0.43	0.18	0.86	0.22	0.71
45. Cutting/Piercing	0.07	0.06	0.07	0.03	0.06	0.04	0.03	0.11	0.08	0.12	0.05	0.10	0.04	0.04	0.01	0.08	0.04
46. Explosion	0.17	0.14	0.15	0.08	0.04	0.27	0.09	0.28	0.09	0.26	0.28	0.11	0.04	0.07	0.19	0.07	0.15
47. Electric Current	0.62	0.75	0.24	0.30	0.18	0.27	0.38	0.56	0.50	0.60	0.56	0.29	0.18	0.21	0.45	0.16	0.42
48. Unintentional Excl. Traffic	25.57	26.65	20.28	17.99	19.35	17.60	21.63	31.55	24.88	29.56	23.00	23.09	17.16	17.27	24.38	18.09	24.35
49. Unintentional (Total)	47.12	50.46	38.93	34.98	33.30	35.38	38.21	59.30	45.14	59.97	42.00	50.31	34.93	31.54	59.60	31.34	48.42
Suicide																	
50. Firearm	9.85	9.98	7.42	6.12	2.65	6.42	5.40	8.05	8.05	11.71	8.39	18.92	6.76	2.74	12.28	2.77	9.02
51. Poison Solids/Liquids	0.87	1.03	1.57	1.12	1.14	1.21	1.14	0.81	1.21	1.27	0.80	2.71	1.17	0.62	1.98	0.88	1.33
52. Motor Vehicle Exhaust	0.56	0.16	1.08	0.55	0.90	1.48	1.63	0.21	1.20	1.53	1.22	1.65	1.39	0.73	1.13	0.66	0.37
53. Hanging	1.21	0.95	1.94	1.85	2.86	1.93	1.77	0.54	1.35	1.95	1.66	2.15	2.10	2.29	2.34	1.90	0.92
54. Drowning	0.24	0.23	0.65	0.22	0.30	0.21	0.27	0.10	0.26	0.09	0.16	0.11	0.22	0.19	0.01	0.22	0.24
55. Cutting/Piercing	0.08	0.11	0.12	0.23	0.19	0.15	0.14	0.14	0.15	0.19	0.13	0.28	0.31	0.21	0.15	0.19	0.12
56. Jumping	0.12	0.08	0.14	0.37	0.44	0.19	0.19	0.07	0.26	0.07	0.11	0.38	0.15	0.42	0.07	0.83	0.05
57. Non-Firearm (Total)	3.27	2.84	5.89	4.89	6.36	5.59	5.75	1.85	4.85	5.36	4.38	7.87	5.65	4.95	5.93	5.20	3.44
58. Suicide (Total)	13.12	12.82	13.31	11.01	9.02	12.01	11.15	9.91	12.90	17.08	10.77	24.79	12.41	7.69	18.21	7.97	12.46
Homicide																	
59. Firearm	5.46	10.40	1.22	5.84	1.62	6.92	1.02	9.03	6.45	2.92	1.70	7.36	1.08	2.87	6.00	6.39	6.43
60. Cutting/Stabbing	0.90	2.50	0.37	2.01	1.09	1.88	0.60	2.19	1.56	0.93	0.74	2.15	0.38	1.76	2.41	2.77	1.71
61. Strangulation	0.19	0.35	0.12	0.41	0.26	0.51	0.17	0.24	0.45	0.25	0.15	1.11	0.09	0.34	0.43	0.57	0.27
62. Other	1.05	1.37	0.64	1.02	0.86	1.46	0.51	1.45	1.35	0.81	0.55	2.10	0.33	1.23	2.07	1.35	1.20
63. Non-Firearm (Total)	2.15	4.22	1.13	3.44	2.21	3.85	1.27	3.87	3.37	1.99	1.44	5.35	0.90	3.33	4.90	4.70	3.18
64. Homicide (Total)	7.61	14.62	2.35	9.29	3.83	10.77	2.29	12.90	9.82	4.91	3.15	12.71	1.88	6.20	10.90	11.09	9.62
65. Legal Intervention-Firearm	0.09	0.14	0.04	0.09	0.08	0.15	0.03	0.17	0.07	0.05	0.03	0.42	0.06	0.08	0.31	0.13	0.11
66. Undetermined-Firearm	0.22	0.19	0.04	0.18	0.06	0.09	0.18	0.71	0.34	0.40	0.37	0.26	0.27	0.07	0.55	0.17	0.19
67. Undet-Poison Solids/Liquids	0.24	0.14	0.24	0.56	0.79	0.52	0.21	0.09	0.32	0.49	0.22	1.14	0.25	0.15	1.29	0.37	0.26
68. Undetermined (Total)	0.84	0.49	0.51	1.47	1.36	1.06	1.01	1.22	1.25	1.60	1.29	2.28	0.93	0.56	3.04	3.17	0.91
69. Injuries (Total)	68.81	78.55	55.15	56.85	47.59	59.40	52.71	83.51	69.19	83.61	57.24	90.54	50.22	46.17	92.10	53.71	71.53

Table 9 (cont.) Death Rates per 100,000 Population by State of Residence, 69 Causes, 1980-1986

Cause	ND	OH	OK	OR	PA	RI	SC	SD	TN	TX	UT	VT	VA	WA	WV	WI	WY
Transportation																	
1. Motor Vehicle-Train	0.42	0.44	0.54	0.18	0.09	0.01	0.35	0.16	0.19	0.45	0.29	0.19	0.13	0.18	0.20	0.30	0.31
2. Motor Vehicle Occupant	16.43	12.43	22.43	17.52	12.74	7.80	19.77	19.52	19.35	19.00	14.32	15.55	13.86	14.81	19.60	12.57	29.52
3. Motorcyclist	1.67	1.02	2.16	2.26	0.69	1.58	2.33	1.61	1.65	1.99	2.00	0.95	0.90	1.75	0.69	2.01	1.56
4. Bicyclist	0.19	0.27	0.31	0.44	0.24	0.16	0.49	0.29	0.22	0.35	0.42	0.27	0.22	0.26	0.15	0.39	0.31
5. Pedestrian	1.57	2.08	3.06	2.88	2.56	2.80	4.24	2.61	2.69	4.07	3.15	2.26	2.72	2.55	2.58	1.98	2.44
6. Motor Vehicle-Traffic (Total)	19.88	15.82	27.97	23.10	16.28	12.39	26.86	24.04	23.95	25.42	19.93	19.06	17.72	19.38	23.03	16.99	33.83
7. Pedestrian-Nontraffic	0.38	0.17	0.34	0.21	0.07	0.09	0.21	0.63	0.26	0.29	0.45	0.14	0.21	0.21	0.22	0.18	0.40
8. Pedestrian-Train	0.25	0.16	0.23	0.12	0.14	0.09	0.35	0.10	0.12	0.19	0.09	0.08	0.21	0.15	0.34	0.08	0.20
9. Aircraft	0.70	0.32	0.84	1.16	0.24	0.21	0.48	1.00	0.41	0.66	1.34	0.24	0.43	1.15	0.28	0.35	2.13
Drowning																	
10. Boat-Related	0.51	0.30	0.41	1.17	0.17	0.45	0.79	0.37	0.48	0.39	0.44	0.76	0.49	1.01	0.46	0.42	0.62
11. Non-Boat	1.74	1.37	2.84	2.68	1.23	1.18	2.92	2.04	2.36	3.00	2.27	1.66	2.01	2.46	2.27	1.57	2.36
12. Drowning (Total)	2.24	1.67	3.25	3.85	1.40	1.62	3.71	2.41	2.84	3.39	2.71	2.42	2.50	3.48	2.73	1.99	2.98
Poisoning																	
13. Opiates	0.04	0.07	0.06	0.17	0.09	0.12	0.12	0.00	0.05	0.19	0.06	0.03	0.23	0.32	0.11	0.08	0.17
14. Barbiturates	0.00	0.04	0.03	0.01	0.02	0.01	0.04	0.02	0.04	0.03	0.00	0.03	0.01	0.02	0.05	0.04	0.00
15. Tranquilizers	0.00	0.04	0.03	0.04	0.03	0.10	0.04	0.05	0.05	0.04	0.03	0.03	0.04	0.07	0.02	0.04	0.06
16. Antidepressants	0.04	0.05	0.05	0.05	0.03	0.04	0.10	0.00	0.09	0.06	0.02	0.00	0.04	0.08	0.05	0.08	0.06
17. Alcohol	0.02	0.07	0.21	0.06	0.07	0.12	0.31	0.20	0.14	0.12	0.03	0.16	1.02	0.11	0.07	0.06	0.11
18. Solids/Liquids (Total)	0.55	1.08	1.11	1.45	1.37	1.67	1.68	0.90	1.47	1.34	0.72	0.90	2.08	1.84	1.15	1.08	1.28
19. Motor Vehicle Exhaust	0.59	0.40	0.15	0.12	0.24	0.22	0.22	0.63	0.15	0.08	0.23	0.30	0.15	0.23	0.37	0.65	0.57
20. Gas/Vapor (Total)	1.14	0.67	0.70	0.30	0.52	0.34	0.39	1.12	0.38	0.41	0.47	0.57	0.34	0.36	0.81	0.85	1.22
Falls																	
21. Stairs	0.72	0.73	0.16	0.53	1.29	1.16	0.23	0.68	0.28	0.10	0.75	0.95	0.56	0.41	0.70	0.86	0.40
22. Ladder/Scaffold	0.19	0.16	0.11	0.18	0.17	0.24	0.11	0.22	0.10	0.13	0.19	0.08	0.16	0.17	0.12	0.21	0.09
23. Building/Structure	0.21	0.29	0.33	0.28	0.29	0.15	0.18	0.16	0.23	0.29	0.22	0.35	0.24	0.29	0.29	0.23	0.51
24. Different Level	0.49	0.42	0.42	0.70	0.35	0.73	0.32	0.53	0.41	0.35	0.65	0.54	0.31	0.75	0.51	0.46	0.65
25. Same Level	0.61	0.25	0.18	0.45	0.13	0.28	0.08	0.47	0.19	0.13	0.23	0.33	0.15	0.28	0.12	0.46	0.23
26. Other/Unspecified	3.70	3.61	4.40	3.64	3.35	3.78	3.18	4.34	3.69	3.02	3.40	3.81	3.81	3.48	3.82	3.12	3.49
27. Fall (Total)	5.93	5.47	5.61	5.78	5.59	6.34	4.09	6.63	4.90	4.03	5.44	6.06	5.24	5.38	5.56	5.34	5.36
Fires and Burns																	
28. Housefires	1.42	1.64	2.14	1.37	1.89	1.41	3.98	1.55	2.53	1.74	0.66	2.64	2.02	1.48	2.80	1.39	0.57
29. Clothing Ignition	0.06	0.09	0.21	0.11	0.16	0.07	0.17	0.06	0.14	0.12	0.03	0.08	0.15	0.11	0.23	0.11	0.09
30. Fires/Burns Excl. Scalds	1.90	1.93	2.87	1.66	2.25	1.65	4.56	2.20	3.25	2.23	1.14	3.02	2.56	1.77	3.26	1.68	1.08
31. Fires/Burns (Total)	1.93	1.99	2.93	1.71	2.30	1.76	4.61	2.28	3.33	2.31	1.21	3.05	2.66	1.83	3.35	1.72	1.16

Table 9 (cont.) Death Rates per 100,000 Population by State of Residence, 69 Causes, 1980-1986

Cause	ND	OH	OK	OR	PA	RI	SC	SD	TN	TX	UT	VT	VA	WA	WV	WI	WY
Other Unintentional																	
32. Firearm	0.85	0.53	1.12	0.67	0.35	0.09	1.30	1.12	1.38	1.38	0.43	0.38	0.63	0.42	0.64	0.40	1.62
33. Excessive Heat	0.08	0.07	0.60	0.13	0.08	0.04	0.36	0.04	0.49	0.24	0.04	0.08	0.11	0.04	0.09	0.07	0.06
34. Excessive Cold	0.72	0.23	0.44	0.38	0.34	0.18	0.76	1.14	0.58	0.18	0.36	0.65	0.65	0.27	0.48	0.46	1.05
35. Exposure/Neglect	0.25	0.08	0.10	0.22	0.06	0.01	0.11	0.24	0.13	0.09	0.06	0.22	0.13	0.17	0.09	0.08	0.26
36. Lightning	0.02	0.03	0.04	0.02	0.02	0.03	0.05	0.10	0.07	0.04	0.09	0.08	0.05	0.01	0.01	0.04	0.03
37. Natural Disaster	0.06	0.04	0.16	0.11	0.11	0.00	0.08	0.06	0.05	0.10	0.11	0.03	0.06	0.18	0.31	0.08	0.48
38. Aspiration-Food	1.06	0.58	0.73	0.55	0.71	0.57	1.04	0.98	0.86	0.76	0.56	0.54	0.66	0.67	0.82	0.57	0.99
39. Aspiration-Nonfood	0.53	0.48	0.99	0.49	0.87	0.57	1.21	0.45	0.87	0.77	0.51	0.73	1.00	0.49	0.78	0.29	0.99
40. Suffocation	0.44	0.29	0.45	0.48	0.26	0.33	0.33	0.39	0.32	0.48	0.66	0.27	0.31	0.43	0.32	0.34	0.62
41. Struck by Falling Object	0.53	0.33	0.53	0.81	0.38	0.16	0.61	0.65	0.52	0.41	0.58	0.76	0.60	0.70	1.15	0.39	0.82
42. Collision with Object/Person	0.04	0.08	0.17	0.35	0.09	0.12	0.13	0.10	0.10	0.12	0.05	0.08	0.11	0.14	0.08	0.23	0.14
43. Caught/Crushed	0.00	0.04	0.12	0.11	0.06	0.06	0.04	0.18	0.02	0.06	0.14	0.00	0.05	0.09	0.03	0.03	0.17
44. Machinery	1.57	0.48	0.92	0.96	0.47	0.12	0.62	2.20	0.93	0.68	0.58	0.87	0.72	0.63	1.05	0.93	1.59
45. Cutting/Piercing	0.08	0.05	0.08	0.05	0.03	0.09	0.09	0.02	0.05	0.07	0.04	0.08	0.04	0.04	0.07	0.06	0.03
46. Explosion	0.15	0.10	0.35	0.07	0.12	0.00	0.19	0.31	0.18	0.25	0.23	0.11	0.09	0.30	0.17	0.08	0.48
47. Electric Current	0.51	0.36	0.96	0.32	0.27	0.22	0.39	0.55	0.43	0.73	0.36	0.38	0.40	0.30	0.66	0.31	0.51
48. Unintentional Excl. Traffic	23.37	18.18	25.67	23.16	19.85	17.32	25.30	26.59	24.00	21.77	20.23	22.49	21.99	21.75	24.01	17.66	28.61
49. Unintentional (Total)	43.24	34.00	53.64	46.26	36.13	29.71	52.15	50.64	47.95	47.19	40.16	41.55	39.70	41.13	47.04	34.65	62.45
Suicide																	
50. Firearm	6.12	6.57	9.86	9.63	6.11	2.80	8.07	7.53	9.46	9.21	8.37	9.46	8.75	7.56	9.51	6.14	14.28
51. Poison Solids/Liquids	0.78	1.17	1.11	1.57	1.24	1.92	0.88	0.77	0.83	0.90	1.76	1.63	1.41	1.79	0.83	1.22	0.74
52. Motor Vehicle Exhaust	1.06	1.39	0.82	1.26	0.88	1.34	0.45	1.16	0.45	0.54	1.33	0.90	0.56	1.51	0.50	1.98	1.79
53. Hanging	1.95	1.62	1.53	1.70	1.93	3.02	1.03	2.73	1.21	1.42	1.48	1.82	1.41	1.86	1.06	2.23	1.59
54. Drowning	0.17	0.25	0.07	0.20	0.28	0.46	0.18	0.14	0.29	0.09	0.05	0.24	0.34	0.31	0.24	0.27	0.09
55. Cutting/Piercing	0.11	0.14	0.11	0.19	0.19	0.22	0.10	0.08	0.09	0.14	0.16	0.22	0.19	0.26	0.11	0.15	0.09
56. Jumping	0.15	0.23	0.08	0.38	0.45	0.55	0.09	0.10	0.15	0.11	0.11	0.14	0.22	0.46	0.18	0.16	0.09
57. Non-Firearm (Total)	4.64	5.20	4.14	5.72	5.46	7.74	2.94	5.22	3.28	3.62	5.07	5.52	4.55	6.45	3.12	6.34	4.80
58. Suicide (Total)	10.75	11.77	14.00	15.35	11.59	10.54	11.01	12.75	12.74	12.83	13.44	14.98	13.30	14.02	12.63	12.49	19.07
Homicide																	
59. Firearm	1.08	3.76	5.89	2.66	3.11	1.68	6.89	1.57	7.07	10.12	1.68	1.50	5.35	2.65	4.35	1.78	2.95
60. Cutting/Stabbing	0.32	0.99	1.45	0.95	1.34	1.06	1.82	0.88	1.70	2.76	0.70	0.38	1.37	1.02	0.74	0.67	0.99
61. Strangulation	0.15	0.24	0.35	0.44	0.25	0.45	0.35	0.20	0.45	0.48	0.19	0.22	0.36	0.40	0.22	0.19	0.45
62. Other	0.42	0.92	1.49	0.95	1.01	1.18	1.40	1.18	1.07	1.55	0.90	0.65	1.02	1.04	0.86	0.57	0.88
63. Non-Firearm (Total)	0.89	2.16	3.28	2.34	2.59	2.68	3.57	2.26	3.01	4.80	1.79	1.25	2.74	2.47	1.82	1.43	2.33
64. Homicide (Total)	1.97	5.93	9.17	5.00	5.71	4.36	10.46	3.83	10.09	14.92	3.47	2.75	8.10	5.11	6.16	3.21	5.28
65. Legal Intervention-Firearm	0.02	0.11	0.35	0.06	0.16	0.16	0.03	0.04	0.09	0.16	0.12	0.03	0.12	0.18	0.09	0.05	0.11
66. Undetermined-Firearm	0.34	0.10	0.23	0.13	0.15	0.03	0.23	0.49	0.83	0.25	0.31	0.08	0.11	0.16	0.34	0.12	0.40
67. Undet-Poison Solids/Liquids	0.11	0.18	0.30	0.94	0.69	0.36	0.12	0.22	0.28	0.16	1.35	0.16	0.13	0.51	0.31	0.22	0.37
68. Undetermined (Total)	1.02	0.71	0.87	1.79	1.70	0.94	0.66	1.75	1.65	0.73	2.31	0.41	0.53	1.32	1.53	0.94	1.28
69. Injuries (Total)	57.00	52.53	78.05	68.51	55.20	45.73	74.33	69.01	72.54	75.85	59.51	59.71	61.77	61.68	67.46	51.34	88.19

319

Table 10. Death Rates Per 100,000 Population by Age and Race, 14 Causes, 1980-1986

Cause	Race	0	1-	5-	10-	15-	20-	25-	30-	35-	45-	55-	65-	75+
MV Occupant	W	4.62	3.32	2.44	3.66	33.12	32.58	21.48	16.69	13.61	12.20	11.68	13.17	17.96
	B	5.11	3.17	2.12	2.24	10.19	18.14	16.30	15.29	13.95	12.47	12.29	11.83	13.15
	NA	12.36	8.16	4.87	5.78	44.61	54.61	50.43	39.30	32.44	27.11	24.14	15.83	35.53
	A	3.31	1.84	1.77	2.39	11.19	14.84	10.46	8.27	8.24	8.55	7.21	8.56	9.86
Pedestrian	W	0.28	2.28	2.70	1.90	3.21	3.33	2.63	2.26	2.17	2.52	2.82	3.88	8.11
	B	0.50	4.80	5.67	1.88	2.22	3.97	4.73	5.01	5.55	6.14	6.96	7.39	9.76
	NA	1.87	5.66	4.57	1.83	10.93	14.78	14.76	14.04	14.16	18.11	14.38	17.11	20.47
	A	0.60	2.47	3.03	1.28	1.39	1.66	1.73	1.15	1.40	2.04	3.56	9.90	16.43
Motor Vehicle-Traffic (Total)	W	4.94	5.73	6.05	7.30	40.96	41.82	28.13	21.39	17.20	15.47	14.93	17.39	26.38
	B	5.60	8.12	8.61	5.40	14.41	25.00	23.23	22.17	20.60	19.09	19.62	19.49	23.21
	NA	14.23	13.82	10.41	9.24	59.13	74.26	67.89	55.29	47.67	45.83	38.85	33.19	56.00
	A	4.06	4.36	5.41	4.40	14.17	17.86	13.02	9.92	9.99	10.92	10.95	19.05	26.55
Drowning	W	2.17	5.00	1.68	1.41	3.76	3.62	2.78	2.18	1.71	1.67	1.53	1.62	2.01
	B	3.13	2.76	3.74	5.06	6.09	5.74	5.09	4.82	3.66	3.20	2.72	2.54	2.17
	NA	5.24	8.82	3.02	3.08	7.26	10.35	10.19	9.64	7.49	5.96	4.96	3.32	4.82
	A	1.35	3.02	2.67	1.88	3.13	3.05	2.04	1.46	1.24	1.13	1.57	2.46	3.92
Poisoning Solids/Liquids	W	0.31	0.28	0.05	0.10	0.64	1.73	2.99	3.07	2.01	1.52	1.23	1.28	2.27
	B	0.76	0.79	0.06	0.04	0.44	1.46	4.10	5.86	5.24	3.12	2.49	2.12	3.32
	NA	0.37	0.54	0.10	0.77	2.27	2.52	2.60	5.37	3.54	2.67	2.65	2.81	5.42
	A	0.60	0.12	0.07	0.03	0.08	0.45	0.49	0.77	0.49	0.45	0.36	0.45	0.63
Falls	W	0.93	0.54	0.19	0.24	0.92	1.32	1.21	1.23	1.45	2.68	4.60	10.18	67.89
	B	2.76	1.32	0.25	0.22	0.34	1.00	1.48	2.53	3.72	5.94	7.78	10.40	33.61
	NA	3.37	0.54	0.39	0.39	1.05	2.09	1.98	3.17	4.53	5.83	6.78	13.79	52.99
	A	0.75	1.18	0.32	0.17	0.41	0.55	0.46	0.30	0.61	1.04	1.94	6.85	36.28
Housefires	W	2.30	3.13	1.24	0.67	0.67	1.04	1.03	0.88	0.88	1.21	1.54	2.25	4.11
	B	9.46	11.64	4.72	1.75	1.02	1.68	2.20	2.71	3.17	4.43	6.09	9.30	19.96
	NA	4.87	6.66	1.85	1.16	1.57	2.78	2.50	3.54	3.38	4.13	2.81	4.09	11.44
	A	0.45	1.14	0.58	0.34	0.38	0.26	0.23	0.33	0.26	0.29	0.54	0.97	1.52
Unintentional Excl. Traffic	W	17.40	14.21	5.65	6.05	12.68	16.01	15.73	14.84	13.85	16.57	20.31	32.02	117.25
	B	42.36	23.13	11.05	9.44	12.00	16.56	20.76	25.11	27.93	33.02	40.95	56.22	130.84
	NA	38.95	29.17	10.71	10.59	25.71	38.96	38.26	40.52	41.91	46.80	50.09	55.15	154.76
	A	8.27	8.16	4.62	3.73	6.26	7.05	5.67	5.11	5.09	5.96	9.37	20.68	72.31

Table 10 (cont.) Death Rates Per 100,000 Population by Age and Race, 14 Causes, 1980-1986

Cause	Race	0	1-	5-	10-	15-	20-	25-	30-	35-	45-	55-	65-	75+
Firearm Suicide	W	0.00	0.00	0.01	0.70	6.31	10.06	9.54	8.77	8.77	9.97	10.70	12.48	13.90
	B	0.00	0.00	0.00	0.26	2.30	5.45	6.14	6.02	5.05	4.14	4.30	5.07	4.78
	NA	0.00	0.00	0.00	0.77	11.28	17.74	14.56	9.78	7.74	5.71	5.46	4.85	3.01
	A	0.00	0.00	0.00	0.17	2.41	3.80	2.76	2.47	2.06	1.88	1.62	1.56	1.64
Suicide (Total)	W	0.00	0.00	0.03	1.23	10.08	16.24	16.71	16.19	16.05	17.55	17.75	19.05	22.42
	B	0.00	0.00	0.02	0.69	4.06	9.83	11.49	11.44	9.23	7.20	6.70	6.84	6.43
	NA	0.00	0.00	0.10	2.70	21.17	29.13	25.37	20.02	16.14	10.82	7.77	6.64	4.82
	A	0.00	0.00	0.04	0.74	6.07	10.55	8.84	7.42	6.57	7.68	9.78	11.46	17.70
Firearm Homicide	W	0.24	0.28	0.29	0.58	3.78	6.74	6.87	6.21	5.50	3.94	2.27	1.49	0.94
	B	0.60	0.72	0.66	1.88	20.66	41.81	45.99	41.37	31.93	21.37	13.84	8.20	5.48
	NA	0.37	0.33	0.49	0.77	5.95	10.78	11.75	10.74	8.65	6.63	3.31	1.53	0.60
	A	0.15	0.24	0.22	0.50	2.94	4.55	4.26	3.68	4.11	4.28	1.85	1.49	0.76
Homicide (Total)	W	4.41	1.69	0.69	1.09	6.11	10.45	10.34	9.13	8.13	6.38	4.30	3.34	3.86
	B	15.95	6.88	2.31	3.17	28.23	58.34	65.40	60.71	48.50	34.80	24.19	17.52	15.63
	NA	8.61	3.81	0.97	1.73	14.08	26.70	25.26	22.58	19.60	18.48	10.25	6.38	9.63
	A	2.56	1.30	1.12	1.01	5.01	7.47	7.14	5.52	6.90	6.58	4.01	4.32	4.68
All Firearm	W	0.27	0.54	0.69	2.39	11.96	18.64	17.82	16.18	15.27	14.76	13.66	14.58	15.39
	B	0.81	1.27	1.17	2.89	25.18	49.84	54.95	49.98	38.92	26.82	19.13	14.10	10.90
	NA	0.74	0.98	1.95	2.99	22.21	37.13	31.62	23.92	19.11	15.55	9.76	7.15	3.61
	A	0.15	0.24	0.30	0.77	5.92	9.19	7.48	6.56	6.37	6.29	3.52	3.12	2.53
All Injuries	W	27.85	21.97	12.52	15.90	70.83	86.25	72.88	63.47	56.87	57.50	58.63	73.01	171.57
	B	69.06	39.63	22.36	19.08	60.17	112.79	125.30	125.00	111.47	97.83	94.52	102.39	179.25
	NA	65.91	47.57	22.29	24.74	123.15	175.39	162.82	144.15	130.42	127.27	111.60	104.95	227.62
	A	15.19	14.17	11.33	9.98	32.19	44.16	35.92	28.87	29.51	32.04	34.88	56.62	124.27

W = White   B = Black   NA = Native American   A = Asian

321

Index of Authors

Index of Subjects

Printed in the United States
862700002B